Photography with a microscope

This beautifully illustrated book describes how to record images viewed through a microscope. Dealing with the principles and practice of photomicrography, it is written for all who take photomicrographs, or who contemplate attaching a camera to a microscope. The book describes techniques which may be applied to many disciplines for teaching, research, archives, or pleasure. Techniques for the improvement of contrast are covered in considerable detail. Besides standard photography, the book describes modern digital techniques, and there is a short chapter on drawing.

In addition to its value as a work of reference, the authors' clear didactic style makes this book suitable for use as a textbook for courses in photomicrography and/or elementary light microscopy.

FRED ROST, author, photographer and artist, has a special interest in the photography of small objects.

RON OLDFIELD is well known as a microscopist and photographer, and has won several awards in the prestigious Polaroid international photomicrographic competitions.

Both authors have been involved in microscopy and photography for many years, and have published other books on microscopy. Both are past Presidents of the Microscopical Society of Australia, and Fellows of the Royal Microscopical Society.

Books by the same authors

Frey, D., Oldfield, R.J. & Bridger, R.C. (1979) *A colour atlas of pathogenic fungi*. 168 pp. Wolfe Medical Publications, London. German edition, *Farbatlas pathogener Piltze*. 168 pp. Schlütersche Verlagsanstalt und Druckerei, Hanover.

Oldfield, R.J. (1970–1994) *Light microscopy lecture notes* (annual editions). Macquarie University, Sydney.

Oldfield, R.J. (1994) *Light microscopy, an illustrated guide*. 160 pp. Wolfe Publishing, London.

Rost, F.W.D. (ed) (1990) *Research and teaching: School of Anatomy, University of New South Wales.* 59 pp. University of New South Wales, Sydney.

Rost, F.W.D. (1991) *Quantitative fluorescence microscopy*. 236 pp. Cambridge University Press, Cambridge.

Rost, F.W.D. (1992; reprinted with addendum 1996) *Fluorescence microscopy,* vol. I. 253 pp. Cambridge University Press, Cambridge.

Rost, F.W.D. (1995) *Fluorescence microscopy,* vol. II. 457 pp. Cambridge University Press, Cambridge.

Tancred, E.J. & Rost, F.W.D. (eds) (1988) *Anatomy class manual for First Year Medicine*. 7th edn. University of New South Wales, Sydney.

Vu, D.H. & Rost, F.W.D. (eds) (1989–1995) *Anatomy class manual for First Year Medicine* (8th–14th annual editions). University of New South Wales, Sydney.

Photography with a microscope

Fred Rost

Emeritus Professor of Anatomy, University of New South Wales
Honorary Visiting Professor, Macquarie University
Sydney, Australia

and

Ron Oldfield

Senior Research Fellow, Macquarie University
Sydney, Australia

CAMBRIDGE
UNIVERSITY PRESS

PUBLISHED BY THE PRESS SYNDICATE OF THE UNIVERSITY OF CAMBRIDGE
The Pitt Building, Trumpington Street, Cambridge, United Kingdom

CAMBRIDGE UNIVERSITY PRESS
The Edinburgh Building, Cambridge CB2 2RU, UK www.cup.cam.ac.uk
40 West 20th Street, New York, NY 10011-4211, USA www.cup.org
10 Stamford Road, Oakleigh (Melbourne), Victoria 3166, Australia www.cup.edu.au

First published 2000

Printed in the United Kingdom at the University Press, Cambridge

Typeface Times New Roman 11 pt. *System* Microsoft Word 5.1

Design (except for this page) and typesetting by the authors

A catalogue record for this book is available from the British Library

ISBN 0 521 77096 3 hardback

Contents

Information on the contents of the parts and chapters is to be found on the title page of each part.

List of plates

Abbreviations and symbols

ANSI	American National Standards Institute
ASA	American Standards Association (film speed rating)
B&W	black-and-white
BFP	back focal plane (of objective)
°C	degrees Celsius
CCD	charge-coupled device
cf	compare with
CI	Contrast Index
CMO	common main objective (of stereomicroscope)
D	depth of field, or optical density
DIC	differential interference contrast
DIN	Deutsches Industrie Norm (film speed rating)
E	exposure increase factor, or light intensity on emulsion, or optical extinction (optical density)
EI	Exposure Index
f/	lens aperture ratio (focal length/diameter)
$\bar{G}$	(*G*-bar) average gradient of characteristic curve
gsm	grams per square metre
H	photographic exposure
Hz	Hertz (cycles per second)
I	intensity of light
IR	infrared
ISO	International Organization for Standardization (film speed rating)
J	joule
K	kelvin (absolute temperature)
log	logarithm
LP/mm	line pairs per mm
LSCM	laser-scanning confocal microscope
M	total magnification
m	metre
max	maximum
min	minutes (of time), or minimum
mm	millimetre
MRD	minimum resolved distance
ms	millisecond (10^{-3} s)
n	refractive index
NA	numerical aperture
nm	nanometre (10^{-9} m)
OTF	off-the-film (metering)
p	reciprocity exponent
RMS	Royal Microscopical Society (microscope objective thread)
rms	root mean square (eg of granularity)
s	second (of time)
sin	sine function of an angle
SLR	single-lens reflex (camera)
T	transmittance
t	time
T_c	corrected time for exposure
T_m	measured time for exposure
T_{max}	peak transmission
TTL	through the lens (metering of camera)
UV	ultraviolet
V	volts
W	watts

Greek letters

α	(alpha) half the angle subtended by the lens as seen from the object
γ	(gamma) contrast ratio
λ	(lambda) wavelength
λ_{max}	wavelength of peak transmission
μm	(mu em) micrometre (10^{-6} m)
μs	microsecond (10^{-6} s)

Preface

This book is intended for all who use or are studying photomicrography. It assumes only a very basic knowledge of how to use an optical (light) microscope. For those who are about to take photomicrographs for the first time, the basic information required is to be found in the first group of chapters (Part I, Chapters 1–5). Those who do not have access to sophisticated equipment will enjoy Chapter 4, which describes how to get the most for the least money. Part II (Chapters 6–8) deals with the microscope. Part III (Chapters 9–13) describes special optical techniques for revealing details of specimens and for photography in stereo. Part IV (Chapters 14–17) deals with advanced photography, including modern digital and video techniques. Part V (Chapters 18–19) describes photographic materials and processing, and also equipment, materials and basic techniques for drawing. Part VI is a series of useful appendices. There is some duplication of material from Part I in Parts II–VI, in order that Part I can stand alone without breaking the logical sequences of Parts II–VI.

For use as a textbook in a course in photomicrography following a course in microscopy, Parts II and III could be omitted at the instructor's discretion. The book could also be used as an elementary textbook of microscopy (to avoid having a second text); a logical sequence would begin with Chapter 2, followed by Parts II and III, Chapters 1 and 3, possibly Chapter 18, and Appendix A1.

We (Fred and Ron) as co-authors have been fortunate in being able to work together amicably on this joint effort. Naturally, our experiences and opinions differ. In some cases, we democratically express our separate opinions.

Fred is grateful for hospitality at Macquarie University; much of the text was drafted while on sabbatical leave there. Ron has been granted privileged access to equipment, laboratories and an office following retirement.

We are grateful to the following colleagues and friends (named in alphabetical order) for reviewing chapters before publication: Professor Anne Ashford (draft equivalent to Chapters 1 and 6), Anne Cartmell (Chapters 5 and 19), Yve Close (Chapter 19), Dr Peter Elliston (Chapters 6, 7 and 8), Arne Müller (Chapter 17), and Dr Virginia Shepherd (Chapters 1–5). The sources of illustrations not made by us are acknowledged in the captions.

Once again we wish to express our appreciation of the collaboration of Dr Alan Crowden and Sandi Irvine of CUP, and we now welcome that of Dr Maria Murphy.

Fred Rost
Ron Oldfield

Sydney, 1999

Part I

Basic photomicrography

This part provides an introduction to photomicrography and associated techniques. The part stands alone, and contains sufficient information for the reader to start making photomicrographs, using transmitted-light microscopy. Chapter 5 includes information on how to assemble a poster or plates for publication.

- Aims: to provide sufficient information for the reader to be able to use a basic microscope correctly, to take photomicrographs in colour or black-and-white, and to include the pictures in a publication or poster.
- Prerequisite knowledge: none.
- Exercises: see Appendix A3.
- Further information: subsequent parts of this book.

1
Introduction to photomicrography

The art and science of taking photographs with a microscope is called photomicrography. This photographic technique is very widely used in science, medicine and engineering (not necessarily in that order). The photographs may be taken for various reasons, scientific, commercial, or artistic.

We (co-authors Fred and Ron) believe that most users of photomicrography will start with a specific need, such as a record of results achieved, slides for a seminar or for teaching, or prints for a thesis or for publication. Therefore, in Part I (Chapters 1–5) we explain how to tackle assignments like these, and how you can get results with simple, easy techniques. The underlying theory, and more specialised techniques, are discussed later in the book.

You (gentle reader) will have a specimen, some film, a microscope, and be eager to start taking pictures. We must ask for your patience while we deal with necessary preliminaries. By the end of Chapter 3, you should be taking photomicrographs!

Plan of this book

The chapters of this book are grouped into five sections (Parts I–V). The first part, Chapters 1–5, describes basic photomicrography, assuming only very elementary knowledge of optical microscopy. Part II, Chapters 6–8, discusses optical microscopy in some detail, and this is expanded in Part III (Chapters 9–13) to include some special optical techniques such as polarisation, interference contrast, fluorescence and stereomicroscopy. Part IV, Chapters 14–17, deals with advanced photomicrography, and assumes previous study of Chapters 1–3 in Part I and Chapters 6–8 in Part II. In Part V, Chapter 18 describes the photographic side of the business. Chapter 19, which we believe to be unique, describes the production of images by drawing with pencil, pen and ink, or computer graphics tablet. Finally, as Part VI there is a group of appendices (including Exercises). There is no glossary, but the comprehensive index should enable the rapid location of definitions.

Definitions

Small objects can be photographed using various types of equipment and techniques. For the photography of progressively smaller objects, you can use close-up photography, photomacrography, or photomicrography, as defined below:

Close-up photography (Fig 1.1) is photography from a distance (measured from the film plane) between 10 times and 4 times the focal length of the lens. This corresponds to magnifications from 0·125× to 1·0× (reproduction ratios from 1:8 to 1:1). The actual dimensions of the field depend upon the size of the film in the camera. The upper limit with the standard 35 mm format is 24 mm × 36 mm, but for a large-format camera using the 4×5 inch (100 mm ×127 mm) format the upper limit is approximately 95 mm × 120 mm.

Photomacrography (Fig 1.2, left) is photography at a magnification of 1× or greater. There is no theoretical upper limit for magnification, but the practical upper limit is about 20×. As before, the actual field size depends on the format: the field size is the same size or smaller than the film format.

Photomicrography (Fig 1.2, right) is photography through a compound microscope, in which two stages of magnification by positive lenses (objective and eyepiece) take place. The objective produces an intermediate image, which is again magnified by an eyepiece to produce the final image for the eye or the camera. You can achieve much higher magnifications by this method. The usual range of magnifications used in photomicrography is (roughly) from 10× to 500×.

To avoid possible confusion, we should add that *microphotography* is the production of a very small photograph. This technique is used, for example, in the production of integrated circuits (as in computer chips, Figs 1.1–1.2).

Magnification is the ratio of the linear size of the image to the size of the object. The magnification is usually expressed as a factor (eg 300×); an alternative is the reproduction ratio (eg 300:1). Dimensions of the specimen are usually measured in *micrometres*, abbreviated µm (µ, pronounced *mew*, is a Greek letter equivalent to *m*). There are 1000 µm in 1 mm. An unofficial alternative name for micrometre is *micron*.

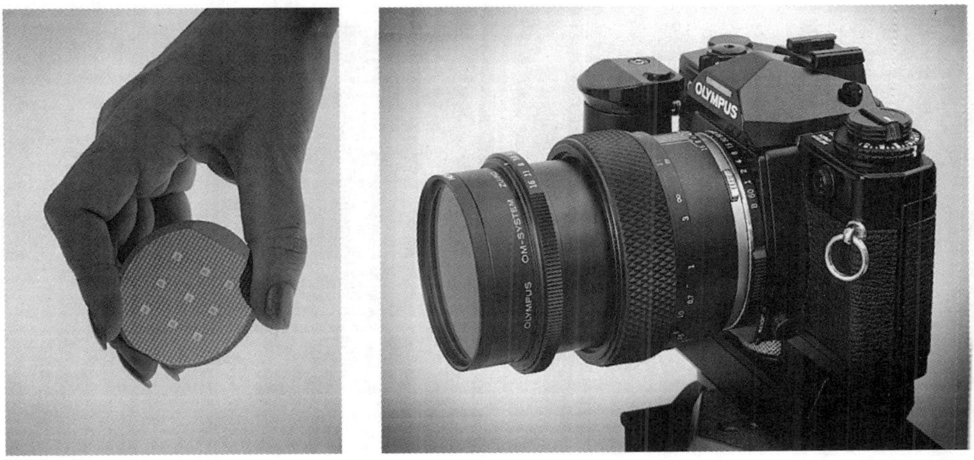

Fig 1.1. Close-up photograph (left) of an integrated circuit (IC) chip, 50 mm in diameter. On the right, the camera with a 'macro' lens which was used to take the photograph. Figures 1.1 and 1.2 illustrate photography of a small object, namely the IC chip, with different techniques for different magnifications: close-up photography, photomacrography and photomicrography. The IC is itself an example of microphotography. The three pairs of pictures each show the equipment used and the corresponding photograph. All techniques employed the same camera body. The object fields shown in Figs 1.1 and 1.2 measure 180 mm × 125 mm, 7 mm × 9 mm, and 0·5 mm × 0·7 mm, respectively.

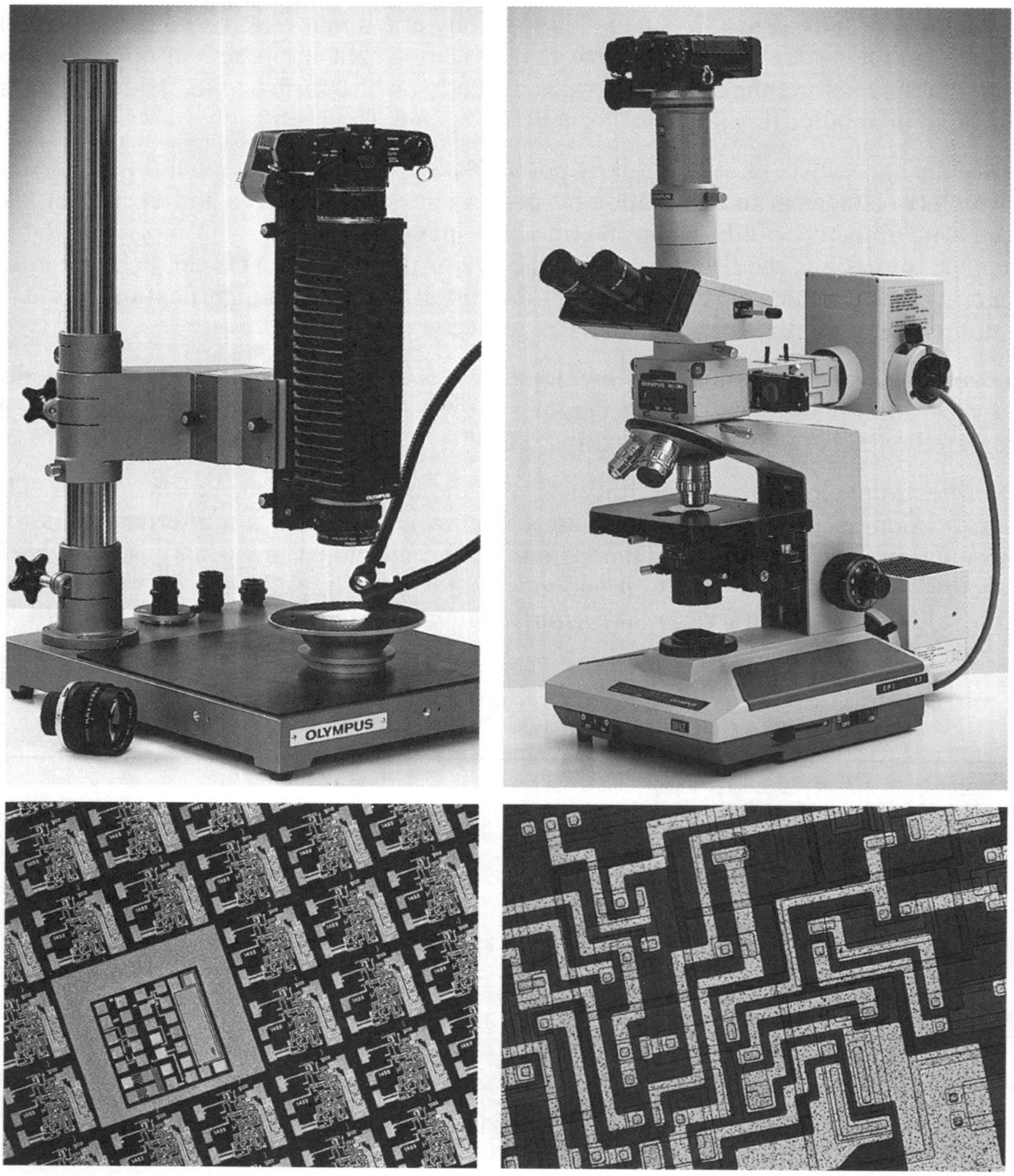

Fig 1.2. The integrated circuit shown in Fig 1.1 has been photographed with specialised equipment (above, left), to produce a *photomacrograph* (lower, left); the field which is shown measures 7 mm × 9 mm. A microscope (above, right) has been used with the same specimen to produce a *photomicrograph* (lower, right); the size of the field which is shown measures 0·5 mm × 0·7 mm. Note that the same camera body can be used for the close-up picture (Fig 1.1), the photomacrograph and the photomicrograph.

Format is the size and shape of the image on the photographic film. In 35 mm film, the individual images (frames) measure 24 mm ×36 mm. A large format sometimes used for photomicrography is 4×5 inches (10×12 cm).

Making a start in photomicrography

For the purposes of this chapter, it is assumed that you have used a microscope before, but have had no previous experience of photomicrography, and have a specific need to take pictures using ordinary transmitted-light microscopy. This and the next two chapters have a logical sequence: the things that you will need are discussed in this chapter; setting up the microscope is described in the next chapter, and basic photomicrography in Chapter 3. Other techniques of microscopy, such as phase-contrast methods and fluorescence, are discussed in later chapters.

Some suggestions for incorporating photomicrographs into publications and posters are given in Chapter 5.

Looking after yourself and the microscope

Long sessions at the microscope should be facilitated by ergonomic seating, and preferably with subdued and carefully directed lighting. Do not assume that uncomfortable binocular viewing, and headaches, are a necessary accompaniment to your task as a microscopist. It is not demeaning to your skills to ask questions of the microscope supplier concerning the appropriate setting of the binocular head to suit your needs.

If you wear spectacle glasses, you will have to decide whether or not to wear them. If you do not suffer from astigmatism, it is usually more convenient to take them off while looking into the microscope; if your eyes have astigmatism, better-corrected vision is obtained by keeping the spectacles on. We recommend that you try with and without spectacles to find out which suits you best. Modern microscopes usually make adequate provision for spectacle wearers, by so-called high-eyepoint eyepieces (oculars), which have sufficient clearance to provide space for spectacles; for an older microscope, you need to acquire a pair of high-eyepoint eyepieces.

To use, for the first time, a modern research microscope, complete with its built-in or dedicated photomicrographic camera, can be a daunting prospect, especially when the instruction manuals are no longer to be found. It is never too late (well, hardly ever) to acquire the manual. The manufacturer is as anxious as anyone to have the microscope used correctly. Only the supplier of photographic film has something to gain by poor microscopy, and that dubious gain is the sale of more film! Do make contact with the manufacturer of the microscope, who will be delighted that a user is interested in gaining proficiency with their instrument. Even if it is a 30 year-old instrument, a photocopy of the file copy of the manual is likely to be made available at small cost. The best advertisement for a microscope is a skilled and happy customer. Instruction courses and microscopical societies are a useful source of practical training.

Before you start photography with a microscope, it is worth spending time ensuring that the instrument is really clean (see Appendix A1). There are certain lenses and surfaces that are particularly prone to the collection and subsequent imaging of dust particles. Before putting the slide on the stage, look at the slide itself and its coverslip. Be especially careful with temporary mounts not to ruin the specimen, but permanent mounts should always receive scrutiny and attention with a mild glass-cleaning solvent. Slowly move the slide while observing the specimen in the microscope. Dust on filters, or on the condenser, will show as stationary flecks; dust and artefacts on the slide will move with the specimen.

Be very critical of the image and appraise it most carefully. Imperfections that can be tolerated when looking through the eyepieces will become quite intolerable when recorded as a photographic print or projected in the conference room as a slide transparency. The concentration and effort that is made to compose and focus the picture may tend to allow the simpler mistakes to be overlooked. The microscope field must be *evenly illuminated*. Uniform lighting, with good contrast over the entire field, is normally guaranteed using *Köhler illumination* (see Chapter 7). However, the lower the magnification, ie the larger the object field, the more difficult it is to attain this apparently simple requirement. Objectives with a magnification of 4× and lower are likely to need special ultra-low or auxiliary condensers (see Chapter 7).

The microscope and camera

The first prerequisite is a microscope. Microscopes are described in Chapter 2, and their optical equipment in more detail in Chapters 6–13. A brief summary is given here. Microscopes designed for photomicrography should be equipped with both a binocular tube for observation and a separate monocular tube to accommodate the camera (Fig 1.2). A sliding mirror or beam-splitting device allows the choice of sending the light from the objective to the observation tube, or to the photographic tube, or to both simultaneously.

To be able to take satisfactory pictures, the microscope should have good lenses and a Köhler illumination system. As regards lenses, at this stage it need only be said that you should use flat-field (plan) objectives if possible (see Chapter 6). The Köhler illumination system is described in Chapter 7.

Cameras for photomicrography (described in detail in Chapter 14) are usually specially constructed to suit the particular microscope, and are mounted on the vertical tube of the trinocular head (Fig 1.2, upper right). In microscopes specially designed for photomicrography, the photographic system may be incorporated into the microscope body or form a substantial module attached to the top of the stand (see Fig 14.3). An ordinary camera can be adapted, as described in Chapter 4. In practice, one of the following will be used:

- A dedicated 'photomicroscope', intended specifically for taking photographs, with appropriate optical equipment.
- A good-quality microscope with a trinocular head and flat-field objectives, and an attached photomicrographic camera unit.
- A microscope of some kind, with an 'ordinary' camera body.

This book deals primarily with the first two cases; the third case is dealt with specifically in Chapter 4, Limited-budget photomicrography.

Choice of film

Format

Most photomicrographic cameras today use the 35 mm format. This film is sold in cassettes, and consists of a length of film with sprocket holes along each edge.

Each cassette has enough film for a particular number of exposures, usually 20, 24 or 36. Polaroid instant film is commonly used in $3^1/_4 \times 4^1/_4$ inch (9×12 cm) and 4×5 inch (10×12 cm) formats. The new APS (Advanced Photographic System) gives smaller negatives (measuring 16·7 mm × 30·2 mm) and can (at present) be used only for colour prints. You can adapt some APS single-lens-reflex cameras to some microscopes (see Chapter 4).

Type

Photographic film is made in several different types for different purposes. The most important types are listed below. Other types, for specialised purposes, are described in Chapter 18.

Colour negative (print) film is probably the most widely used for general pictorial purposes. As its name implies, it is used mainly for the production of prints. From a single negative, as many prints as needed can be printed, at any desired size. The film is colour-balanced for daylight, and requires the use of a blue filter on the microscope.

Colour transparency (slide, diapositive) film is the most widely used for scientific and technical purposes. As its name implies, it is used mainly for the production of transparencies, which can either be projected, or used for publication. Excellent prints can also be made from transparencies, but the cost is considerably greater than when using negative film. The film is usually colour-balanced for daylight, and therefore usually requires the use of a blue filter on the microscope. There are also other types of film, variously known as 'artificial-light' (type A or type B) film, which do not require a blue filter (see Chapter 8); however, our experience is that they are usually less suitable for general use.

Black-and-white (B&W) negative (print) film was the first type of film, but is now used mainly for special purposes. As its name implies, it is used for the production of B&W prints. From a single negative, as many prints as needed can be printed, at any desired size. The film can be used with any kind of light, and does not require the use of a blue filter. Contrast can be controlled by filters and/or chemical processing.

Speed and resolution

Films are made with differing degrees of sensitivity to light, for different purposes. Film speed is measured in ISO units; other units, that have been used in the recent past and are still referred to on some camera systems, include ASA and DIN. These systems are explained in Chapter 16. Slow films (ISO less than 100) usually give the sharpest, clearest pictures, and are usually the most suitable for photomicrography. Medium-speed films (typically ISO 100) are the most widely used for general photography, and are quite suitable for photomicrography. Fast films (ISO 200 or more) require shorter exposures, and are useful for photographing moving objects and for fluorescence (Chapter 11). They tend to be less sharp and give less contrast.

So which film?

Many workers shoot colour transparency (reversal, positive) film, this being usually the most convenient, the cheapest, and giving slides for projection or reproduction. Transparencies are preferred for reproduction, one reason being that the printer can check the printed colours against those of the transparency.

If colour prints are needed, there are several possibilities. Firstly, you can make excellent, but expensive, prints from transparencies using an enlarger and appropriate paper (eg Ilfochrome). Secondly, you can take the photomicrographs directly on colour negative film. In this case, it may be helpful or indeed essential to have transparencies as well so that the operator making the prints can be shown the correct colours. Thirdly, prints can be made from an internegative made by rephotographing the transparency with colour negative film; Fred has found this method quite satisfactory for most purposes, using a fine-grain negative film and having the developing and printing done at the local mini-lab. Fourthly, transparencies can be copied onto Polaroid print film. Finally, transparencies or miniprints can be scanned and printed digitally (see Chapter 17).

For B&W prints, obviously B&W negative film is best. However, the choice of film may be influenced by access to a darkroom and to competent darkroom technicians. Small prints for reproduction in journals, etc, can be made from colour negative film, and from transparencies via a B&W internegative.

For photography without a darkroom, you can either rely on commercial processing, or use Polaroid instant materials. Alternatively, digital imaging and computer processing can be carried out without a darkroom (see Chapter 17).

The film

Photomicrographs for record purposes are often taken on colour transparency (slide) film.

Slides for a seminar or for teaching are best taken on colour transparency (slide) film.

Prints in colour for a thesis are most cheaply taken on colour negative (print) film.

Prints in black-and-white for publication or a thesis are best taken on black-and-white negative film.

Pictures for publication in colour should be taken on colour transparency (slide) film.

Digital imaging is becoming an important alternative.

Getting started

We will assume that your first assignment is taking some photomicrographs of a specimen on a slide, using conventional transmitted-light microscopy.

The materials and equipment that you will need are:

- A microscope (described in Chapter 2, and in more detail in Chapters 6–8).
- The specimen.
- A camera, built-in or attachable. Cameras are described in Chapters 14 and 4.

The procedure for taking the picture is described in Chapters 2 and 3 (and in more detail in Chapter 15). It can be can be summarised as follows.

- Adjust the microscope for optimal performance (see Chapter 2).
- Load the camera, with an appropriate film (chosen according to principles described below, and in Chapter 19).
- Select the area of the specimen to be photographed (Chapters 3 and 5).
- Decide what filters, if any, to use (see Chapters 3 and 8).
- Set the lamp current to the correct value (colour film only; see Chapters 3 and 8).
- Determine the correct exposure (see Chapter 3; for difficult conditions, refer to Chapter 16, Exposure measurement.
- Operate the camera shutter to make the exposure, possibly also taking additional ('bracketed') photographs at different exposures (see Chapter 3).
- Record details of the film, subject, magnification, etc. Co-author Ron recommends photographing a stage micrometer (see Chapter 3) on every roll of negative film as a record of the magnification(s) used.
- Process, or have the film processed, or developed and printed, as appropriate (see Chapter 18).
- Mount the print to make a plate for publication or a poster, if required (see Chapter 5).

Extending the same procedure to more complex forms of microscopy, such as fluorescence, interference contrast and polarisation, usually only requires setting up the microscope for the appropriate mode of microscopy (see Part III, Chapters 9–12). There are, however, some special problems associated with darkground and fluorescence microscopy, which are discussed in the appropriate chapters (9 and 11).

The special techniques of photomicrography with a stereomicroscope are described in Chapter 13.

Aims of photomicrography

What is to be included in the picture? What aspects are to be brought out? Does it matter if the colours are altered? How much resolution and contrast are required?

You are using a microscope because of the *detail* that it produces in the image. The magnification that you employ in the microscope and camera is to make that image detail visible. There are very basic principles involved in the ability or inability of the system to *resolve* that detail, which are discussed in Chapter 6. The most suitable magnification is sometimes obvious, for example when you wish to illustrate a complete organism or structure. However, aesthetic considerations (Chapter 5) may sometimes dominate the choice. Avoid too large a magnification. More often than not an objective one step lower in magnification than the one chosen for visual examination is appropriate for photography, because you will select for the photograph only a part of the field viewed in the eyepiece.

Aesthetic considerations

Photomicrographs can be very beautiful. Even for a photograph intended only as a record of a specimen, not for publication, a little additional time and care in composition may yield rich dividends in beauty. Artistic considerations are of even greater importance in the production of pictures intended for publication or public presentation, the latter including lectures to students. These matters are dealt with in Chapter 5.

Fidelity of reproduction

The representation of the object in the photograph can differ from the original object in colour, contrast, definition, and shape.

Colour reproduction cannot be expected to be exact, because of limitations of the film. Neither will it be constant, because of differing batches of film and (with long exposures) differing reciprocity failures of the three photosensitive layers of the colour film. In stained specimens, the exact shades of overall colour are very seldom significant, and therefore it is a waste of time worrying about small variations in colour. In particular, there is little point in using the colour correction filters recommended by the manufacturers to compensate for reciprocity failure.

Contrast is, roughly speaking, the ratio of the brightest to the darkest parts of the picture. This will depend upon the film, the development process, and the exposure, as well as the specimen. For example, *Kodachrome* film has higher contrast than *Ektachrome* film; contrast varies with the developer type and development time, and highest contrast is normally obtained with the 'correct' exposure. Control of contrast is discussed in Chapters 10, 15 and 18.

Definition or resolution in the photograph relates to the amount of fine detail that can be shown; it usually depends mainly on the optical system, and otherwise on the nature of the film and the manner of development. The resolving power of the optical system is determined by the numerical aperture (NA; see next paragraph) of the objective and of the condenser (except in fluorescence and darkground microscopy, where the NA of the condenser does not affect the resolution of the microscope). In practice, the resolution of the film is unlikely to be a limiting factor in the detail shown by the photomicrograph, although with high-speed film graininess will be apparent. Definition is discussed in detail in Chapters 3 and 6.

Numerical aperture (NA) is (roughly speaking) a measure of the diameter of a lens, such as an objective, compared to its focal length. NA is related to the *f*-number of a camera lens. For small NAs, the NA is approximately equal to half the reciprocal of the *f*-number.

Troubleshooting

Hints on dealing with faults that may be found in photomicrographs are given in Appendix A2.

2
The microscope

Good photomicrography is nine-tenths good microscopy and one-tenth good photography. It is essential to have a good-quality optical system and to adjust the microscope as finely as possible (see Fig 2.1). This chapter gives an outline of the structure and function of microscopes, sufficient to enable the reader to understand the next chapter, in which the procedure for taking photographs is outlined. Readers who are already expert microscopists may skip to Chapter 3.

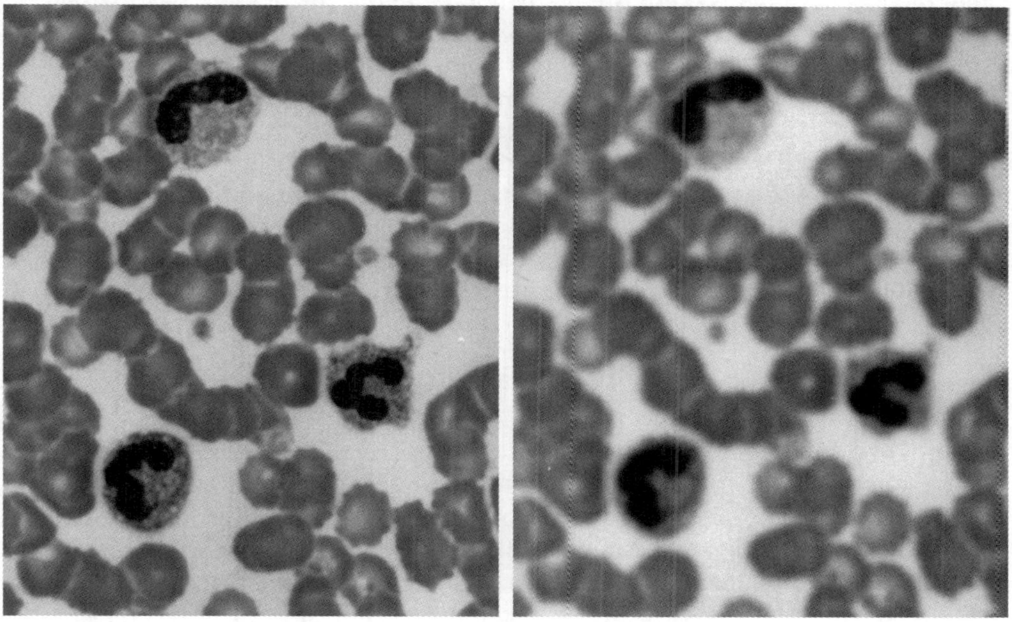

Fig 2.1. Blood smear, Leishman stain. Excellent and poor pictures of same subject, same 1000× magnification, field size 80 µm × 65 µm. Left, using 40× oil-immersion objective, NA 1·00, combined projective and enlarger magnification 25×. Right, using 10× objective, NA 0·25, combined projective and enlarger magnification 100×. Note increased resolution with higher NA (on the left). Zeiss *Universal* microscope, Olympus *PM-10ADS* 35 mm photomicrographic camera, Ilford *Pan F* film developed in *ID11* developer.

For further information on microscopy, see Part II (Chapters 6–8), Oldfield (1994), and Inoué & Spring (1997). Excellent booklets, of general interest but oriented towards particular manufacturers, include those of Anon (1984a, Olympus), Kapitza (1994, Zeiss), and Schade (1995, Leica).

The type of microscope under consideration, the compound microscope, has a two-stage magnifying system. There are two lens systems, the *objective* and the *eyepiece* (ocular), mounted at opposite ends of a tube (the *body tube*). The objective is composed of several lens elements that form an enlarged real image of the object being examined (Fig 2.9). This image is called the *intermediate image*. The intermediate image is further enlarged by the eyepiece. The observer, looking through the eyepiece, sees an enlarged *virtual image* of the intermediate image. This final image, situated at infinity, can be examined by the eye or photographed by a camera. The *total magnification* of the microscope is determined by the focal lengths of the objective and eyepiece. The body tube, the specimen and an illumination system are supported by a *stand*. This has a flat *stage* for holding the specimen to be examined, and a *focusing mechanism* for moving specimen and microscope tube towards and away from each other so that the specimen can be brought into focus. Typically, specimens for microscopic examination are translucent and are viewed by light shone through them. The stage is therefore pierced with a hole for the passage of light, and carries on its underside a condensing lens (*condenser*) to concentrate light rays onto the specimen. Illumination is provided by a *lamp*, the light of which is usually focused into the condenser by another lens or system of lenses.

The basic function of a microscope is to reveal details too minute to be visible with the naked eye. Therefore, the essential characteristics of the optical system are *resolution* and *magnification*. The magnification of a microscope is produced jointly by the objective and the eyepiece. The resolution (minimum resolved distance, MRD) of a microscope can be defined as the ability to separate minute details that are very close together. This is usually measured as the least distance between two minute circular objects of high contrast at which they can still be seen to be separate. Resolving power depends primarily on the objective's numerical aperture (NA; see Chapter 6); higher NA gives improved resolution.

If the light rays from the specimen do not fully fill the aperture of the objective, its theoretical resolving power is not obtained. It is the function of the condenser to provide a cone of light that passes through the specimen and which has an angle sufficiently wide to fill the aperture of the objective. The condenser must be adjusted properly or else the quality of the image suffers.

To complement the magnifying system, a microscope has an illuminating system (Fig 2.2), which usually is used to shine a powerful beam of light through the transparent specimen from beneath (opaque specimens require a different system, for which see Chapter 7). The characteristics of the illumination are important in achieving the resolving power appropriate to high magnification.

In the illumination system, light is generated by a light source (lamp). Light from the lamp is collected by a collector lens in the lamphouse and focused through a field diaphragm into the condenser, which focuses the light onto the specimen. Somewhere in the illumination system, a filter may be inserted to select the appropriate wavelengths for illumination. The illumination and observation systems are similar, and symmetrical about the object. In principle, they are to some extent interchangeable – the objective can be used as a condenser, and vice versa. The basic transmitted-light illumination system will be described first, because it is the most widely used. However, the same principles apply to metallurgical microscopes. Illumination is discussed in more detail in Chapter 7, and specialised methods of

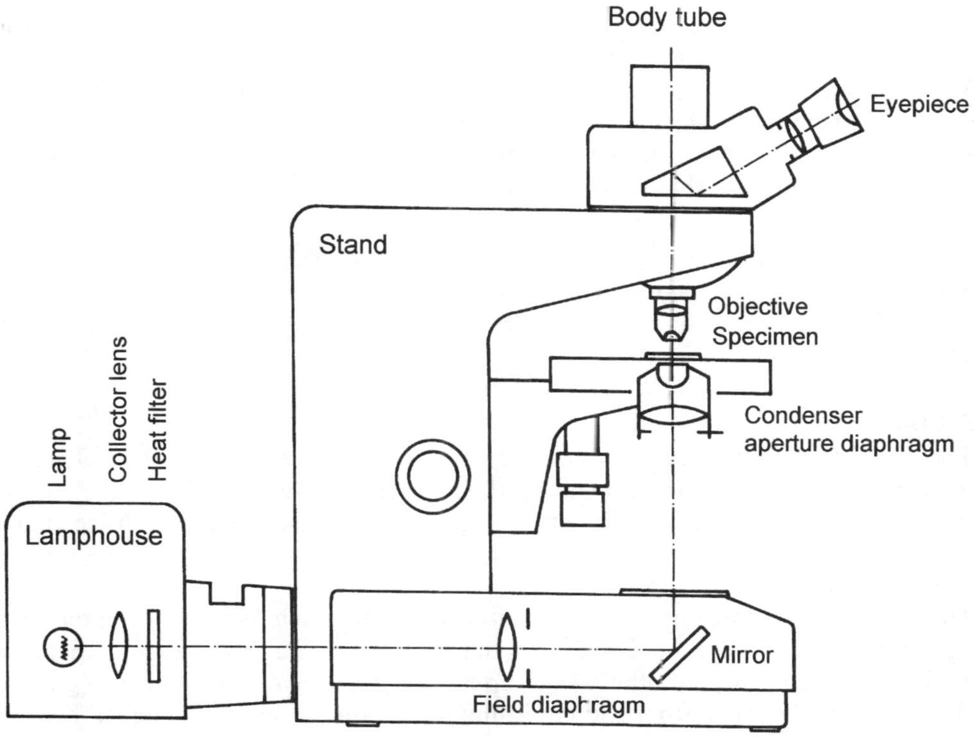

Fig 2.2. The optical system of a microscope (using transmitted light) similar to that shown in Fig 2.3.

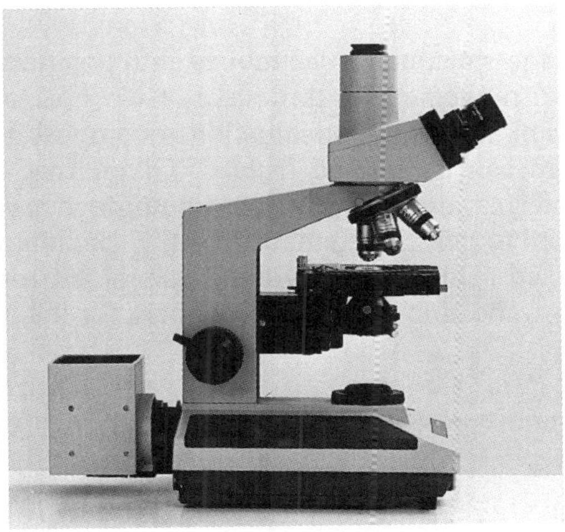

Fig 2.3. A typical basic microscope. Olympus *BH* series, with trinocular tube for a camera (which is not shown). Cf Fig 2.2.

Anatomy of a microscope

We recommend that you read the remainder of this Chapter with a microscope in front of you, if possible. A typical microscope is illustrated in Fig 2.3. Functionally, there are three main parts: the optical magnifying system, the illumination system, and the mechanical parts that hold everything together.

Mechanical components of the microscope

The main mechanical components of a microscope consist of the stand, body tube, nosepiece for objectives, and stage and substage for supporting the specimen and the substage condenser.

The stand

The stand is the part that supports the body tube, stage and substage. There are three main types of stand: upright (normal), inverted and stereo. In the upright type, the body tube is situated above the stage, and the condenser underneath, so that the specimen is viewed from above and illuminated from below. In inverted microscopes, the situation is reversed.

The stand must be strong and sufficiently resistant to vibration, both external and that generated internally, eg by the camera shutter. The best way to deal with external vibration is to place the whole apparatus on a heavy, solid base (granite is said to be best) separated from the environment by spring supports (eg rubber feet). The heavier and more rigid the stand, the better it is from the point of view of photography.

The stage

The stage (Fig 2.4) usually serves the following functions:

- It supports the object.
- It has provision for the specimen to be moved into position to be examined. This requires translational movement in three axes (two horizontal, one vertical for focusing), and rotation about the optical axis (to compose the picture) unless the camera or the image can be rotated instead. Given that the specimen can be reversed end-for-end, or (alternatively) the photograph turned round, only 180° of rotation is required to permit orientation of the specimen at any required angle with respect to a fixed camera. If the stage cannot be rotated through at least 180°, it is necessary to be able to rotate the camera (or the image, using an image-rotating device).

There are several main types of stage (Fig 2.4), each with respective advantages and disadvantages.

The plain rectangular stage is the simplest and cheapest. It has a flat top, pierced by a hole for transmitted light (if relevant), and its only movement is up-and-down for focusing. A plain stage accepts objects of all kinds, including glass slides, Petri dishes and rock samples. The object must be moved by hand, but unlimited translational and rotational movements are possible. Such movement by hand requires practice, particularly as a conventional microscope reverses the image, and is difficult under high magnification. A plain rectangular stage with no hole and no substage is used for opaque specimens.

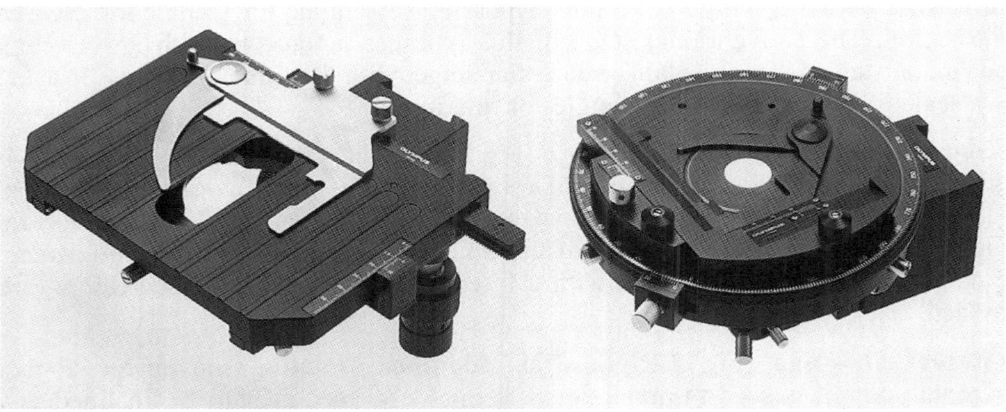

Fig 2.4a. Typical microscope stages. Left, rectangular mechanical stage. This one has a grooved surface designed for oil immersion use. Right, centrable rotating stage, graduated in degrees, with attached mechanical stage. See also Fig 2.4b.

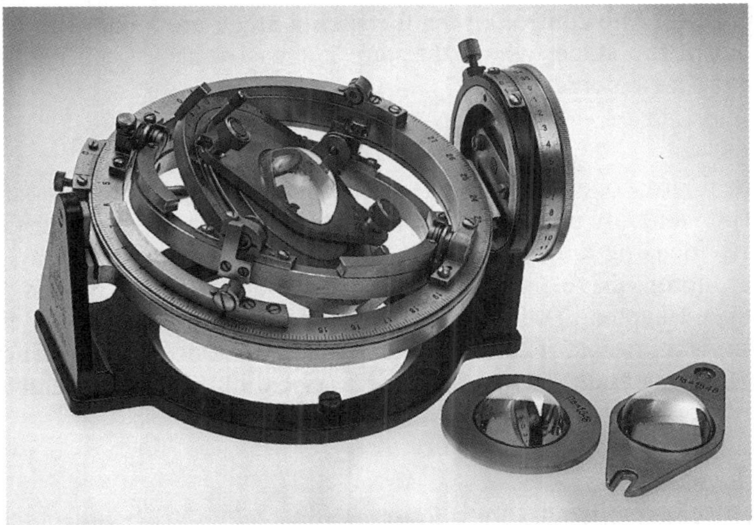

Fig 2.4b. A special 'universal' stage, capable of rotation about three axes, with specialised optical components for examining crystals. Cf Fig 2.4a.

A rectangular mechanical stage (Fig 2.4a) is most commonly fitted to biological and general-purpose microscopes. This accepts rectangular slides, and gives the best and most convenient *X–Y* positioning of the specimen. The controls are usually placed below the stage in a convenient position. (Co-author Fred would prefer such controls on the left side, as he is right-handed, and operates the microscope with his left hand while writing notes with his right.) The slide clip must be removed to accommodate Petri dishes etc. There is often some provision for rotation, but this is seldom adequate (ie it is less than 180°). In laboratories in which condenser immersion is routinely employed, a stage with channels (Fig 2.4a) is useful to prevent oil sticking the slide to the surface of the stage.

A circular rotating stage is desirable, possibly essential, for techniques involving polarisation. The conventional stage of this type has a flat top, with an attachable mechanical stage as for the plain rectangular stage, with the same problems. It usually has a scale of degrees to measure angles of rotation.

A centrable circular rotating stage (Fig 2.4a, right) is similar to the above, but has provision for moving the centre of rotation, for alignment with the optical axis of the objective. Under some circumstances this movement can be used for final delicate adjustment of the position of the object. The actual rotating movement is not as precise as that of the type with a fixed axis, and a scale of degrees is rarely provided.

A universal stage (Fig 2.4b) has an additional rotating movement about a horizontal axis; it is used in mineralogy, to enable a specimen to be inclined at an angle to the microscope axis so that the optical axes of a crystal can be located.

An accessory mechanical stage (see Fig 2.4a) is a device for holding and moving rectangular slides and to provide a range of fine movement controlled by rack-and-pinion mechanisms. It can be fitted to any stage that does not have a similar mechanism built-in. The control knobs for such a stage are small and inconveniently situated on top of the stage, where they are not easily accessible and may foul the objectives on the nosepiece.

Focusing

In modern microscopes, focusing is accomplished by moving the stage (carrying the specimen) up and down. Separate controls for coarse and fine adjustments are the norm. The fine-focusing knob commonly has a scale, for measurements of specimen thickness. A motor drive is sometimes incorporated, particularly in confocal microscopes (see Chapter 17). In older microscopes, the stage is usually fixed, and the body tube is moved instead. If an experimental technique demands instrumentation on the stage (eg for injection), a fixed stage is essential, and is typically provided in inverted microscopes.

Trinocular heads

Most microscopes intended for photography have the usual binocular observation tubes and a third tube (the phototube, Figs 2.5 and 2.6) extending vertically for the camera. A sliding mirror directs light from the objective either to the binocular tubes or to the photographic apparatus as required. Commonly, a beamsplitter is fitted to provide a third possibility (Fig 2.6, centre), whereby part of the light is directed in each direction. Changing the separation of the eyepieces, to adjust for the interpupillary distance of the observer's eyes, affects the focusing, unless an automatic (and expensive) compensating device is also provided. Without such compensation, correct focusing of a camera using an eyepiece graticule may not be achieved. Trinocular heads that offer the choices of 100% light through the observation tube and 100% up to the camera (Fig 2.6, right) are preferred for observation and photography of dim light, such as fluorescence. Some microscopes have multiple ports for cameras, typically for one or two 35 mm cameras and a large-format camera or a video camera.

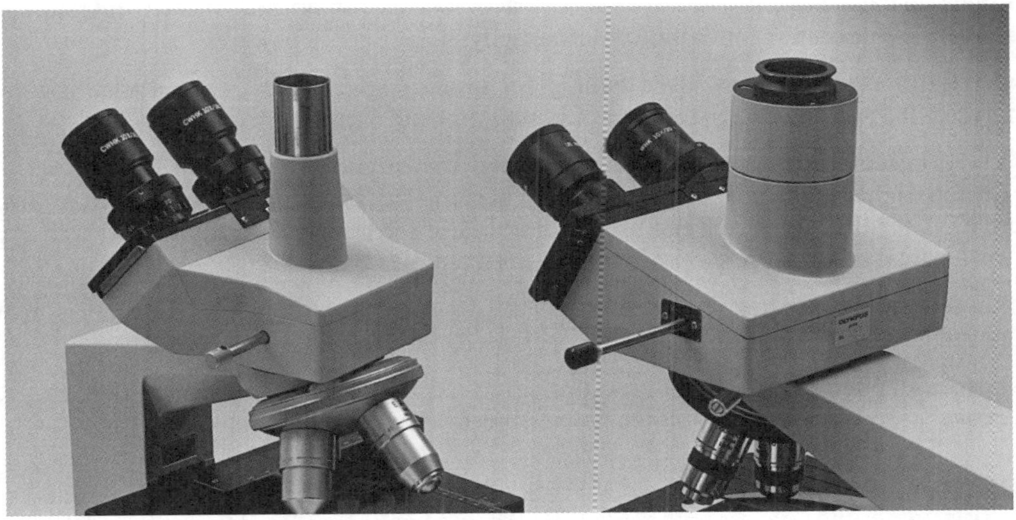

Fig 2.5. Trinocular body tubes on Olympus microscopes. On the left, a simple version which accepts standard eyepieces in the phototube. The binocular eyepiece tubes are capable of being adjusted individually to the correct tubelength when their separation is varied. On the right, a trinocular tube with a specialised mount for Olympus cameras. The eyepieces have automatic compensation for tubelength.

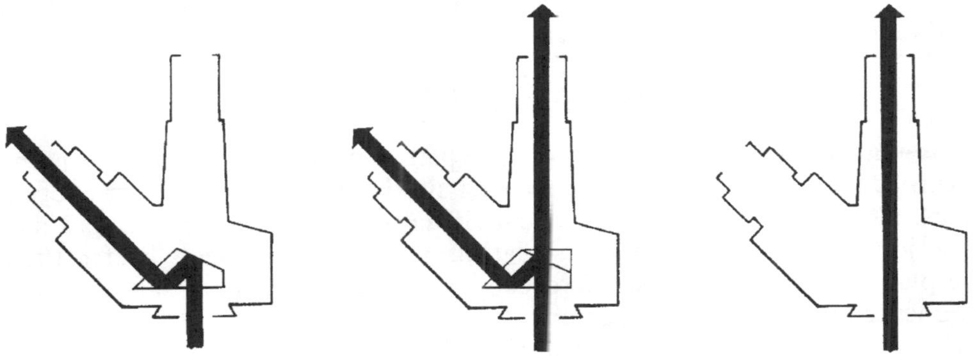

Fig 2.6. Trinocular body tubes illustrating settings of the beamsplitter. Left: all light to the eyepieces. Centre: light split between eyepieces and camera. Right, all light to the camera.

Types of microscope

Modern microscopes are normally designed and manufactured on a modular basis, with a basic stand and a variety of interchangeable modules and accessories for different purposes. The following basic types are usually recognised:

Biological microscopes are general-purpose upright microscopes. All but the simplest usually have provision to accept accessories for phase contrast, interference contrast, fluorescence, and photomicrography.

Polarising microscopes, used mainly for mineralogical work, have a polariser and analyser in their optical system (see Chapter 10) and a circular rotating stage.

Metallurgical microscopes, used mainly for studies of opaque specimens by reflected light, have an epi-illumination system (to illuminate the specimen from above). The stage may lack the usual central hole for transmitted light. Research-type metallurgical microscopes are often built inverted (see below).

Inverted microscopes (see below) are designed for viewing specimens from underneath.

Stereomicroscopes have a double optical system, one system for each eye, to give stereoscopic vision of three-dimensional objects. They are discussed in Chapter 13.

Inverted microscopes

It is sometimes necessary to examine the specimen from underneath, and for this purpose an inverted microscope is used, in which the objective is underneath the stage and the condenser above. Such an arrangement is advantageous for investigations of living cells, eg tissue cultures (where the cells are on the bottom of a culture vessel) or for microinjection studies, where the inverted microscope provides more space for a micromanipulator above the stage.

In the majority of inverted microscopes, the whole of the viewing system (including the binocular head and the camera) is below the level of the stage (Fig 2.7). In some Leica inverted microscopes, the light path of the viewing system is taken up to the top of the microscope so that a standard binocular or trinocular tube is fitted in the conventional position, and the camera sits on top.

The optical magnifying system

The viewing system of a microscope is the part of the optical system that produces a magnified image of the object. The viewing system includes the objective, eyepiece (ocular), intermediate magnifying system (if any), and the camera. It may include accessories such as an analyser (for polarisation microscopy, see Chapter 10) or a phase plate (for phase-contrast microscopy, see Chapter 10) or a barrier filter (for fluorescence microscopy, see Chapter 11).

The objective produces a real, magnified image (the intermediate image) in the plane of the diaphragm of the eyepiece. The eyepiece further magnifies this image, producing a virtual image at infinity, behind the specimen. This virtual image is seen by the eye, the lens of the eye converting the virtual image to a real image on the retina. In the camera, the camera lens acts similarly to produce a real image in the film plane. Note that the virtual image produced by the eyepiece used to be regarded as being 250 mm in front of the eye, that being regarded as the nearest comfortable focusing distance of the eye; the magnification of the eyepiece is still calculated on the assumption that the image is in that position. In classical microscopes, the intermediate image is situated approximately 150 mm above the objective (Fig 2.9, left); in some modern microscopes, the objective produces a parallel beam of light, from which the intermediate image is brought to a focus by a *tube* (*Telan*) *lens* (Fig 2.9, right). In the later case, the objectives are said to be *infinity corrected.*

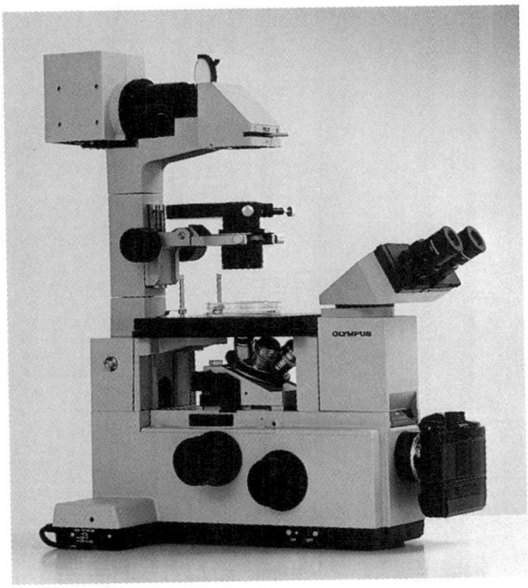

Fig 2.7. An example of an inverted microscope, the Olympus *IMT–2* with attached camera (bottom right). Cf Fig 2.8.

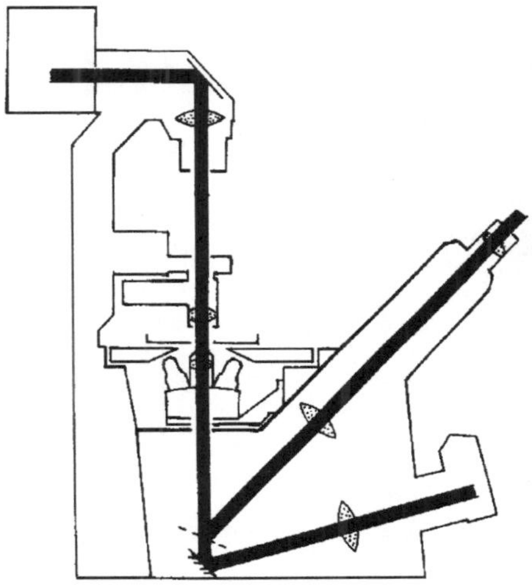

Fig 2.8. Optical diagram of the Leica inverted microscope. Cf Fig 2.7.

The overall magnification is determined jointly by the objective, the eyepiece (for the eye) or projective (a kind of eyepiece used by the camera), the intermediate magnifier (if any), and the camera lens. Numerically, the overall magnification is equal to the product of the respective magnifications of the components named above. Given that the first three components are changeable, it follows that any given overall magnification can often be achieved in more than one way, using different combinations of magnifications of objectives, intermediate lenses, and eyepieces.

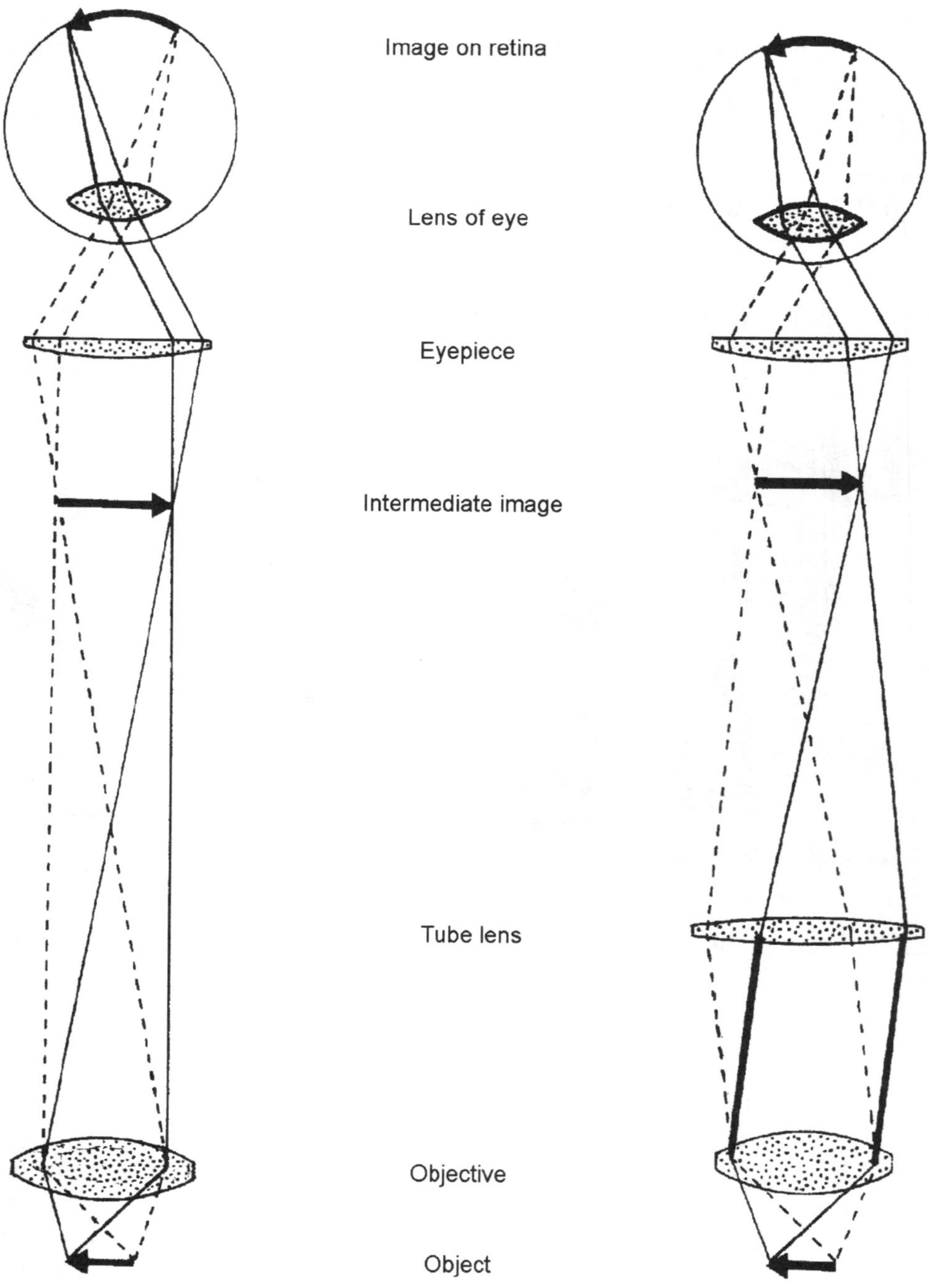

Fig 2.9. Microscope optical systems. Left, the optical system of a conventional microscope. Right, the optical system using an infinity-corrected objective. Note the additional tube lens, and the parallel ray paths (shown as heavy lines) between the objective and the tube lens.

The objective

The prime purposes of the objective (Fig 2.10) are to resolve detail in the object and to provide initial magnification. The brightness of the final image is also determined in part by the objective. Objectives have markings similar those shown in Fig 2.10. These matters are explained in more detail in Chapter 6.

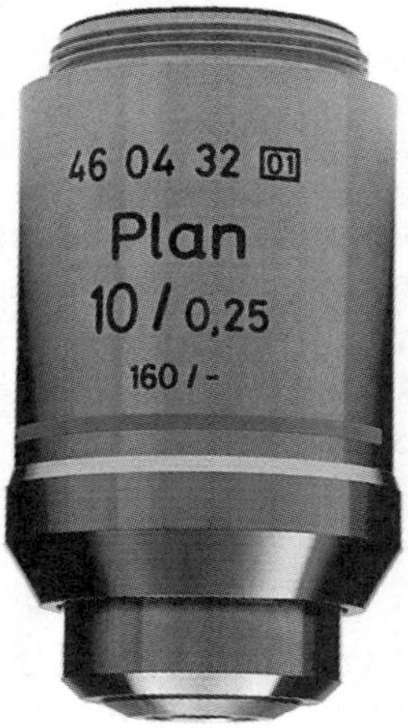

Fig 2.10. Photograph of a typical objective. Zeiss 10× magnification, 0·25 numerical aperture (NA), dry (non-immersion) objective.

Typical markings for objectives; some are shown in the figure (left).

'Cambridge'	The name of the manufacturer.
46 04 32 01	Manufacturer's catalogue number (or, on older objectives, a serial number, which is much more useful).
'Plan'	The type of objective: in this case, a flat-field achromatic objective.
'10' or '10×'	The magnification.
'0·25' or '0,25'	The numerical aperture.
160	Tubelength in mm (if applicable).
∞	Infinity correction.
'0·17' or '0,17'	The thickness of coverslip for which the objective is designed. '–' here means that the coverslip thickness is unimportant.
Coloured ring	Colour-code for magnification.
A black ring	If present, denotes an oil-immersion objective.

The magnification of an objective is determined by its focal length; the shorter the focal length, the greater the magnification.

The numerical aperture (NA) of a microscope objective corresponds to the *f*-ratio or *f*-number of a conventional camera lens. The NA is (roughly speaking) a measure of the diameter of a lens, such as an objective, compared to its focal length. For small NAs, the NA is approximately equal to half the reciprocal of the *f*-number.

The resolution of the optical system (ie its ability to resolve and reproduce fine detail) depends primarily on the NA of the objective. Objectives with a numerical aperture greater than about 0·9 require that the space between the object and the objective be filled with a liquid medium, such as immersion oil or water. The consideration of immersion objectives is deferred to Chapter 6.

The parfocal distance is the distance between the focused plane of the specimen and the shoulder of the nosepiece into which the objective is screwed. Modern objectives usually have a parfocal distance of 45 mm; old ones (to about 1970) commonly used

37 mm. Objectives are said to be parfocal if they have the same parfocal distance. It is inconvenient, and sometimes dangerous to the specimen, to mix objectives that are not parfocal.

Magnification-changing devices

Magnification-changing devices can be added as accessories to several types of microscope, to enable the optimal magnification to be obtained for observation or photography. These normally consist of a rotating turret carrying a choice of lenses that can be turned into the optical pathway. Alternatively, a zoom system may be used.. They assist considerably in composing the picture for photomicrography.

Eyepieces (oculars)

Eyepieces serve to magnify the intermediate image produced by the objective, and to produce either a virtual image below it (for examination by the eye) or a real image above it (for photography). Optically, they contain two major components: a diaphragm that serves to limit the field of view, and a lens system to provide the required magnification. In many microscope systems, the eyepiece lenses also help to correct aberrations introduced by the objective.

Lens aberrations and corrections

All lenses are subject to imaging faults known collectively as lens aberrations. It is the skill and art of the optician to design systems of lenses to minimise these inherent defects. The higher the degree of correction, the higher is the cost; for this and other reasons, objectives are commonly sold with varying degrees of corrections. It is not necessary for the photomicrographer to know much about these aberrations; however, it is useful to have at least a general understanding of them, so that one can choose the most appropriate equipment for a particular purpose, or to get the best possible result from a given set of optical equipment. From a practical point of view, for photomicrography it is almost essential to have flat-field (plan) objectives. Aberrations are discussed in Chapter 6.

The illumination system

The purpose of the illumination system is primarily to illuminate the specimen with sufficiently intense light of an appropriate wavelength range, and (in the case of transmitted-light microscopy) to adequately fill the aperture of the objective. In addition, the illumination system may be required to provide alternative forms of illumination, such as darkground, phase-contrast, or fluorescence excitation, for special forms of microscopy discussed in Chapters 9–12.

The illumination system (Fig 2.11) consists essentially of a lamp, a collector lens in front of the lamp to concentrate the light onto the condenser, and a condenser to concentrate the light onto the specimen and fill the angular aperture of the objective.

Direction of illumination

The classical form of illumination produces a beam of light that passes through the specimen into the objective. This is known as transmitted-light illumination, or transillumination. For opaque objects, and in some other circumstances, the light is directed downwards, around or through the objective onto the specimen. Illumination from the same side as the objective is often referred to as epi-illumination.

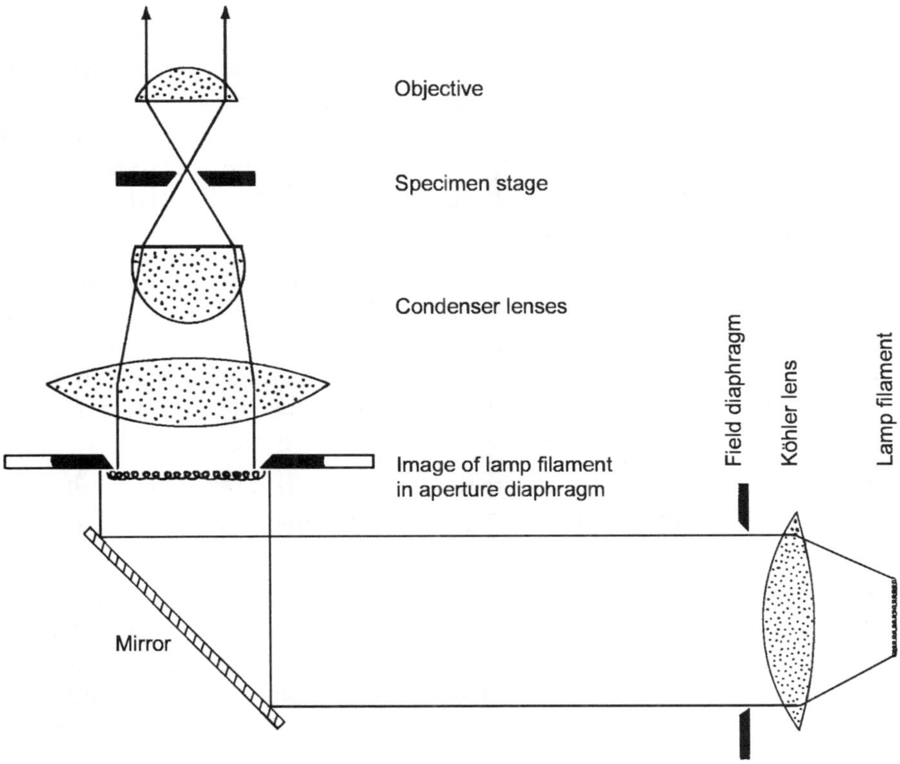

Fig 2.11. The basic illumination system (Köhler illumination) for transmitted-light microscopy.

The lamp or illumination source

Tungsten–halogen lamps are the most common on modern microscopes. The lamp is supplied with current regulated by a rheostat. There should be a meter (ammeter) to measure the current passing through the lamp, or a voltmeter to measure the voltage across the filament (measurement of current is said to be preferable, but we have no evidence about it). Some modern microscopes have an array of luminous diodes; these are more robust than a meter but if there are only a few diodes in the array, the current can only be set to a limited number of values, corresponding to the values at which the next diode is not quite lit.

Electronic flash systems are preferable for living, motile specimens and have some advantages for general use, but they are expensive and surprisingly little developed for microscopy.

Mercury arc lamps are typically used in fluorescence microscopy (see Chapter 11). They are not suitable for general microscopy because of their discontinuous spectrum, expense and (except for very recent models) lack of intensity control by a transformer or rheostat.

Illumination optical system

The best illumination is provided by a Köhler illumination system, described in detail in Chapter 7. Light from the lamp is collected by a collector lens in the lamphouse and focused through a field iris diaphragm into the condenser, which focuses the light onto the specimen; the light passes through the specimen and enters the objective. The condenser has an important iris diaphragm, which controls the angle of the cone of light that illuminates the specimen.

The field diaphragm limits the area of the specimen that is illuminated. This diaphragm is an iris diaphragm, usually placed near the collector lens on the side away from the lamp. The field diaphragm is used as a virtual source of light and is imaged by the condenser onto the specimen. To minimise stray light that may reduce the contrast of the image, the field diaphragm should be adjusted to illuminate an area only slightly larger than the area of interest.

The condenser focuses light onto the specimen, and (in normal transmitted-light work) is so arranged that light passes through the specimen and fills the aperture of the objective.

The aperture iris diaphragm is usually located underneath the condenser and regulates the angle of the cone of light passing through the specimen and entering the objective. It is adjusted to maximise resolution or contrast as required (see Chapter 7). An image of the lamp filament should be focused into the plane of this diaphragm.

Setting up and adjusting a microscope

This section is intended primarily to give practical information relevant to the routine operation of laboratory microscopes. Further details are to be found in standard texts of general microscopy such as that of Oldfield (1994), in booklets supplied by the manufacturers of microscopes, and (in relation to techniques such as polarisation, darkground, fluorescence, etc) Chapters 9–12 of this book.

When a microscope is properly adjusted it gives its best performance, and it is least likely to cause eyestrain and headache for the operator. It is convenient to provide a checklist near each microscope, especially to assist staff in training. The following is an example of a general checklist; it may require modification to suit individual types of microscope. It assumes the type of stand in which the stage moves up and down for focusing rather than the older variety in which the body tube moves and carries the objective and the eyepiece.

It must be noted that there are two diaphragms to be adjusted, namely the field diaphragm and the aperture diaphragm. The former is usually situated on or within the base of the microscope and determines the diameter of the field of illumination. The aperture diaphragm is usually located underneath the condenser and regulates the angle of the cone of light passing through the specimen and entering the objective. Their respective actions can be demonstrated by placing on the stage a block of fluorescent glass or plastic (Fig 2.12) or a small beaker containing a solution of a fluorescent dye such as Fluorescein or Rhodamine B.

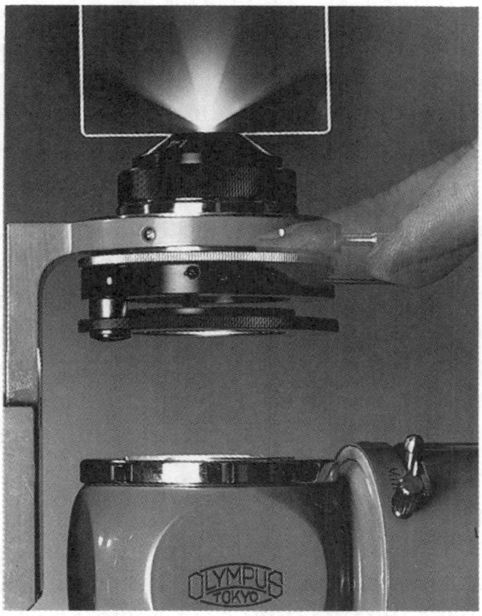

Fig 2.12. The cone of light produced by the condenser, and the effect of altering the aperture diaphragm. The beams of light are demonstrated by fluorescence inside a block of fluorescent plastic, placed on top of the condenser. The device at the bottom contains the mirror to reflect light up into the condenser. The stage is not shown. Double exposure photograph, showing the operator's fingers altering the aperture diaphragm, and the corresponding cones of light issuing from the top of the condenser.

Setting up the microscope

The procedure for adjusting a microscope with Köhler illumination is set forth below.

1. **Power supply:** Plug in and switch on the power supply (there may be a separate switch on the microscope base). Adjust the rheostat until the lamp gives a suitable brightness (this may require readjustment later).

2. **Check the condenser**: Rack the substage condenser up fully. The top lens (swung in if necessary) should generally be only slightly below the level of the stage; if it does not reach this level check whether the condenser has slipped down in its holder (it is usually held by a knurled screw). Open the condenser aperture diaphragm fully. Check whether a filter is present in the filter holder; if there is one of the frosted variety, remove it temporarily or replace it with a clear one.

3. **Select low-power conditions**: There may be a movable condenser top which must be swung out or an auxiliary lens which usually has positions marked L and H for low and high powers, respectively.

4. **Nosepiece**: Swing the lowest-power objective (usually 4× or 10×) into place, ensuring that the nosepiece clicks into position.

5. **Specimen**: Lower the stage and place a slide on it. This usually involves opening a clip, inserting the slide, and allowing the clip to swing gently back to hold the slide. Do not allow the clip to spring back sharply because this will probably break or chip a corner of the slide. Ensure that the slide is sitting flat on the stage with its

coverslip uppermost. Bring the specimen into the centre over the top lens of the condenser.

6. **Focus the specimen**: Rack the stage up with the coarse-focus knob while looking at the stage to make sure that the specimen does not strike the objective. Continue until the specimen is closer to the objective than the distance that you expect it to focus at (say about 10 mm for the usual 4× objective). Next look through the eyepieces and rotate the coarse-focus knob in the opposite direction until the specimen comes into focus. This procedure ensures that the objective does not hit the specimen, avoiding damage to both specimen and objective.

7. **Focus the condenser**: Close the field diaphragm on the base of the microscope until its image is smaller than the field of view. Focus its image into the same plane as the specimen by turning the condenser focusing knob while looking down the eyepiece. Sometimes colour fringes are visible, that change with focusing up and down: they indicate poor colour correction in the condenser. Check that the diaphragm image is central in the field of view; if it is not, adjustment is usually by centring screws in the condenser mount. Open up the field diaphragm until its image (including coloured fringes, if any) is just clear of the field of view.

8. **Check that the light source (lamp filament) is centred**: Some modern microscopes have no provision for centring the filament; others provide centring screws. An image of the lamp filament can sometimes be made visible by moving an auxiliary lens (if the H position gives source-focused illumination) or by removing the eyepiece. Alternatively a white card can be held just below the condenser to show an image of the lamp. Some manufacturers provide a ground-glass to be placed on the base of the microscope under the condenser.

9. **Adjust the condenser aperture**: At this stage any frosted filter previously removed can possibly be put back, but only if it is essential for uniform illumination. Remove the eyepiece and look down the body tube. The rear of the objective should appear illuminated. Adjust the condenser aperture diaphragm until only about two-thirds to seven-eighths of the objective aperture is illuminated. Replace the eyepiece. This adjustment should be repeated each time the objective is changed.

10. **The binocular head**: One or both eyepieces should be adjustable for focus. If there is only one adjustable eyepiece, close the eye that is looking through it; otherwise close either eye. With the eye that is open, focus the specimen sharply. Close that eye and open the other, and with it focus the specimen by adjusting the second eyepiece. The specimen should then be in focus for both eyes. Adjust the interocular distance as required until clear binocular vision is obtained.

11. **Oil immersion**: When it is known that the oil-immersion objective lens will be used and the highest possible resolution is required, it may be helpful to oil the condenser before placing the slide on the stage, in order to obtain the full aperture (NA) of the condenser and objective. This procedure is not normally required if the aperture of either the condenser or the objective is 0·9 or less. Put a few drops of oil on top of the condenser, place the slide on the stage, and very gradually raise the condenser until the oil touches the lower surface of the slide. Avoid air bubbles in the oil; if any occur, remove the slide, wipe off the oil, and start again. Focus the condenser as described above.

Find the area of interest in the specimen and focus it with the highest-power dry objective. Turn to the lowest-power objective (which is short and well clear of the oil on the slide, as well as adjacent to the oil-immersion objective), place one large drop of oil on the slide over the condenser and gently rotate the nosepiece to bring the oil-immersion objective into place. Some spring-loaded objectives can be locked in the up position, brought over the specimen and lowered gently into the immersion fluid. Avoid passing the 40× objective over the oil because it will get oil on its front surface. Focus carefully with the fine-focus knob. If the object was focused for the high dry objective, the oil-immersion objective is usually almost in focus or requires focusing upwards slightly with the fine adjustment. Remove an eyepiece and adjust the condenser aperture diaphragm; replace the eyepiece. Make final adjustments of the aperture and field diaphragms to give the most suitable resolution, contrast, and depth of field. The field iris diaphragm is set to the camera field, which is smaller than the eyepiece field.

When the observations are finished, wipe the slide, the objective, and the condenser (if oiled) with appropriate solvent on a piece of clean lens-cleaning tissue (or cotton cloth, or really soft facial or toilet-paper tissue which is the most economical).

For best results, the immersion oil recommended by the microscope manufacturer should be used. Some years ago a number of immersion oils were found to be carcinogenic and so old stocks should be discarded. In some cases glycerol can be used instead; its refractive index is 1·47 compared with 1·52 (see Chapter 6, Table 6.2) and its advantages are economy and ease of cleaning because it is miscible with water.

After oil has been put on the slide, returning to the high dry objective can present problems. In haematology and other fields that require scanning at medium power and frequent changes to high power, it is advantageous to have two oil-immersion objectives, one with high magnification and another with medium magnification (for instance 100× and 50× or 63×).

3
Basic photomicrographic technique

This chapter explains the basics of taking a photomicrograph (such as those shown in Plates 8 and 9) using conventional transmitted-light microscopy.

The steps to be taken, in general, for basic photomicrography in transmitted light are the following:

- Setting up the microscope.
- Loading the camera with appropriate film.
- Examining the specimen, and selecting the field of view to be photographed.
- Choosing a filter, if required.
- Focusing the camera.
- Determining the exposure.
- Making the exposure.

These procedures are summarised in Table 3.1 for black-and-white (B&W) photography, and Table 3.2 for colour.

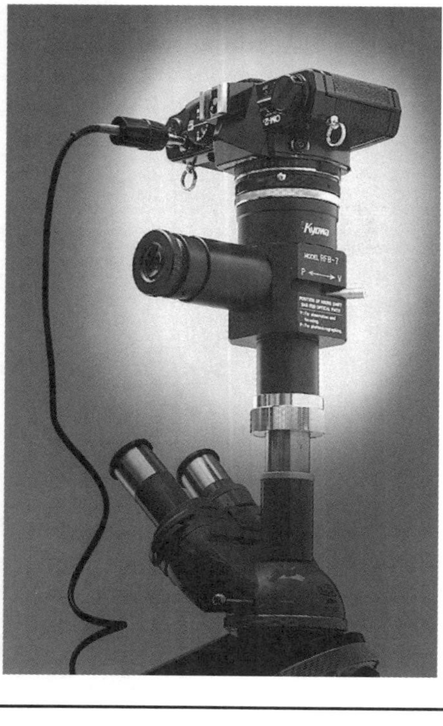

Fig 3.1. An attachment photomicrographic module (Kyowa *RFB-7*) with a 'telescopic' viewfinder. A graticule in the telescope is in a plane optically conjugate (equivalent) to the film plane; an aerial image from the microscope is brought into the same focus as the graticule (see Fig 3.2). Note also the pneumatic shutter release.

Table 3.1. Steps for basic photomicrography in black-and-white

Setting up the microscope

Check that the microscope is correctly set up (see Chapter 2), and that the optics and stage are clean.

Loading the camera

Select a suitable B&W film (see Chapter 1).

Load the film in the camera, following the manufacturer's instructions.

Set the film speed rating (ISO, EI, ASA, DIN) on the camera's exposure meter or control box.

Record the date and film type in your logbook, notebook, or computer.

Examining the specimen

Turn the nosepiece to a low-power objective (4× or 10×), ie one with a reasonably long working distance.

Place the specimen slide on the stage, specimen towards the objective, and centre the specimen to the objective.

Examine the specimen with the low-power objective.

Locate the area to be photographed.

Decide the magnification to be used, and select the appropriate objective.

Adjust the Köhler illumination to optimal conditions (see Chapters 2 and 7).

Select a filter (if required) (see Chapter 8).

Selecting the field of view to be photographed

Look in the viewfinder, and move the specimen until the desired composition is obtained (see Fig 3.2 and Chapter 5).

Check that the magnification is appropriate. If necessary, change the objective and/or projective. Record, in your logbook, notebook, or computer, the specimen, subject, and optical combination.

Focusing the camera

Focusing is usually achieved by adjusting the microscope's fine focus until an aerial image of the subject, as seen in the viewfinder (or focusing telescope) coincides with a graticule.

Adjusting the illumination

Check the Köhler illumination for the objective in use (see Chapters 2 and 7).

Adjust the field diaphragm until its image is just clear of the area to be photographed.

Determining the exposure

The recommended exposure is read, using either full-frame or spot metering.

Compensation may be necessary in some circumstances (see Chapter 16).

In manual systems, the chosen exposure is set.

Making the exposure

Check that the light path is set to the camera, and press the button, avoiding vibration.

If in doubt of the exposure, bracket the exposures, usually at 1 stop (2×) intervals.

On each roll of film, co-author Ron recommends photographing a stage micrometer with each optical combination used, to indicate the magnification(s).

Record the exposure(s) given, and check details of specimen and microscope technique.

Table 3.2 Steps for photomicrography in colour

Setting up the microscope

Check that the microscope is correctly set up, and that the optics and stage are clean.

Loading the camera

Select a suitable colour film (transparency or negative; see Chapter 1 for brief help, or Chapter 18 for details).

Load the film into the camera, following the manufacturer's instructions.

Set the film speed rating (ISO, ASA, DIN, EI) on the camera's exposure meter or control box.

Record the date and film type in your logbook, notebook, or computer.

Examining the specimen

Turn the nosepiece to a low-power objective (4× or 10×), ie one with a reasonably long working distance.

Place the specimen slide on the stage, specimen towards the objective, and centre the specimen to the objective.

Examine the specimen with the low-power objective.

Locate the area to be photographed.

Decide on the magnification to be used, and select the appropriate objective.

Adjust the Köhler illumination to optimal conditions (see Chapters 2 and 7).

Selecting the field of view to be photographed

Look in the viewfinder, and move the specimen until the desired composition is obtained (Fig 3.2 and Chapter 5).

Check that the magnification is appropriate. If necessary, change the objective and/or projective. Record, in your logbook, notebook, or computer, the specimen, subject, and optical combination.

Focusing the camera

Focusing is usually achieved by adjusting the microscope's fine focus until an aerial image of the subject, as seen in the viewfinder (or focusing telescope) coincides with a graticule.

Adjusting the illumination

Check the Köhler illumination for the objective in use (see Chapters 2 and 7).

Adjust the field diaphragm until its image is just clear of the area to be photographed.

Check that the blue colour-correction filter is in place (assuming daylight-type film) and that no other colour filters are present (unless a special effect is required).

Turn up the lamp current to the preset value.

Determining the exposure

The recommended exposure is read, using either full-frame or spot metering.

Compensation may be necessary in some circumstances (see Chapter 16).

In manual systems, the chosen exposure is set.

Making the exposure

Check that the light path is set to the camera, and press the button, avoiding vibration.

If in doubt of the exposure, bracket the exposures, usually at $^2/_3$ to 1 stop (1·6× to 2×) intervals.

On each roll of negative film, co-author Ron recommends photographing a stage micrometer with each optical combination used to indicate the magnification(s).

Record the exposure(s) given, and check the details of the specimen and microscope technique.

Photomicrographic cameras

Cameras for photomicrography are usually specially constructed to suit the particular microscope, and are mounted on the vertical tube of a trinocular head (shown in Fig 2.5). In microscopes specially designed for photomicrography, the photographic system may be incorporated into the microscope body (Fig 14.3) or form a substantial module attached to the top of the stand (Fig 14.1; see also Fig 3.1). An ordinary camera can be adapted if necessary (see Fig 1.2 and Chapter 4). Photomicrographic cameras are described in detail in Chapter 14; the following paragraphs are a summary.

A photomicrographic camera is basically similar to an ordinary camera, the microscope system serving as the lens. There are two main kinds of system used for forming an image on the film. In all cases, objectives are used in the normal manner. However, whereas for observation the eyepiece produces a virtual image and the lens of the eye converts this to a real image on the retina, in the photomicrographic system a real image is required on the film plane and, therefore, one of the following is needed:

- The normal eyepiece is supplemented by a lens equivalent to the lens of the eye.
- The normal eyepiece is replaced by a projective (photoeyepiece; a special projection eyepiece) that produces a real image on the photographic film.
- The microscope is re-focused to produce the required real image in the film plane.

In some photomicrographic cameras, the camera contains lenses that completely replace the eyepiece (see Chapter 14). Some manufacturers employ a system that has an eyepiece at the top of the phototube, and the camera sitting above that with additional lenses to form a real image. A similar effect can be obtained by using a conventional camera, complete with lens, arranged to look through the normal eyepiece; the object will be in focus if the lens of the camera is set to infinity and provided also that the lens of the camera is not too close to the eyepiece, ie is held at the eyepiece exit pupil (see Chapter 4).

Setting up the microscope

Stability

The microscope bench itself must not vibrate. This problem is usually related to the floor on which the bench is located, a product of too-close positioning to ventilation or air-conditioning plants, or of heavy street traffic. If a large dish, bowl or bucket of water is placed where the microscope is to be positioned, any rippling of the water surface (best observed by reflecting light off it onto a white screen) is a certain sign of floor or table vibration. If there is a problem, see Chapter 15 for suggestions.

Cleanliness

The microscope should be maintained in a clean, dust-free and functional condition. Surfaces that, when dusty or dirty, are particularly likely to create imaging problems are the objective front lens, and all glass–air surfaces, even the internal ones, of the photographic eyepiece. Ask a technician to show you how to clean lens surfaces; any trained salesperson will be delighted to encourage such care by one of their customers. Further information on this important topic is given in Appendix A1.

Basic adjustment of the microscope

The main steps involved in setting up a microscope are described in Chapter 2. We will now assume that the microscope has been set up ready for use.

Choice of film

Selection of film type according to the desired product (eg prints or projection slides) was discussed in Chapter 1, and finer points of photographic materials are discussed in Chapter 18.

Loading the camera

The film is loaded into the camera, following the manufacturer's instructions. The film speed rating (ISO, ASA or DIN; or EI, see Chapters 16 and 18) is set on the camera's exposure meter or control box; this rating is not necessarily that marked on the packet (see Chapters 16 and 18). The date and film type should be recorded in the logbook (notebook or computer).

Selecting the field of view to be photographed

The specimen

A perfect specimen is the best starting point for a perfect photograph. This implies a thin, flat section or smear, good contrast, lack of specimen movement, and control of coverslip/mountant thickness. These are important considerations all too frequently beyond practical control. Opaque specimens are usually highly polished to achieve a flat surface.

Action: one turns the nosepiece to a low-power objective (4× or 10×), ie an objective with a reasonably long working distance, places the specimen slide on the stage, and centres the specimen under the objective. The specimen is first examined with the low-power objective, to locate the area to be photographed.

Selecting the field of view to be photographed

The 10× objective is the normal starting point for focusing. One must then decide the magnification to be used, and select the appropriate objective. Experience may be needed to determine the best magnification to use; beginners are inclined to overdo the magnification, by choosing an enlargement that is greater than that which best illustrates a given feature. Aesthetic considerations in choosing the field are discussed in Chapter 5. Look in the viewfinder, and move the specimen until the desired composition is obtained. Besides movement in the *X* and *Y* axes, this process may include rotating either the specimen or the camera to an appropriate angle.

Determining the magnification

In many cases, the overall magnification on the film can be calculated by multiplying the magnification of the objective by the camera magnification factor, which is given by the manufacturer.

A *stage micrometer* is a glass slide on which is engraved a scale, usually one or two millimetres long, with graduations every 0·01 mm (10 µm). If this is photographed, the overall magnification to any print or transparency can easily be determined. Co-author

Ron recommends photographing a stage micrometer with each optical combination used on any roll of negative film, so that the magnification of the prints can easily be calculated, even if the enlarger magnification is unknown.

Records and imprinted data

One should now record, in the logbook, notebook, or computer, the specimen, subject, and magnification. If a data imprint function is available, set it as required. Some microscopes have provision for superimposing a scale bar on the film.

Focusing the camera

Focusing is usually achieved by adjusting the microscope's fine focus until an aerial image of the subject, as seen in the viewfinder (or focusing telescope, Fig 3.1) coincides with a graticule or reticle (Figs 3.2, 3.3). Moving one's eye from side to side should not produce any relative movement of the subject and graticule. Such relative movement will be observed in one particular direction if the aerial image is below the graticule, and in the other direction if the image is above the graticule. This is called *aerial image focusing*. Focusing with a single-lens-reflex (SLR) camera is described in Chapter 4.

Unexpectedly, there is likely to be more difficulty in the focusing of low and very low-power magnifications than with the medium to high powers. An auxiliary magnifier may prove useful, the magnifier being attached to or held against the viewfinder/telescope eyepiece. Special auxiliary magnifiers are available. Zeiss recommend their 8×30 monocular; any similar monocular is suitable, or, at a pinch, one can use one side of a pair of low-power binoculars. Co-author Ron shuns these devices!

Depth of field and depth of focus

Depth of field is the thickness of the specimen that is acceptably sharp at a given setting of the focus control; *depth of focus* is the range over which the image plane (eg film) can be moved while maintaining acceptable sharpness of a specified object plane. The depth of field is approximately inversely proportional to the numerical aperture (NA) of the system, and is decreased somewhat by increasing the total magnification. The depth of field can be increased by closing down the condenser diaphragm. This achieves an increase of depth of field at the expense of resolving power. However, for photographic purposes this may occasionally be a legitimate trade-off. Depth of field is discussed in more detail in Chapter 6, and its practical control described in Chapter 15.

Adjusting the illumination

The illumination system

The ideal form of illumination is that called Köhler illumination, which is dealt with in Chapter 7. Application of the principles of Köhler illumination is usually a matter of consulting and interpreting the microscope manual. For the moment, first check that the condenser is fully raised. Then take out an eyepiece and look down the tube from a short distance; close the aperture diaphragm (of the condenser) until the bright central disc is reduced to about two-thirds of its maximum diameter. Replace the eyepiece, and check that the field appears evenly illuminated. The image of the field diaphragm should be clear of the field (preferably by only a small distance). If colour film is being used, check that the appropriate colour correction (blue) filter is in place (see below, Colour photomicrography).

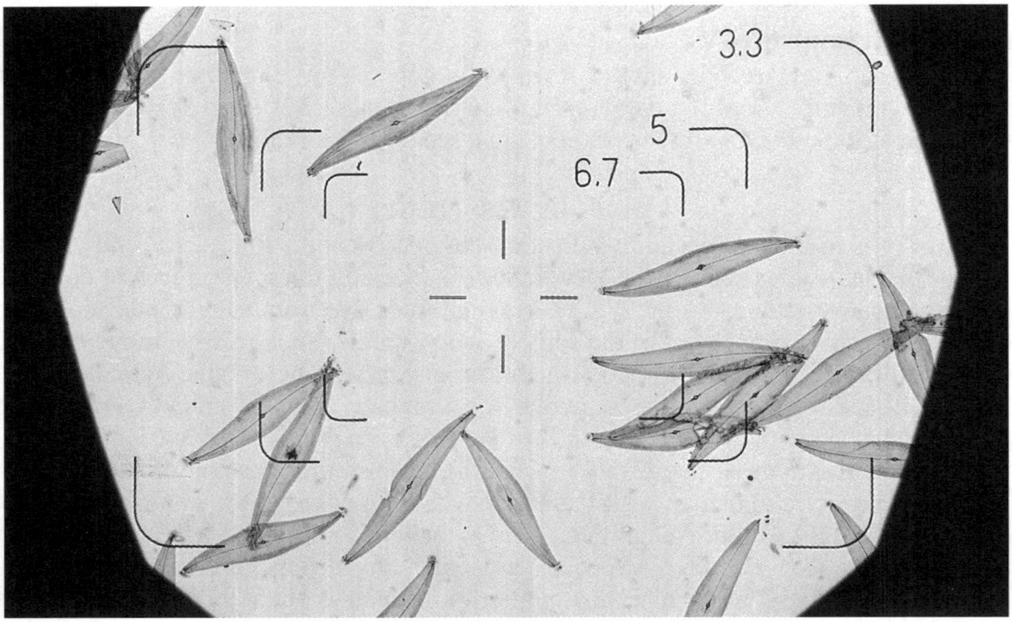

Fig 3.2. View through an Olympus viewfinder eyepiece: the graticule (reticle) in focus, the specimen in focus, and the dark edge of the field diaphragm visible at the periphery but outside the area to be photographed. The field which will be photographed depends on the magnification of the projective; borders are shown for projective magnifications of 3×, 5×, and 6·7×. The centre of the graticule has pairs of closely spaced lines (not seen to be separated in this photograph) for focusing the eye (see Fig 3.3).

Fig 3.3. Double lines in the focusing graticule (Fig 3.2) appear sharp (right) when correctly focused for the eye.

Condenser immersion

If the condenser has an NA greater than 0·9, it is specifically designed to be immersed to the slide. Immersion is essential if the full NA of the condenser is required, eg for optimum resolution, for an immersion darkground condenser, or for differential interference-contrast (DIC) systems. Most users, understandably, will prefer to avoid this immersion process, and, since it is necessary mainly for use with oil-immersion lenses, we defer consideration of it to Chapter 15.

Colour filters

Filters are used to adjust the colour of the light (for colour photography) and for increasing contrast of stained material using B&W photography.

The filter needs to be placed in the light path of the microscope, usually between the specimen and light source. Filters are typically placed either in a holder below the condenser, or in a slot in front of the lamp. If neither of these positions is available, filters can generally be placed on the base of the microscope where the light comes out, below the condenser. In this position, however, because of proximity to the field diaphragm, any dust on the filter may appear in the image and be photographed. Since the field stop is superimposed on the plane of the specimen, the inevitable dust on the filter will be more or less sharply imaged on the specimen, quite unacceptably so. It may be useful practice to use a clear glass filter as a deliberate trap for the dust that falls on this field iris plane, but careful and frequent cleaning of the filter is then appropriate.

Colour photomicrography

It is usually necessary to use a special blue filter (see below) to obtain the correct colour rendition. No other colour filter can be used, unless correct colour rendition is specifically not required.

Colour temperature. To a first approximation, it may be said that colour film records the amounts of red, green and blue light in the image. The light used for illumination must therefore contain red, green and blue light in the correct proportions.

In an incandescent lamp, the proportions of light emitted at various wavelengths (colours) vary with the temperature of the filament. The hotter the filament, the more blue is emitted; at lower temperatures, more red is emitted. It is therefore convenient to express the spectral distribution of a light source in terms of its temperature. Because the spectral distribution from a practical light source is affected by the nature of the material from which it is made, instead of the actual temperature, a so-called colour temperature is referred to. The temperature of the filament depends upon the amount of current flowing through it.

Daylight contains relatively more blue than can be obtained from an incandescent tungsten filament, because the filament cannot be heated hot enough (it melts first). Therefore, to achieve a daylight-like quality, a blue filter is used. To achieve the correct colour, the current through the filament needs to be set to an appropriate value.

A blue filter is normally supplied as standard equipment, to convert the colour temperature of the lamp to that of daylight – at least approximately. If you have any trouble with this filter, buy another from a photographic supply house. Photographic filters are made and sold in large quantities, so it is possible to obtain a better filter, with coated surfaces, in a metal mount, much more cheaply. Use Tables 8.1–8.3 to determine which filter(s) you need. The normal choice, using a halogen lamp at its full rated current, is Wratten 80A; such filters can be purchased from any camera supply house, as well as from the microscope manufacturers (who usually seem to charge more). For further details, see Chapters 7 and 8.

Obtaining the correct colour. Before embarking on a programme of photomicrography, it is desirable to calibrate the light source. This involves photographing a typical subject, or an empty microscope field under various conditions, to determine those conditions that produce the correct balance of colour temperature, resulting in a neutral-grey photograph (see Colour rendition, Chapter 15). Colour transparency (slide) film must be used, because prints from colour negatives are subject to additional filtration and cannot be relied on for judgement. There are in principle two possibilities: either, with a given blue filter (or possibly no filter, given artificial-light film), one takes a series of pictures with varying values of lamp current; or, if the lamp current is fixed (eg by the lamp being run at maximum), the series of pictures is taken with a series of blue filters or filter combinations. If the camera has a colour temperature meter, it is only necessary to confirm that the meter indicates the colour temperature required for the film type in use.

Black-and-white photography

In B&W photography, a coloured filter may be used to adjust the contrast of a coloured or stained specimen, or to emphasise or subdue one particular colour. Filters suitable for this purpose are discussed in Chapter 8, and their applications in Chapter 15.

Determining the exposure

The correct exposure time is determined by a combination of many factors. These may be summarised as: the brightness of the specimen, the magnification of the image onto the film, the effective NA of the objective, the amount of light losses in the optical system, and the sensitivity of the film under the prevailing circumstances. These factors are discussed in more detail in Chapters 15 and 16. The exposure is usually determined by using an exposure meter to measure the overall brightness of the image, from which the duration of the required exposure is calculated having regard to the sensitivity of the film and the type of specimen.

Factors which affect the required exposure

With a particular microscopical technique, the exposure required will depend on:

- The brightness of the light used for illumination.
- The optical transmission (transparency) of the specimen (or reflectivity or fluorescence, as the case may be).
- The amount of light gathered by the objective.
- The overall magnification from the specimen to the film.
- The sensitivity of the film.
- The desired tone (darkness or lightness) of the photograph.

To complicate matters, the reading given by the camera's exposure meter will be affected by the proportion of the field occupied by the specimen. It is necessary to distinguish two types of image, both of which will give erroneous readings on an exposure meter and need to be handled differently. Firstly, there is the type of image that consists of bright patches on a dark background, as is typically the case in darkground and fluorescence microscopy. Under these circumstances, the exposure meter overestimates the exposure, because of the dark areas. Secondly, there is the type of image that consists of dark patches on a light background. In this case, the exposure meter underestimates the exposure. Compensation for these conditions is discussed in Chapter 15. Additional problems associated with low light levels are discussed in Chapter 16.

Exposure measurement

Correct exposure is discussed in detail in Chapter 16. For the present, we give a summary. We will assume for the present purposes that the photomicrographic camera used has a built-in exposure meter, as is usually the case these days. Many systems offer a choice of *full-field* (*integrated*) or *spot* metering (Fig 3.4). For the person in a hurry and for the beginner, it is probably best to rely on full-field metering. Spot metering is fine if the spot can be made to coincide with a typical part of the subject.

For an attachment camera, the film speed rating that is stated by the film manufacturer for pictorial work is excessive for conventional bright-field photomicrography. Our experience is that for an attachment camera, $^2/_3$ stop more exposure should be given than for pictorial work, ie the ISO film speed rating should be reduced by $^2/_3$ stop). We understand that in the Olympus photomicrographic cameras, an allowance of $^1/_3$ stop is made.

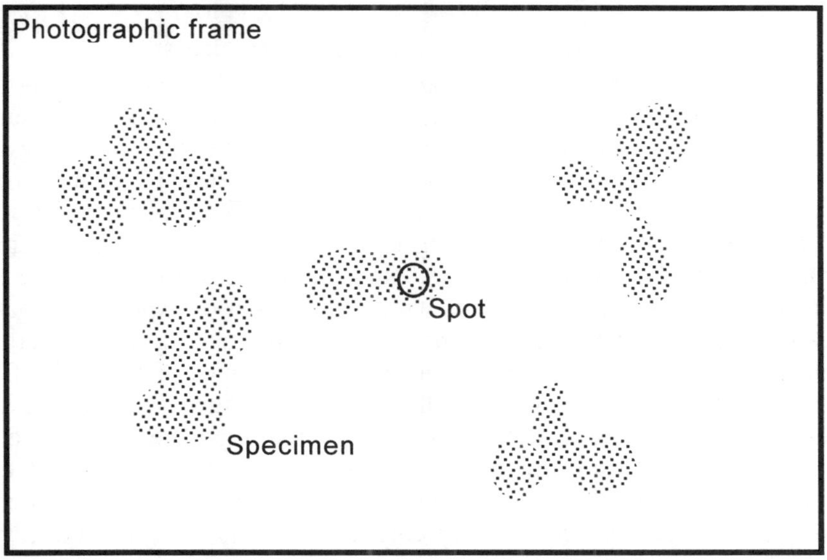

Fig 3.4. Use of a spot meter for exposure measurement: the measuring spot (measured area) is represented by the small circle in the middle. Note that if the arrangement of the object in the field is fixed, it may not be appropriate for the measuring spot to be in the centre of the field (see Fig 16.1). On such occasions, either the spot must be movable or else the measurement be made before moving the object into the right position for photography. Integrated metering measures from the full field, and may give an incorrect result with a specimen of this type.

Despite having an accurate photometer, some manual compensation is usually required, based on experience. We recommend keeping a detailed record of all pictures taken. The record should include the ISO film speed set, the photometer reading, the compensation settings (if any), and the length of the exposure given. Afterwards, when the pictures have been developed, note the ones that were correctly exposed. It may be useful to make, from these data, a graph of photometer reading versus optimal exposure. It is normal to find up to a $^1/_2$ stop variation in exposure calibration due to changes in film batches and processing runs of colour transparency films.

There are special problems associated with very long exposures, particularly those required for fluorescence microscopy. These problems, and methods to deal with them, are discussed in Chapters 15 and 16.

Obtaining a white background for colour pictures

The first and most important point to remember is that the background will come out white if, and only if, the film is sufficiently exposed. Even if the light is not correctly colour-balanced, so long as the exposure of background areas exceeds the latitude of the film, they will appear white. If the exposure is too short, the background will appear one of several colours: grey, if the light is correctly balanced; blue, if the lamp current is too high; amber, if the lamp current is too low; or some other colour, at long exposures, due to the addition of a colour cast induced by reciprocity failure (see Chapters 16 and 18).

Making the exposure, and bracketing

Check that the light path is set to the camera, and press the button. If in doubt of the exposure, or with unusual material, it is accepted wisdom to *bracket* exposures. With B&W or colour negative film meant for pictorial photography, the bracketing should be at 1 stop intervals (ie a factor of 2 between successive exposures). Usually two or three different exposures will be sufficient, but in extreme cases five exposures at $^1/_2\times$, $^1/_4\times$, $1\times$, $2\times$, $4\times$ will be required. Even with quite normal specimens it is a useful practice to take two exposures, one at the estimated correct exposure and a second at $2\times$ the estimated exposure. This is a safety measure against wrong judgement of exposure (negatives that are too dark being preferred to negatives that are too light), and against the rare but very annoying darkroom mishap of scratching of one of the frames of film. The film is the cheapest part of photography. Films with higher contrast, such as *Technical Pan*, and colour transparency films are described as having little exposure latitude, ie they are intolerant of even minor exposure inaccuracy. For these films, bracketed exposures should be at $^2/_3$ stop intervals, but for critical work, such as for publication, $^1/_3$ stop intervals gives a range in which acceptable results can be guaranteed, with the expectation of one perfect shot and another very acceptable one. With colour transparencies, one slightly light transparency for projection, and one slightly dark transparency for publication, are ideal.

If the specimen is not going to be available for a re-shoot if necessary, take an additional exposure just in case of accidental damage to the negative or transparency. In these circumstances, and if the specimen is very important, co-author Fred is never happy unless he has at least two shots on each of two separate rolls of film taken with different cameras!

Record, in your logbook, notebook, or computer, the exposure(s) given.

The cable release. Camera shake is a very real threat to sharp pictures in photomicrography. If the camera is not electrically controlled from a separate control box, a remote release should be used to avoid transmitting movement of finger or hand to the camera. Remote releases exist in three varieties: electric, pneumatic and cable. For reducing camera shake, their effectiveness is in the order given.

Quality control

We recommend that, when using equipment for the first time, or after any significant alteration, you check the illumination system by photographing a blank (empty) field. This should be accomplished by first focusing on a specimen, and then either (for high power) moving the specimen out of the field (leaving the slide in place), or (for low powers) replacing the slide with a clean blank one (without specimen). The resulting picture should be a uniform grey all over. An uneven grey will indicate an optical fault, probably in the illumination system. With colour film, any colour (ie not a neutral grey) will indicate a mismatch between the colour of the illumination and the requirements of the film, or else a fault in processing and printing the film (colour negative film has almost always a yellow 'mask', which is eliminated in printing).

Troubleshooting

If the microscope does not give a good image, see Appendix 2 for possible causes. If the pictures do not come out well, or cannot be taken at all because of technical difficulties, the fault may lie in the microscope, the camera, the film, or the processing of the film. Again, see Appendix A2.

Happy shooting!

You should now be able to take good photomicrographs, using transmitted-light microscopy, with the information given in these first three chapters. The next chapter tells how to manage on a very limited budget, and Chapter 5 gives some hints on the finer points of composition, and what to do with the photograph. We recommend that, if you have not already done so, you get some experience of these basic techniques before proceeding to Part II of the book (which begins at Chapter 6). You may wish to try also some of the exercises in Appendix A3.

4
Limited-budget photomicrography

This chapter is intended for young people, students, school teachers, research scientists in unfashionable disciplines, and all others who wish to take photomicrographs on a minuscule budget. In all other chapters in this book, the emphasis is on achieving the highest possible photographic quality, using dedicated photomicrographic equipment. This chapter describes the use of an 'ordinary' camera, how to take useful pictures with minimal equipment, and how to make the best of unsatisfactory equipment. In practice, given a microscope and a camera, the main problem is usually that of coupling the two together. Actual photography using equipment as described below follows the procedures described in Chapter 3.

Equipment

The required equipment consists essentially of a microscope and a camera. The microscope may be one of two types:

- A modern-type microscope in which the body tube is fixed, and focusing is done by moving the stage up and down. The body tube may be monocular (vertical or inclined), binocular or trinocular.
- An older microscope in which the body tube moves up and down for focusing. This kind of microscope can usually be tilted from vertical to horizontal if required. The body tube may be monocular (vertical or inclined) or binocular.

The microscope may be combined with any of three types of camera:

- A single-lens-reflex (SLR) camera with interchangeable lenses, used without lens.
- An SLR camera with built-in lens or used with the lens in place, or a 'compact' camera with a built-in lens.
- A view or field camera, normally used without lens, possibly used with lens.

The possible combinations, in approximately decreasing order of preference, are:

- Microscope with fixed vertical body tube; camera body without lens and with correct adapter (Figs 1.2, 4.4). This is easy to manage and should give perfect results.
- Microscope with fixed vertical body tube; camera body without lens and supported independently (Fig 4.6). This should give perfect results.
- Microscope with fixed body tube; camera body with lens (Fig 4.3). This is more difficult to arrange.
- Microscope with focusing body tube, vertical; camera body without lens. The camera must be supported independently, otherwise the weight of the camera tends to force the focusing tube down, out of focus and onto the specimen.
- Microscope with focusing body tube, vertical; camera body with lens. This combination is very awkward to use. The camera must be supported independently, otherwise the weight of the camera tends to force the focusing tube down, out of focus and onto the specimen.

- Microscope with focusing body tube, horizontal; camera body without lens. This may be difficult to arrange but should give excellent results.
- Microscope with inclined body tube; camera body with or without lens (Fig 15.3). This is difficult to manage.

Camera

Any single-lens-reflex (SLR) camera or view camera, and some compact cameras, can be used to take photographs through a microscope. The 35 mm format is the most economical to buy, to run, and to buy accessories for. The Advanced Photographic System (APS) format is only suitable for small prints, and cannot produce slides because there is no transparency film available for it. If you are buying a camera, buy a 35 mm SLR camera with interchangeable lenses if possible. Avoid brands with a fixed lens, and those for which second-hand accessories are as rare as hen's teeth, in case you want to do close-up photography or other photography as well. Avoid, also, those which rely entirely on expensive and scarce batteries, and obtain instead one that requires only the common AA batteries, or a small battery for metering only. A built-in through-the-lens (TTL) meter is very desirable but not absolutely essential for routine or repetitive work.

Single-lens-reflex (SLR) cameras

SLR cameras (Figs 4.1, 4.2 and 4.4) are such that a mirror behind the lens reflects an image onto a ground-glass screen that corresponds to the film in size and optical distance from the lens. Therefore any image that appears on the screen will also appear on the film. For focusing and composing, the image on the screen is viewed through a magnifier and (usually) a pentaprism that yields an erect, laterally correct image. Meanwhile, the film is protected from exposure by a shutter immediately in front of it (a focal-plane shutter). When the shutter release is activated, the mirror swings up against the screen, thereby both moving out of the light path to the film and blocking the entry of light from the viewfinding system; the shutter opens for the required exposure, closes, and the mirror swings down again.

Exposure is usually determined by a built-in metering system that takes readings through the lens (TTL metering). In TTL metering, measurements of light intensity are usually made from the screen, before exposure. Sometimes, for spot measurements only, light transmitted by a partly transparent region in the middle of the mirror may be metered. Measurements for TTL flash (strobe) control, and sometimes for control of shutter opening time actually during the exposure, are made from light reflected from the film during exposure (the 'off-the-film' or OTF method).

Modern camera bodies intended for use with autofocus lenses may not be able to offer their full range of metering options when connected to a microscope (which the camera regards as a manual-focus lens). In some cameras, the meter may not work at all without an autofocus lens, and even the shutter may not work. In these cases, the camera can be used only with its lens attached. SLR focusing and composing are still possible.

A data-back or multifunction back is available for many SLRs, which will imprint the date and/or time, or a serial number, on the film (on the frame and/or between frames) if desired.

The normal focusing screen of SLR cameras is adequate for ultralow and low-power photomicrography only. In those SLR cameras with interchangeable focusing screens, a clear glass (or plastic) screen with cross-hairs of twin lines as in a photomicrographic graticule (cf Fig 3.2) is preferred for medium- and high-power photomicrography. Modern laser-cut screens are much preferable to the older ground-glass, in which fine detail cannot be seen. Nikon type *M* screens (with a clear Fresnel lens all over, and lines for focusing) are ideal, type *C* (matte with a central clear area and crosslines for focusing) is next best (possibly better for low powers). Co-author Fred has also used types *F* and *U*, which are normally intended for mirror lenses and very long-focus telephoto lenses respectively. A magnifier is very useful (but not according to co-author Ron!); this may be attached to the camera eyepiece, or one of the special high-power magnifying heads available for some professional-type SLRs (such as the Nikon *F3*, *F4* and *F5*). A right-angle viewfinder attachment or a 'vertical' viewfinder enables one to focus and compose the picture more easily, otherwise one has to stretch up and look downwards into the camera.

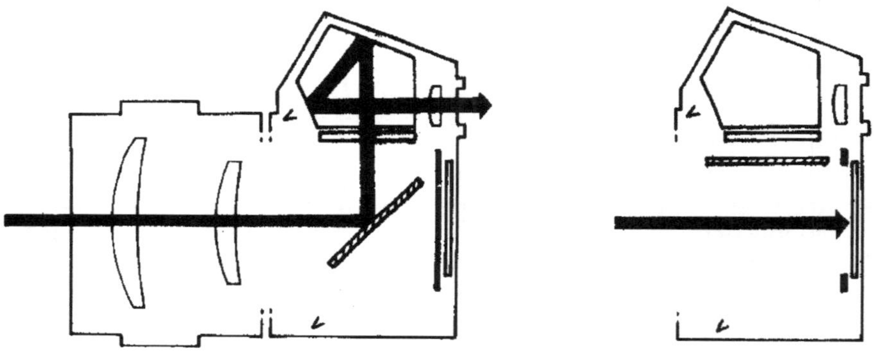

Fig 4.1. Diagrams of SLR camera. Left, with lens attached, and the mirror down for focusing. A light path is shown through the lens and reflected by the mirror onto the focusing screen. An image of the screen is reflected around the pentaprism and through the eyepiece. Two alternative positions for a photometer for TTL metering are shown: one in the pentaprism, and another in the camera body for OTF metering. Right, mirror up, for exposing film. The light path is shown passing though the opened shutter onto the film.

The shutter

SLR cameras usually have a *focal-plane shutter* consisting of two roller blinds just in front of the film. These blinds are arranged on either side of the film opening so that one blind opens to expose the film and is followed by the other blind, moving in the same direction, to close the shutter. The length of the exposure is determined by the interval between the opening and closing of the two blinds. For shorter exposures, the second blind follows closely behind the first so that, in effect, a slit between the two blinds passes in front of the film, each part of the film receiving an exposure whose length depends on the width of the slit as well as on the speed with which the slit traverses the film. The blinds may move either longitudinally or transversely with respect to the axis of the film. In some cameras, the cloth blinds are replaced by one or more thin sheets of titanium. Focal-plane shutters are very reliable, but may generate a substantial amount of vibration as the first blind is brought to a halt. Some focal-plane shutters are better than others – eg that in the Nikon *F4* is excellent. Some Nikon SLRs have manual shutter speeds adjustable in increments of $^1/_3$ stop, which is very helpful.

A *leaf shutter* mechanism has very light moving parts, symmetrically arranged, so that it generates hardly any vibration when opening and closing. If there is a choice of shutter, a leaf shutter is to be preferred to a focal-plane shutter, creating less vibration. In a camera with a focal-plane shutter, it may be possible to arrange a supplementary leaf shutter, to be used for the actual exposure while the camera's focal-plane shutter is held open.

Shutter release

To avoid vibration, one should avoid touching the camera immediately preceding and during the exposure. After all manual operations are complete, the camera and specimen should be given sufficient time for all vibrations to die down before the exposure is given. This implies the use of a remote release system. In order of preference, these are:

- An electric release. These are available only for cameras with electronically controlled shutters. Their advantage over the self-timer (see below) is that the moment of exposure can be chosen by the operator. As an aside, we wish that there was an internationally agreed and accepted standard socket for such releases, as there is for mechanical ones.
- The camera's self-timer, particularly if it is electronic (no moving parts). The self-timer may also (in some cameras) pre-release the mirror of an SLR. The time delay, although possibly wearying for the operator, also ensures that all vibrations have died down before the shutter opens. Several SLR cameras have variable self-timer delay times, down to 2 seconds.
- A pneumatic release (Fig 3.1). This gives good isolation of the camera from the operator, and (unlike the self-timer) the moment of exposure can be chosen by the operator. The pneumatic tube should be long enough for a substantial length of it to lie firmly on the table; it should not merely dangle between the shutter and the operator's hand, or some vibration will be transmitted.
- A cable release. In our experience, such releases tend to be much too short and too stiff; and some operators find it difficult to hold the cable loosely and to avoid jerking it. A length of about 500 mm is required. It should be as flexible as possible. As Blaker (1989) remarked, the more the cable resembles a piece of limp spaghetti, the better! We can confirm Blaker's experience that the cheaper ones are often the best in this respect.

Long exposures

There are special problems associated with long exposures for photography of dim images; these problems are discussed at length in Chapters 15 and 16. In the present context, it is only necessary to point out that some SLR cameras have quite sensitive TTL metering, and that many modern SLR cameras have shutters that can give very long exposures (sometimes using a special multifunction camera-back).

Mirror pre-release

The SLR mirror is a significant source of camera vibration; as it is released, it swings up, and stops suddenly. Therefore, under critical conditions such as photomicrography, the mirror should be released (pre-released) before the shutter mechanism is actuated, if the camera has provision for this procedure (as in, for example, the Nikon *F4*). In some cameras, such as the Olympus *OM4* series and the Nikon *FM2*, the self-timer pre-releases the mirror at the beginning of the countdown.

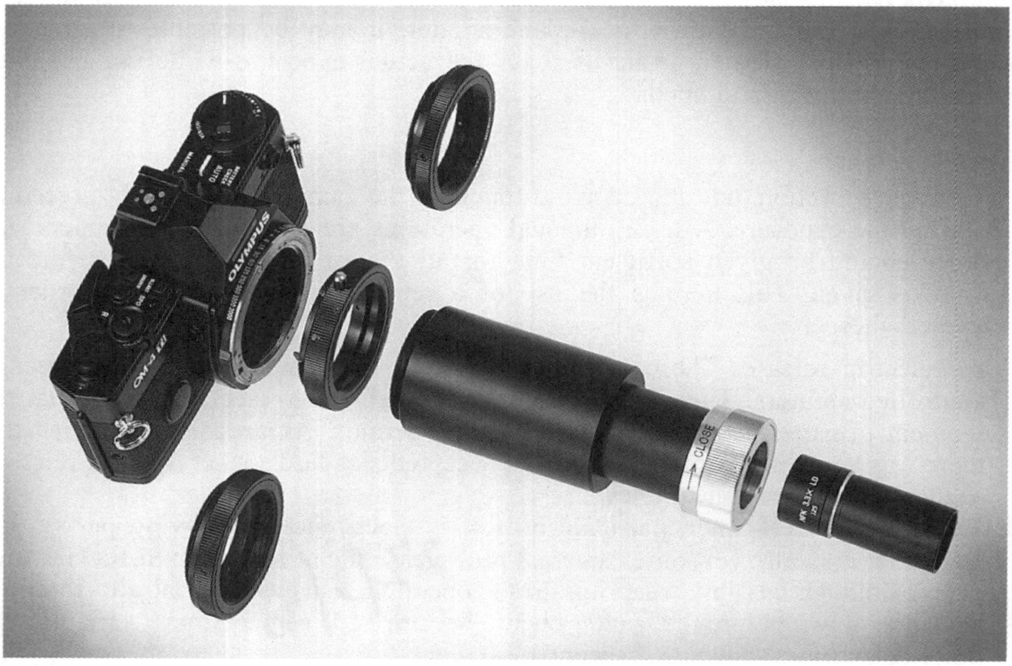

Fig 4.2. Microscope adapter, showing a range of T-mount adapters to various cameras.

Coupling of camera to microscope

Cameras with lens attached

It used to be possible to take photomicrographs with a compact camera by setting it at infinity focus, and holding or fastening it over the eyepiece (Fig 4.3). Figure 4.5 shows one of co-author Fred's first photomicrographs, taken with a very simple camera held against the microscope eyepiece. Unfortunately, most modern compact cameras cannot be used, because they have a shutter that is operated only by an external (ie not TTL) lightmeter, with no manual override. There are a few exceptions with manual exposure settings and/or TTL metering, but these are the most expensive ones (such as the Leica *M* series).

The camera must be mounted so that its optical axis coincides with that of the eyepiece. The best way to attach the camera firmly is to have an adapter made, which will screw into the filter thread of the camera lens and attach to the microscope (eg by slipping over the eyepiece tube). If the camera is used with its lens attached, an ordinary eyepiece must be used, rather than a projective. The eyepiece produces an image at minus infinity, which is brought to a focus on the film plane by the camera (with lens focused at infinity). The aperture stop of the camera lens should be left fully open, otherwise vignetting (obstruction of the corners of the image) will occur.

The height of the camera's lens above the eyepiece is critical; above or below the optimal position, a good image may not be obtained, and there may be vignetting.

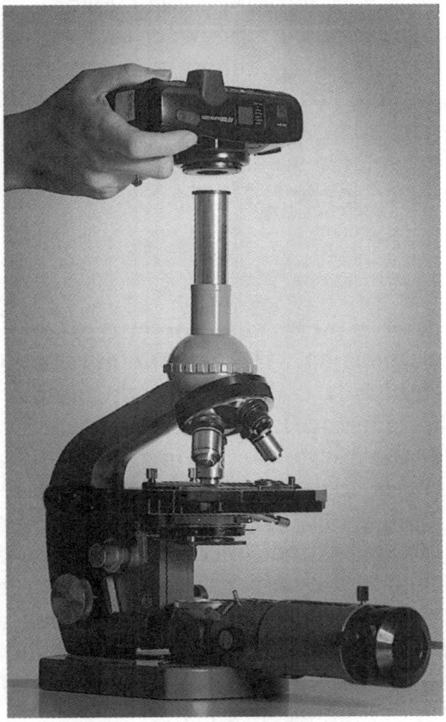

Fig 4.3. Compact camera on microscope. Olympus model *E* microscope from about 1970.

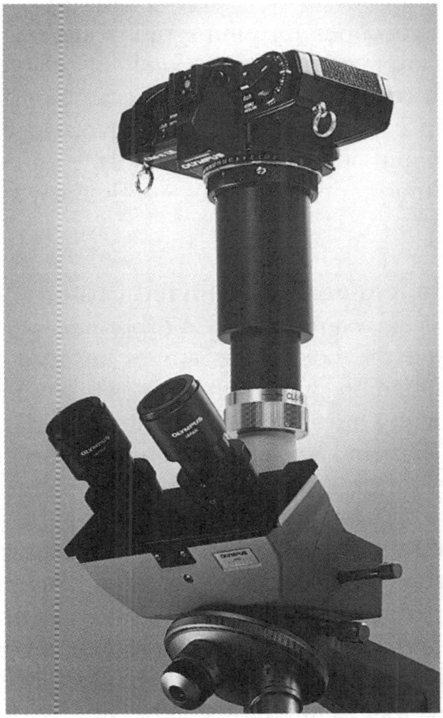

Fig 4.4. Olympus *OM*-type SLR camera, mounted on the trinocular head of an Olympus *CH-2* microscope using a Kyowa photographic adapter tube.

The microscope is focused normally by eye, the camera lens is set to infinity, and the camera aperture (iris diaphragm of the camera lens) is left open – although the actual setting is not particularly relevant and does not have the usual bearing on the exposure determination. The camera lens surface should be at the exit pupil of the eyepiece. The problem with this technique when using a standard lens on the camera is that the whole field of the microscope eyepiece, possibly some of it out of focus through curvature of field, may occupy less than half of the area of the film, and be much too small to be useful. This problem can be corrected by using a camera lens with longer-than-normal focal length, for example an 80 mm rather than a 50 mm lens for a 35 mm camera. Wide-angle lenses are therefore not suitable, and some zoom lenses cannot be used because of the position of their entrance pupil.

Commercial adapters to SLR camera body

The best equipment coming within the purview of this chapter consists of a microscope with trinocular head (see Chapter 2), an SLR camera body (without lens), and the appropriate adapter to couple the two. Used in conjunction with a projective (instead of an eyepiece) in the photographic tube, this apparatus is capable of professional-quality photographs.

Adapters for SLR cameras (Figs 4.2, 4.4, 15.3) may be available from the manufacturers of the microscope and/or camera. Leica market such an adapter for attachment to the camera port of a range of Leica microscopes and macroscopes (microscopes for photography at very low magnifications, of the order of 1× to 20×). We are aware of some excellent adapters that were made by Mamiya and Pentax for their respective 35 mm cameras. Similar photographic adapter tubes may be available from camera supply houses. Non-specific adapters for generic microscopes and with T-mount adapters (see Fig 4.2) to suit most SLR cameras are sometimes advertised in photographic magazines, particularly those published in the UK and USA.

Independently supported camera

This method (Fig 4.6) is necessary for heavy cameras and for microscopes in which the body tube moves up and down for focusing. The weight of a camera mounted on such a tube causes the tube to sink gradually under the weight, unless the focusing movement is very stiff (which is another nuisance). Therefore, in such a case the camera should be supported independently of the microscope. Some kind of light-trap to minimise stray light entering the camera is required; it is not necessary to have an absolutely light-tight coupling. The coupling must of course allow the body tube (and the eyepiece with it) to move up and down. A traditional coupling is a pair of concentric cylinders, painted black, one attached to the body tube and the other to the front of the camera. Kodak used to make a number of cylindrical lenshoods, in Series sizes, and it was possible to obtain two such that would fit one inside the other, with one screwed into the camera lens and the other attached to the eyepiece tube. Otherwise, something can be improvised using tin or aluminium cans.

A camera extension bellows can be used as a light-trap coupling. Bellows are very expensive to buy new, but sometimes available second-hand, or can be taken from an old folding camera. It is tedious but not very difficult to make one's own from black cloth and cardboard. A bag-type bellows may be sufficient; this consists of a tube of opaque cloth or leather. A piece of black cloth wrapped round and held by rubber bands is a simple alternative.

Horizontal bellows

Many older microscopes can be tilted to the horizontal if required. This can be convenient in conjunction with an independently supported camera, particularly if bellows are employed. The whole system (light source, microscope, bellows, camera) can be assembled on a standard optical bench bar, to facilitate alignment and adjustment of distances. These older microscope stands often have a screw thread underneath (intended to hold them in a wooden case) that can be used to bolt the stand firmly onto a base.

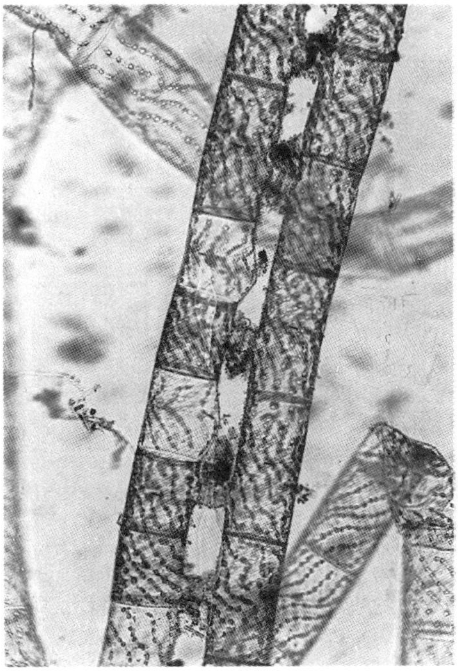

Fig 4.5. Photomicrograph taken in 1952 with compact camera on microscope in First-Year Botany class, University of Sydney. Conjugating *Spirogyra. Jiffy Kodak* camera (1940s vintage), *f*/8 lens at full aperture, Kodak *Verichrome Pan* B&W film roll film (127 format; later cropped to 35 mm format). Microscope unknown, probably about 1935.

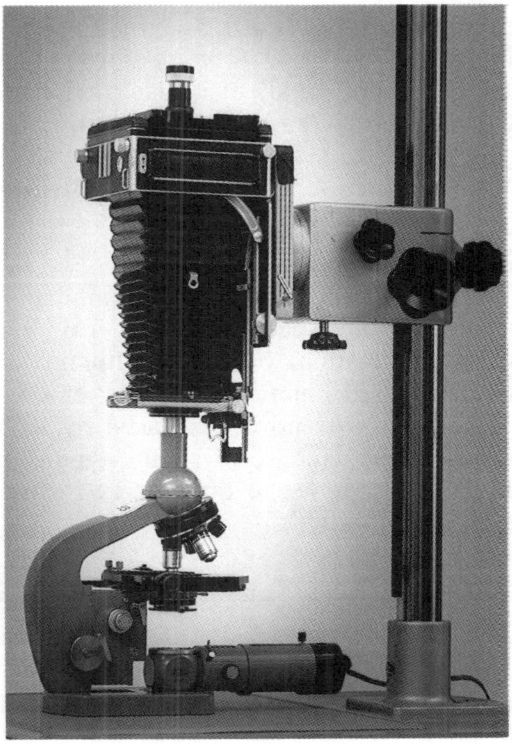

Fig 4.6. Camera independently supported over a microscope. Linhof *Technika V* 4×5 camera (from the 1950s) on Linhof copying stand, Olympus model *E* microscope (from 1960s) .

The microscope

The objective

The performance of the objective is crucial. Therefore, if there is any choice, get the best objectives you can afford, or at least one good one for photography. Flat-field objectives are best for photomicrography; this means that the photographer should try to obtain at least planachromatic rather than ordinary achromatic objectives (we assume here that planapochromats are too expensive).

For black-and-white (B&W) photography, the performance of achromatic objectives can be improved spectacularly by use of a green filter in the illumination path. This restricts the wavelengths of the light to those for which the objective is best corrected, and minimises chromatic aberration. A green filter will also improve the contrast of red–blue stains. Unfortunately, curvature of field is not improved by the use of monochromatic light, so a flat-field (plan) objective is still desirable.

For colour photography, one should consider reducing the wavelength band as much as possible. If using daylight as the light source, an ultraviolet-excluding (UV) filter should be used (obtained from photographic sources – often available very cheaply second-hand). It is also a wise precaution to reduce infrared (heat) radiation with a Schott KG1 filter or equivalent.

Illumination

Source-focused illumination

Early microscopists used illumination systems in which the light source was imaged into the specimen plane. This was known as critical illumination, Nelson–Abbe illumination, or Nelson illumination, and is now more descriptively called source-focused illumination. In better-class microscopes, source-focused illumination has been almost entirely replaced by Köhler illumination (described in Chapter 7). However, the expense of Köhler-type illumination techniques militates against their universal adoption, so that source-focused illumination is often used, especially in teaching laboratories.

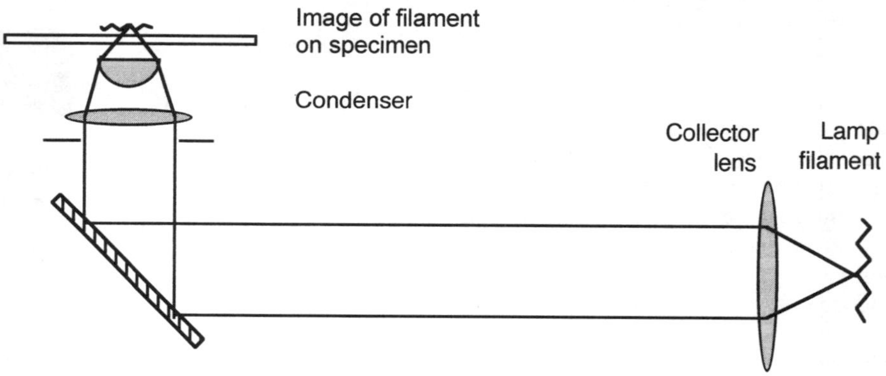

Fig 4.7. Source-focused illumination. The collector lens is optional. A frosted or opal glass diffuser (not shown) is usually placed in front of the light source.

In source-focused illumination, the light source is imaged onto the specimen by the condenser. Some systems add a lamp collector lens (as in Fig 4.7), enabling the use of smaller primary light sources. In this form, source-focused illumination gives high photometric efficiency (efficient use) of a light source when exceedingly high microscope magnifications are required. With high magnifications, the area of observation is very small, and the demands for uniformity of intensity can be more easily met.

Because the light source is imaged onto the specimen, both the specimen and the light source are said to be in field planes. In older microscopes, a field diaphragm is provided immediately below the specimen. The condenser iris diaphragm controls the

NA of the system, and is therefore said to be located in an aperture plane of the microscope. A study of these different planes in the microscope is further developed in the section on conjugate planes in Chapter 6, but it needs to be recognised that the location of the field and aperture planes is not the same in the source-focused and the Köhler methods.

If the illumination source is to be imaged onto the specimen, as source-focused illumination demands, there is a need for a light source with a large surface area, certainly no smaller than 30 mm diameter, of uniform intensity. This is usually provided by some sort of diffusing screen between the primary light source and the microscope substage condenser, the diffuser acting as a secondary light source.

Most cheaply, a conventional electric light bulb of about 40 W rating, with matte glass or opal glass construction, can be used as a light source. The glass of the bulb is focused onto the specimen, while looking through the microscope, using the focusing mechanism of the condenser. An object such as a pencil or pair of forceps held next to the glass surface will facilitate focusing of the bulb surface onto the specimen. If the bulb is frosted (matte), rather than opal, the image will have to be defocused a little so as not to show the ground-glass pattern. The area of the bulb with trade markings must be avoided or else all markings must be removed from the relevant surface of the bulb (by workshop buffing; this, however, may weaken the glass). General-purpose bulbs have their markings at the top; photographic enlarger bulbs have their markings elsewhere, to avoid precisely this problem. Co-author Fred, who had to use a system like this for about eight months during his postgraduate training, found that the concave surface of the mirror gave a better and brighter illumination than the flat side.

There are two objections to the procedure described in the previous paragraph. Firstly, the light source, and therefore the illuminated field, is seldom uniform in intensity distribution. The system was designed for use with oil lamps, which gave a relatively large and uniform source. At low magnifications, the uneven field makes photomicrography impossibly difficult. Frosted glass still transmits a reasonably high percentage of light without deviation, so it is not entirely effective as a diffuser. To achieve better diffusion of the light source an opal glass may be interposed, but an opal glass will diffuse light through a full 360° circle, and this seriously affects light intensity, or at least the efficiency of use of the available light intensity. If a separate diffusing screen is to be used, it should be placed either in a field plane (close to the light source) or in an aperture plane (close to the condenser iris diaphragm).

Secondly, for all but the lowest magnifications, there is excessive flare in the image plane. This is because the diffused secondary source as imaged in the specimen plane is much larger than the area of the specimen that is being observed. The image is soft, lacking contrast, compared with that obtainable by Köhler illumination. To reduce this flare, it is possible to control the size of the illumination area of the specimen by incorporating an iris diaphragm into the system, immediately adjacent to the diffused source. When imaged on the specimen, this diaphragm can adjust the illuminated area of the specimen to that which is accepted by a particular objective, thus considerably improving the contrast.

Adjustment of the condenser

There may need to be a compromise between sufficient aperture to obtain the objective's full resolution, and stopping down as much as practicable to minimise glare and aberrations. For B&W, a coloured (eg green) filter will minimise chromatic aberration.

Ground-glass surface on filters

With cheaper microscopes, some microscope manufacturers supply a filter that has a ground-glass surface, intended to ensure that the microscope field is evenly illuminated. The ground-glass evens out the light intensity, but at the expense of image contrast. See Chapter 7.

Very low magnification

When objectives of magnification of 10× or less are used, some special problems arise. The field is so wide that a typical condenser gives adequate illumination only for a central area, leaving the periphery of the field relatively dark. Ideally, a special ultralow-power condenser (see Chapter 7) should be used with objectives having a magnification of less than 10×. If this is too expensive, there are alternatives. Properly, the top lens of the condenser should be removed (see Fig 4.8), and the condenser re-focused. Alternatively, it may be possible to adapt another lens (eg a photographic enlarging lens) as a low-power wide-field condenser. A less sound but more practical alternative in the classroom is to interpose, between lamp and mirror, a good-quality diffusing screen of large size, approximately 100 mm × 130 mm. Some of the modern instruments with the lamp built-in to the foot of the microscope, and without a filter carrier beneath the condenser, present a difficulty in this respect.

If the above methods prove impracticable, it may be possible to obtain adequate illumination with the condenser removed. Older microscopes, without a built-in light source, provided a concave mirror specifically for use with low-power objectives without the condenser.

Cheap sources of illumination

Daylight is the cheapest, requiring only a mirror to reflect it up into the condenser, and running costs are zero. Unfortunately daylight is not always available: the sun works to a strict timetable and will not even consider working overtime, and may be obscured. The colour (see Chapter 7) of daylight is variable, from the orange of the low sun to the blue of a cloudy sky.

The next cheapest is probably a large opal bulb. If a slide projector is available, it makes a high-intensity light source. Battery-operated lamps are not recommended – they are too expensive to keep supplied with batteries.

Fluorescent lighting generates less heat but is not suitable for photomicrography in colour. It gives a green cast (due to the mercury line at 546 nm) that is difficult to correct with filters, even though commercial filters for this purpose are available from camera supply houses.

Darkground illumination

Darkground (darkfield) microscopy is the simplest form of microscopy other than transmitted-light microscopy. Normally, one uses either a special darkground condenser (see Chapter 9) or a multifunction condenser with darkground facilities.

Patch stop. A brightfield condenser can be converted to a low-power darkground condenser quite easily, by means of a patch stop (Fig 4.8). It requires only a stop in the condenser blocking out the central rays of light that would enter the objective while allowing the peripheral rays to illuminate the object. The aperture diaphragm of the condenser must be fully open. Only those rays reflected, refracted or diffracted by the object enter the objective and hence the object is seen as bright against a black background.

The simplicity of this modification, and the fact that patch stops are not sold by the more prestigious instrument manufacturers, should not deter you from making and using a patch stop.

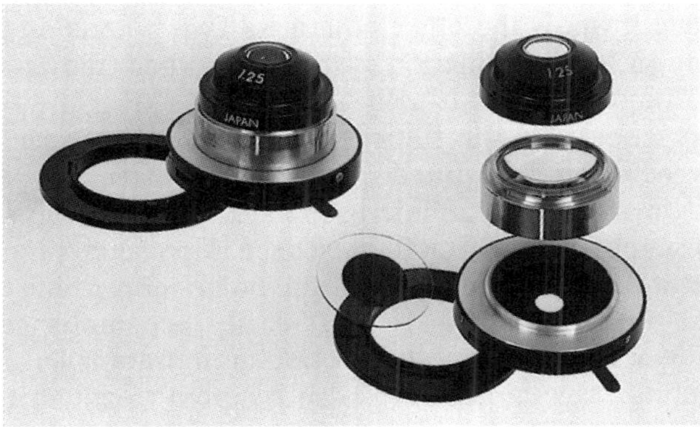

Fig 4.8. A two-lens Abbe condenser with patch stop for darkground illumination. Right, disassembled to show component parts. The patch stop is the clear disc with opaque centre (centre of picture), which fits into the filter carrier.

The patch stop is made from an opaque disc, typically about 18 mm in diameter, made of black paper or metal (a coin of about this size can be used), supported on a transparent disc (a clear glass filter, clear film or foil, etc.). This size works satisfactorily for objectives with a numerical aperture (NA) of up to 0·7. The ideal disc size will vary for different objective NAs, higher NA objectives requiring larger diameter discs than lower NA objectives, but the disc sizes are not critical. The optimum diameter is found by trial and error or by measurement. In the latter case the aperture field diaphragm is closed down until its aperture is just greater than that of the objective: the diameter of the stop should be slightly larger than that of the diaphragm opening thus obtained. The method of construction of a patch stop filter has particular significance for photomicrography when the same principles are applied to Rheinberg filter techniques (see Chapter 9).

In use, first set up the microscope in brightfield, carefully centring the illumination system; then open the aperture iris fully. The patch stop is then inserted. The focusing of the condenser is critical, because only the margins of the condenser aperture are used, and the correct condenser position for Köhler illumination is unlikely to be the best (brightest) position for darkground, due to spherical aberration of the condenser. The possibility of condenser immersion should be recognised, but only if its NA exceeds 1·0 (the objective NA is not relevant in this consideration); because oiling is a messy procedure, it is often avoided. The lamp intensity should be increased to maximum, or nearly so.

Polarisation

Polarisation microscopy (see Chapter 10) requires, as a minimum, two pieces of Polaroid material. It should be possible to buy a small sheet quite cheaply, or maybe an old pair of Polaroid glasses can be sacrificed. Small discs of Polaroid are commonly sold with Polaroid sunglasses, one of which can be placed over the eyepiece. Polarising filters intended for conventional photography can sometimes be obtained second-hand, and usually make excellent polarisers. Linear polarisers are recommended. Circular polarisers, used in SLR cameras with autofocusing, are to be avoided here, because they unnecessarily complicate the situation. If used, it is essential to note that the two sides of a circular polariser are different, and that the correct side must face towards the other polariser. Two polarising discs are required: one (the polariser) to fit the illumination system, the other (the analyser) to fit over or in the eyepiece. The polariser is usually placed either over the field diaphragm on the base of the microscope or in the filter holder under the condenser. The analyser, in a binocular microscope is best fitted in the body tube under the prisms of the binocular head, and in a monocular microscope is most conveniently fitted in the eyepiece. In a microscope intended for fluorescence microscopy, it may be possible to use a barrier-filter slot. Either the analyser or the polariser (or both) must be left free to rotate; for visual observation this is most easily accomplished by rotating the eyepiece, carrying the analyser with it, but in photomicrography it is easier to rotate the polariser. A rotating stage is generally also required to adjust the orientation of the specimen.

Fluorescence microscopy

The photographic equipment described above can be used for fluorescence microscopy, but the camera's TTL metering system is unlikely to be sensitive enough to measure the required exposures, which therefore can only be determined by trial-and-error. Fluorescence microscopy is described in Chapter 11.

Illuminating solid objects

Opaque objects are typically lighted using an epi-illuminator, which illuminates the specimen through or around the objective (Chapter 7). Alternatively, light can be directed onto the specimen from some external source, eg using fibre optics. This is always relatively difficult (see Chapter 13, Stereomicroscopy). A reading-lamp is the most likely to be available. The best are those with a low-voltage halogen lamp. Fluorescent lamps are suitable only for B&W, unless a green overall colour is acceptable. Usually two lamps are needed, one as a main light and the other to fill in the shadows; alternatively, a reflector of white card or crumpled aluminium foil can be used for fill-in. The light can be intensified by using a magnifying glass to concentrate the light on the object; this lens (known as a bullseye condenser) will need to be mounted on a stand or attached to the microscope (Fig 4.9).

Exposure determination

There are three methods for exposure determination: trial-and-error, through-the-lens (TTL) metering with the camera, and metering with a separate meter.

Trial-and-error is described in Chapter 16, and is not generally to be recommended.

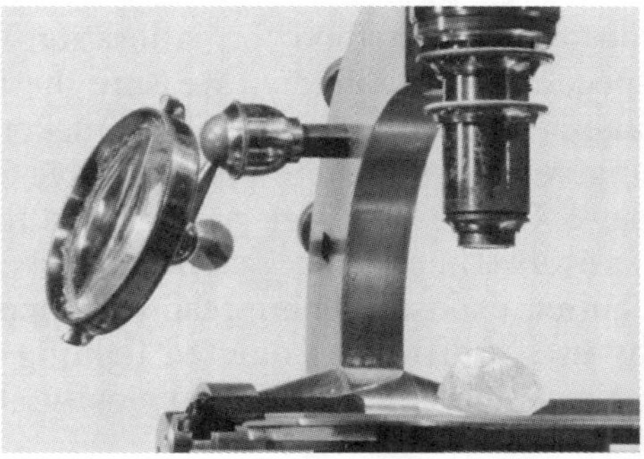

Fig 4.9 (above). A bullseye condenser for illuminating a solid object, attached by an arm to the microscope stand. Microscope and accessories by Smith & Beck, London, about 1850. The specimen is a lump of fluorite. Modern epi-illuminators are shown in Figs 1.2 and 11.2.

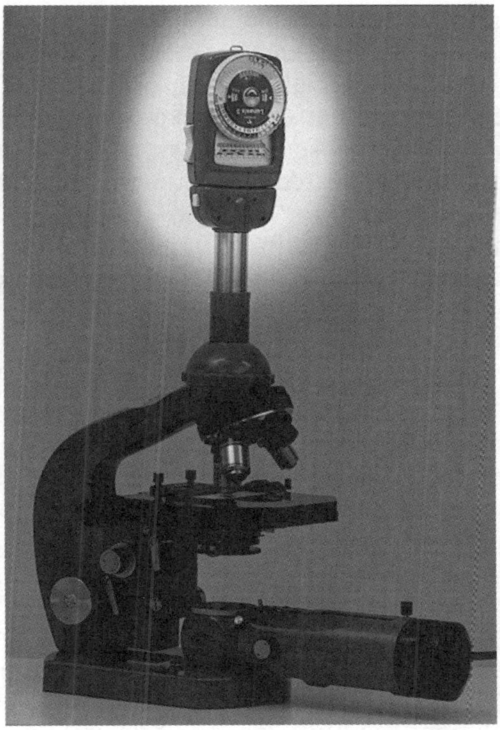

Fig 4.10 (right). Gossen *Lunasix* exposure meter with 'micro' attachment, on an Olympus model *E* microscope.

TTL metering with an SLR camera is relatively easy. For transmitted-light pictures, usually the required exposure is about $^2/_3$ stop more than that indicated by the meter (see Chapters 3 and 16). Note that some interchangeable focusing screens affect the exposure meter, typically causing overexposure. For example, the Nikon type *M* focusing screen (ideal for focusing, as described above) cannot be used for exposure metering with the pentaprism; in the *F4* and *F5* cameras, spot metering (which is not affected by the focusing screen) must be used instead. In the Olympus *OM2n* and *OM4*, metering is off-the-film (OTF), and there is therefore no problem, although the pre-exposure measurement and the actual (correct) exposure may differ.

A hand-held meter may be held over the eyepiece to obtain a reading. Special 'micro' accessories are available for some of the more expensive meters, such as the Gossen *Lunasix* series. This attachment (Fig 4.10) clips onto the meter, and has a snout that is the same diameter as a standard eyepiece, which it replaces during measurement. The meter can be used in three ways.

1. One eyepiece can be removed temporarily, and the meter inserted in its place.
2. The meter can be held over the top of an eyepiece.
3. The meter can be applied to the ground-glass or pentaprism viewfinder of the camera.

The meter will need to be calibrated by trial-and-error, to determine what *f*-stop mark on the meter corresponds to the required exposure. The method for calibration is as follows. Set the exposure meter for the film speed in the usual way. Measure the light by the chosen method (1, 2, or 3, above). Take a series of photographs (bracketing; see Chapter 3) at various exposures, bracketing widely. After the pictures have been processed, choose the one with the best exposure. On the exposure meter, note the *f*-stop that appeared opposite the correct exposure time. This *f*-stop is used as a reference point for all future readings, the required exposure being read off opposite this *f*-stop. The calibration may be affected by use of different coloured lighting or a different type of specimen. For method (3), the *f*-stop calibration is typically about *f*/1·4.

Photographic processing

For B&W, the cheapest procedure may be to develop and print oneself. In the absence of a darkroom and enlarging facilities, B&W negatives can rather easily be developed, using a changing bag to load the film into the developing tank. The processed negative can be sent for commercial printing. Chromogenic film is processed by the same process as colour negatives. B&W prints can be made from B&W negatives by colour mini-labs using the same paper as for colour prints: the resulting prints cannot be expected to win competitions nor to be as permanent as proper B&W prints, but may be quite adequate for many purposes. The same labs generally offer enlargement to about 15×18 cm (6×8 inches). Further advice on photographic processing is offered in Chapter 18. In the absence of a darkroom and enlarging facilities, the use of Polaroid material in the 4×5 inch (10×12 cm) or $3^1/_4 \times 4^1/_4$ inch (8×10 cm) formats can be considered, but here in Australia the film is too expensive for routine use.

Digital photography (Chapter 17) avoids all these processing problems. In any case, given one print or a reasonably large negative, and appropriate equipment, scanning and digital modification and printing is the cheapest and quickest way of obtaining prints (especially labelled prints) for publication.

Further reading

Old books (rather than modern ones) are often the most helpful to the impecunious microscopist, because the older books describe how things were done before the days of modern (expensive) optoelectronics. Old books often have good ideas on how to make suitable accessories for oneself. It is probably not much use us giving a list of books long out of print, but some may be found in institutional libraries. Those that have come our way include those of Hind & Randles (1913), Lawson (1972), Loveland (1970), Shillaber (1944) and Walker (1971). More recent books include that of Delly (1988).

5
Presentation: aesthetic and related considerations

This chapter deals with two main topics: the composition of satisfying pictures, and the assembly of a group of photomicrographs and text into a unit such as a plate for publication or a poster. We also discuss the projection of slides, and the labelling, indexing and storage of photographs.

Composition

Aesthetic considerations

Photomicrographs can be very beautiful. Even for a photograph intended only as a record of a specimen, not for publication, a little additional time and care in composition may yield rich dividends in beauty. Artistic considerations are of even greater importance in the production of pictures intended for publication or public presentation – the latter including lectures to students. If one looks at close-ups and photomicrographs in scientific publications, and even in at least one book on scientific photography, one commonly sees pictures that, although technically acceptable, appear lifeless and unappealing, devoid of artistic inspiration. Admittedly, in scientific photography, accurate representation comes first, and sometimes the subject is such that even Leonardo da Vinci would have been puzzled as to how to make an artistic representation of it!

A photographer who approaches picture-making from the technical, rather than the artistic, side will need specific training to look for beauty and to produce harmonious compositions. It helps greatly to examine really good pictures (see, eg, Ross & Romrell, 1989). However, it is also instructive to look at any set of photomicrographs (as in an atlas of histology) and to decide which pictures are excellent and which are less satisfactory, and the reasons for this. Some may have been printed too small for reasons of economy, many have the wrong colour temperature . . . Besides photographs, one should look at paintings, particularly abstracts and still-lifes (the closest analogy to photomicrographs that one is likely to see). In paintings, one can generally assume that artistic considerations were paramount. Some hints for achieving a good composition are given in the Box on the next page, Basic rules for composition.

Format, aspect ratio. Most cameras have a rectangular format, and most conveniently take pictures with the long axis horizontal (Figs 5.1, 5.3). This is sometimes known as *landscape format,* as distinct from *portrait format* in which the long axis is vertical (Fig 5.2). It is a sign of a good photographer that both formats are used (Fig 5.3). If in doubt, for a particular subject, it is usually best to take some pictures each way, if possible. For the front cover of a magazine, vertical format is essential.

Basic rules for composition

- Fill the frame as much as possible.
- Omit irrelevant areas.
- Place the principal subject, if possible, about one-third of the way from one side and one-third of the way from top or bottom.
- Make the principal subject stand out from the background.
- If photographing several items together, choose an odd number (such as 3 or 5) rather than an even number.
- Choose beautiful shapes both for the subject areas and for the spaces between and outside (negative spaces).
- Avoid having strong lines leading to a corner.

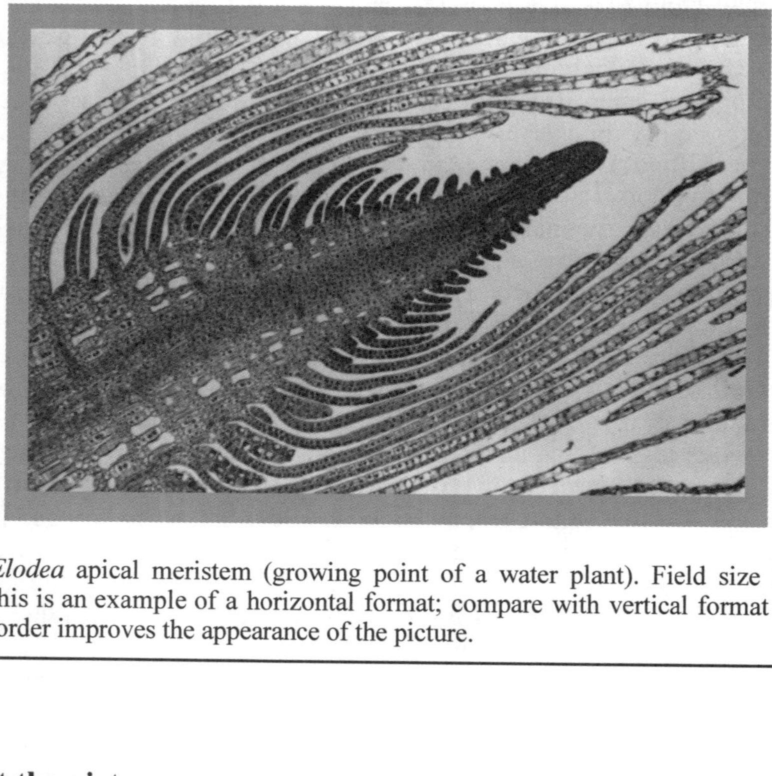

Fig 5.1. *Elodea* apical meristem (growing point of a water plant). Field size 2·2 mm × 1·2 mm. This is an example of a horizontal format; compare with vertical format in Fig 5.2. The grey border improves the appearance of the picture.

Looking at the picture

The first thing is to have a good look at the subject of the intended picture. This means looking at it all over – middle, sides and corners – not just in the middle. This procedure, and artistic judgements of the composition, are often made a little more difficult by the typical photomicrographic viewfinder, which may be cluttered by graticules indicating formats for different projectives, a cross in the middle for focusing, and the irrelevant part of the image outside the format (film) frame. Co-author Ron has some difficulty in assessing the artistic merit of a composition within lines of a graticule, and finds it helpful to have a special graticule in which areas outside the photographic frame are blanked out. Composition may be easier with an SLR as described in Chapter 4, provided that one chooses one with a plain screen and without scales, meter needles, etc, obtruding into the picture area.

Containing the subject in the picture. Sufficient magnification should be used to fill the frame with the relevant object area. Co-author Ron's experience is that beginners may choose too high a magnification, forgetting that the camera records only part of the image as seen in the eyepiece. On the other hand, co-author Fred thinks that there may be a tendency to have the magnification too low, in an attempt to include too much in the one picture. However, the photographer must be careful to avoid unintentional omission of parts at the periphery, such as feet and antennae. It is necessary to train oneself to look around the periphery of the camera field and to plan the picture, from the beginning, so that the peripheral parts of the subject will be included.

Composing the picture is accomplished primarily by first choosing the magnification, and then moving the specimen until a suitable composition is found. When using a spot-measuring photometer operative only in the centre of the field, measure the exposure first if possible, then adjust the composition.

The most prominent object in the field should not normally be placed exactly in the middle of the field, and neither should any division in the specimen divide the field into two precisely equal halves. A good traditional place for the most prominent object is approximately one-third of the distance from side to side and top to bottom (strictly, at the point of the Golden Section, which is more exactly 0·384 of the distance, or slightly more than one-third).

Often, a composition can be improved by no more than turning the specimen (or the camera) to obtain the most harmonious arrangement within the field (see Fig 5.2). Rotating the picture is usually achieved by turning either the stage carrying the specimen, or the body tube plus camera, or the camera alone, in about that order of preference. An optical system to rotate the image (introduced by Leica some years ago) is even more convenient. Since the photograph or slide can always be turned end-to-end, only 180° of rotation of the stage or camera (90° in each direction) is strictly necessary, but less than this is unacceptable for photomicrography.

Obtaining an excellent composition involves conscious or unconscious consideration of aspects such as symmetry, balance, rhythm, tensions, flow, unity, and variety. A full discussion of these topics would entail more space than is available here; some interesting books are listed in the Further reading section at the end of this chapter.

The background

In transmitted-light pictures of sections, the background is formed by the transmitted light. In a colour transparency, this should normally come out as either a very pale grey or pure white. This requires light at the correct colour temperature, and the correct exposure. A much overexposed background of any colour will turn out white. In a print of a similar object, the background should normally come out as a very pale grey.

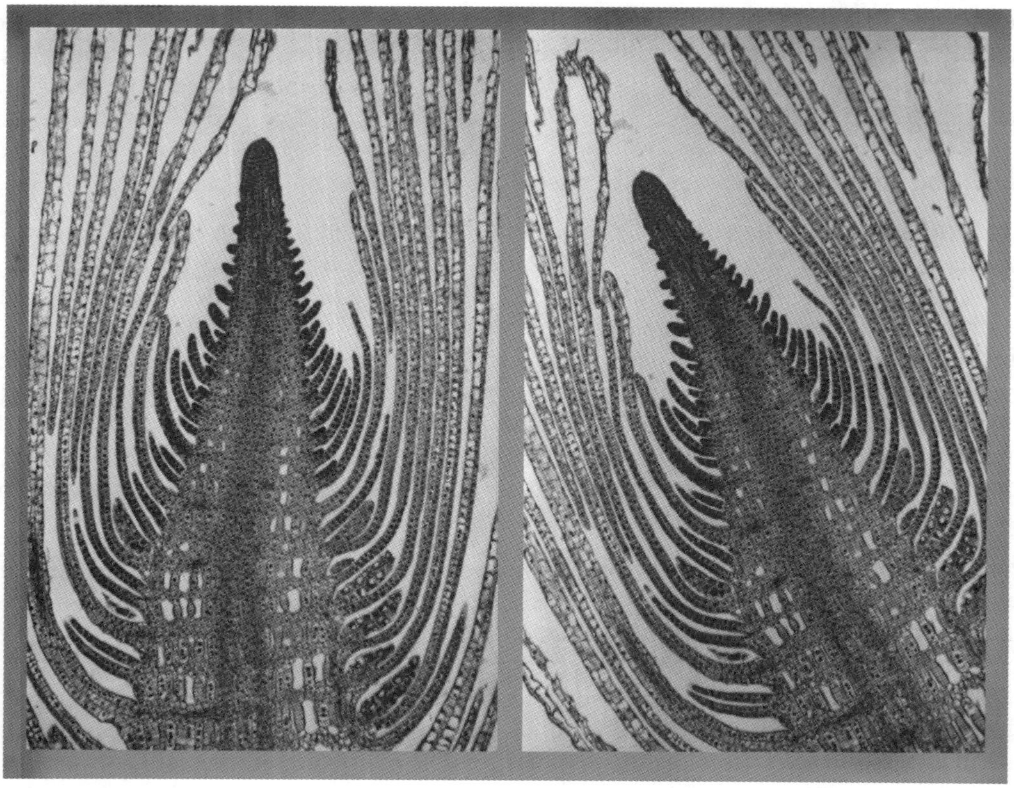

Fig 5.2. Same as Fig 5.1: *Elodea* apical meristem (growing point of a water plant). Field size 2·2 mm × 1·2 mm. The classical 'scientific' vertical orientation on the left, a freer and more artistic expression on the right. Compare with the horizontal format of Fig 5.1.

The spaces between and around the areas of interest are known as *negative shapes.* These should be considered as part of the composition. Awkward negative shapes should be avoided. For the front cover of a magazine, provision should be made for the masthead (name of magazine, etc) at the top, and (commonly) for other printing at the bottom. This provision can be either space (light or dark) or unimportant and unfussy parts of the subject.

Adding colour

Colours in photomicrographs can be very beautiful, particularly those with several fluorescent colours or with two different techniques in harmonising colours. If there is no colour in the picture, one may choose to make the background a specific colour, such as the green obtained by using the same green filter as one would use for black-and-white (B&W) photography. Co-author Fred particularly likes the combination of fluorescence and simultaneous coloured phase-contrast (Plate 7, and Chapters 10 and 11). The most colourful effects are obtainable with Rheinberg illumination (Plate 4 and Chapter 9).

The presentation of projection slides (transparencies)

At a scientific or technical meeting, when slides (transparencies, diapositives) of photomicrographs are shown, there are certain steps that can be taken to enhance the presentation.

Precious slides must be properly protected, preferably in a glass mount. Some projectionists, both professional and amateur, seem unable to avoid putting their fingerprints on slides, and only glass mounts give sufficient protection.

The audience will always appreciate a clear indication of the scale of the picture. This is best shown by a scale bar on the picture itself. With the Nikon *Microphot-FXA* it is possible to photograph a scale bar directly on the original film. Otherwise, it is possible (but not usually practicable) to mark the bar directly onto the transparency (on the emulsion side): only a duplicate transparency should be risked in this procedure. A dark bar may be added in black ink using a fibre-nib pen; a light-coloured bar can be made by scratching a line in the emulsion. To avoid damaging the original slide, a scale bar can be photographed on a second film and the two films mounted together, emulsion sides towards each other so that both will be in focus simultaneously in the projector. Alternatively, a print from the original slide can have a bar drawn on it and then be re-photographed; unfortunately this procedure loses much of the tonal range of the original, due to limitations of the print.

The standard size ('35 mm') mount for projection is 50 mm (not quite 2 inches) square and of undefined thickness. This latter may be a problem. Projectors in the USA tend to be designed for thin slides, and thicker slides stick; projectors in Europe tend to be designed for thicker slides, and thinner ones may not transport properly in the machine. Mounts are available in this size (50 mm × 50 mm) with different sizes of window, or with two or three small windows to enable immediate comparison of different pictures. Portions of medium-format film can be mounted in the larger windows (particularly SuperSlide format, 38 mm square). It is possible to mask a transparency to a smaller size. Aluminium masks of various sizes and shapes can be purchased, and can be mounted with the transparency in the slide mount. Apart from that, any temptation to block out unwanted areas of the picture should be resisted. It always shows, and will make the audience doubt your intellectual honesty.

Larger standard sizes of slides are 85 mm square (the old 'lantern slide' format; which accepts film from 6×7 cm, 6×6 cm and 6×4·5 cm formats), and 70 mm square (specially designed for the 6×6 and 6×4·5 cm formats). Slides measuring 80 mm ×100 mm, for horizontal slides only, are used in the USA. Still larger projectors exist, for formats up to 4×5 inches, but are expensive and rarely available.

Labelling of slides

Slides are conventionally marked with a prominent dot in the bottom left-hand corner, looking at the slide the correct way up (Fig 5.3). The slide is inserted into the projector upside down, with the dot facing the projectionist (ie the rear) and in the top right-hand corner.

Dark (low-key) pictures

Some pictures tend to be very dark overall: these include many photomicrographs taken using fluorescence, darkground and polarisation. Such very dark pictures are commonly shown in a dark auditorium. In these circumstances, the audience's eyes should be given an opportunity to adapt both before and after showing the very dark slides. First, prepare the audience by showing a somewhat less dark slide: a coloured photograph or a diazo slide (white on blue or red; see below). Then, after the very dark slides, a relatively dark slide will enable the audience to become accustomed to the light gradually. One should avoid using a black-on-white diagram or table immediately before a fluorescence or other very dark slide: the audience will not be able to appreciate the very dark slide which follows the bright one. If necessary, the offending bright slide can be sandwiched with a sheet of coloured gelatine, but it is better to have a new diazo slide made.

Diazo slides are rarely made nowadays, but there are two modern alternatives. One is a computer-generated image photographed on ordinary transparency film. Another way is to photograph a black-on-white printout of the desired text, through a coloured filter, onto colour positive (transparency) film, and have the film processed as colour negative film. This will reverse the tones of the image, of course, giving light-coloured letters on a darker background.

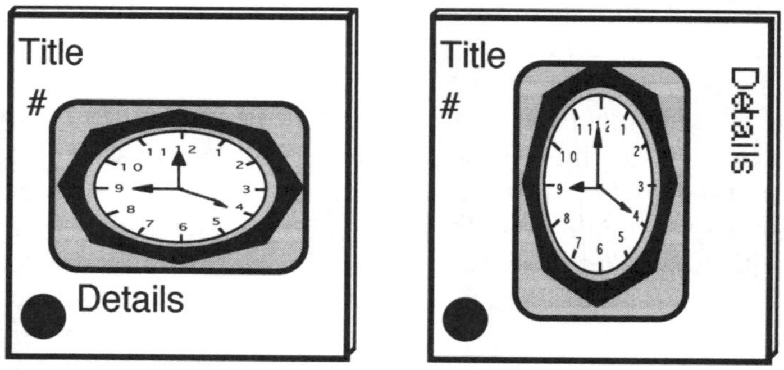

Fig 5.3. Labelling of slides for projection.

Duplication of transparencies

Duplication of pictures is particularly relevant to biological photography, for two reasons: the best photographs may be unique and unrepeatable, and poor ones which are too dark but otherwise valuable can be reproduced somewhat lighter and thereby made more suitable for projection. Transparencies can easily be duplicated, using a single-lens-reflex (SLR) camera (see Chapter 4) and one of the many duplicating devices (which are of variable quality) or with a photomacrographic apparatus. Some loss of detail and colour balance is to be expected. In general, high-contrast films such as *Kodachrome* film should usually be duplicated onto relatively low-contrast films, eg *Ektachrome* film, otherwise the resulting contrast will be extreme. Special duplicating films are available. Commercial duplicating services exist, but may not be able to carry out special procedures such as making a transparency lighter. Copying to a larger or smaller format is possible. For further information, see Young, Benson & Eaton (1985).

Prints for publication

Prints for publication should be printed on glossy paper, at least the same size as the intended printed figure. Colour pictures are better reproduced from transparencies than from prints. When a print is reproduced as a half-tone (like the photomicrographs in this book), the print is subjected to a process which breaks the image up into dots. Fine detail tends to be lost in this process, so greater magnification is required than for an ordinary print.

Prints must be identified. To avoid damaging the picture, identification should be either written on a label which is then stuck on the back, or written with a low-pressure device such as a felt-tipped overhead-projection marker (permanent kind) or a soft pencil. Write your name and the figure number.

For further suggestions, see Luey (1987).

Labels

For publication, the publisher's 'Instructions to Authors' should be consulted as to the typeface and size of type to be used. The same options exist as for scales (see below).

Scales

When prints are prepared for publication, it is usual to add a scale bar (Fig 17.1). One can photograph a stage micrometer under identical conditions of magnification (microscope and print), to determine the length the bar should be. The bar itself is usually most easily applied using Letraset. Alternatively, it may be drawn on a separate piece of paper, in black ink or produced with a laser printer, and glued in position. A one-unit length (eg 10, 100, or 1000 μm) is preferred; if a two-unit or five-unit length is used, ticks at unit intervals are recommended. The addition of a scale bar to transparencies is too tricky (unless superimposed at the time of taking the original photograph), and is best avoided. Some photomicrographic systems have provision for superimposing a scale bar on the original photomicrograph. For scale bars in digital systems and image processing, see Chapter 17.

Multiple figures: making and labelling a plate

For publication, a group of photographs is commonly assembled as a plate (eg Figs 1.2, 1.3, 17.8). The width of the plate is normally the width of the printed column in the journal, or somewhat less. The height should not exceed the height of the printed (text) page, and it is best to allow room for the caption on the same page. The various component pictures should be chosen with care, and thought given to the layout. Ideally, the pictures on a plate should have similar tone value, otherwise the odd one out may not reproduce well. A small space is usually left between individual photographs; if the author cannot do this tidily, the space can be inserted by the blockmaker. Lettering, if not put on by the author, should be indicated clearly on a photocopy or other duplicate of the plate. The assembly of the plate can be done by hand (as in Figs 1.2, 1.3) or by computer (see Chapter 17).

Making B&W prints from transparencies

Making B&W prints from transparencies requires the making of an *internegative*, which is a negative made from the original transparency and from which the required print can be made. Internegatives are easily made by copying (re-photographing) the transparency onto B&W negative film. Colour filters can be used to bring out the desired features (see Chapter 15).

Making a poster

The following are some suggestions to help you make a poster incorporating photomicrographs. For further suggestions, consult Briscoe (1990).

Format. Ascertain the exact size required or permitted for the poster, including whether the format is vertical or horizontal.

Design. The illustrative material for a poster presentation should involve rather more preparation than a series of projection slides that might be used for a 20 minute talk. Unless the viewer is attracted to the poster, possibly by the excellence of the illustrations, it is too easy for the poster to be ignored. Whereas it is an expectation to write, correct, amend and rewrite the script over and over again, it is common practice to accept the first available photographic print. Whether a poster is worth stopping to read may well be judged on the quality of just one or two illustrations. A decision to include a photomicrograph or other illustration should be undertaken with the same care with which the script is reviewed.

Impact! The audience will most likely be attracted either by the title or the pictures, so both should be as striking and well-presented as possible. Someone attracted by the pictures will probably next read the captions, which should be informative enough to stand on their own, and interesting enough to stimulate the reader to examine the poster in more detail.

Assembly. A poster is usually assembled upon a stiff backing, such as coloured cardboard or foam sheets. The classical method is to make it in demountable sections (for transport), which can if necessary be rearranged to suit the space actually available if this differs from that specified in the conference instructions. If the poster is to be laminated, a stiff backing is not required.

Adhesives suitable for mounting photographs onto the poster backing include a spray adhesive, rubber cement ('milliner's glue'), or ideally, dry mounting tissue. Care should first be taken that the mounting medium does not damage the print. Temporary displays put together in a hurry, or trial versions, can be assembled with double-sided tape or Velcro discs. Laminating the poster is strongly recommended.

For digital assembly (strongly recommended), pictures can be scanned into a computer, assembled and text added by desktop publishing software. Such a service is commercially available but may be expensive. The final product is a giant printout, which can be laminated and rolled up into a tube for transport.

Prints. Colour prints are highly desirable, and a well-chosen colour background to the print will ensure that the poster demands attention. The print itself will usually be larger than commonly available from the local photo shop. A first-quality A4 size print will cost up to a hundred times more than the standard postcard-size print which suffices for thesis or home album. The highest-quality colour print is derived, expensively, from a well-exposed transparency. An enlargement from colour negative film is much cheaper, and is likely to be quite acceptable, provided the printer can be advised of the correct background colour (normally a neutral grey). Cheaper but poorer-quality alternatives to a colour print are a photomechanical transfer (a positive print made without a negative) or an enlargement effected by a colour photocopier. The latter can be made from a transparency (best) or a print.

Because of the poor lighting arrangements from which most poster displays suffer, glossy prints will give unpleasant reflections; matte surfaces are a safer alternative, but will lack the depth of colour which gloss surfaces permit. If the poster is to be laminated, use glossy prints – the lamination will give a glossy surface which will reflect anyway. The poster will be viewed from a distance of at least one metre, so that the normal rules concerning empty magnification, which pertain to a viewing distance of 25 cm, can be relaxed accordingly.

Graphs. These are usually best made by computer using *CricketGraph*, etc. See Tufte, 1983, 1990, 1997.

Lettering. This may be computer generated and printed, rub-on *Letraset*, etc. The poster should have your name, address, possibly photograph, and date.

Captions. See examples in this book.

Hanging. Make provision in the layout for hanging. Take your own thumb tacks and/or *Velcro* dots!

Care of photographs

Since photographs may be the only permanent record of experimental work, it is important to take good care of them. This section provides a summary of the main considerations. For detailed information on the care of photographs, see the books by the Editors of Time-Life Books (1972) and Anon (1988).

Labelling

All photographs should be clearly labelled. Negatives are usually stored in sheets which should be labelled at least with the serial number of the roll, and/or the date. Transparencies are often numbered when returned from processing; the roll number should be added. Co-author Fred finds that permanent-ink projection-transparency pens are best, the next best being blue ball-point ink.

Slides and prints should bear an identification number, corresponding to that in your notebook. There are three basic systems:

- Numbering each roll, and then each frame. (For example, 100/15, meaning the 15th frame of the 100th roll). This is probably the easiest.
- A serial number for each picture, from 1 to as many as you take in a lifetime!
- A number for each project, and a serial number within that. The advantage of this is that *all* material related to the project can carry the project number, which is advantageous if you have a lot of material.

There exist computer programs for indexing slides and printing out of labels for the slides; presumably these can be used for prints too.

Storage

Transparencies can be stored in boxes, projector magazines, or plastic files in loose-leaf books or filing-cabinets. Prints should be stored in files of acid-free paper. Negatives are usually stored in loose-leaf transparent sheets.

Co-author Fred finds that the biggest problem is humidity, leading to growth of mould (fungus; foxing of prints) which may occur as one of the disadvantages of a pleasant climate such as that of Sydney. Of course, it is much more of a problem in the tropics. The first thing is to find a reasonably dry place for storage. If there is any problem with damp, in Fred's experience the only satisfactory solution is to install air conditioning or a dehumidifier (which is equally effective and cheaper). Both help to purify the air, the air conditioner by filtering, the humidifier by drawing it past ice-covered cooling coils, which tend to trap particulate matter, possibly including fungal spores.

The American National Standards Institute (ANSI) Standards for Photography (of which a catalogue is published annually) indicate the recommended procedures and materials for the storage of film, plates and paper prints. Since the matter is of particular concern to museum and other archive conservators, some effort has been made to research the subject.

Caution is given here that plastic filing sleeves, envelopes and folders which are made from polyvinyl chloride (PVC) invariably contain phthalate plasticisers; these plasticisers have a disastrous affect on the organic dyes of colour transparencies and colour prints. Such PVC sheeting should not be used to construct storage containers. Because they are relatively stable and inert, it is preferable to use uncoated polyesters and uncoated cellulose acetate – the same materials from which film supports are manufactured. Wilhelm & Brower (1993) recommend the choice of polypropylene and high density polyethylene filing sheets; they warn against the more generally available low density polyethylene.

Further reading

Many books on the practical aspects of art and photography have sections on composition, and there are numerous books on composition and related topics. The Kodak book *Mastering composition and light* (Anon, 1984b) is a good discussion of composition for the photographer, profusely illustrated in colour. 'Mastering' is a perhaps a bit optimistic for so brief a discussion. Clements & Rosenfeld's (1979) *Photographic composition* is an excellent book on artistic aspects of photography. Parramón's (1984) *Composition in painting and drawing* is excellent, with a very clear text. Poore's (1967) *Composition in art* has a lot of information not found in other books. Smith's (1985) *Designing a photograph* is a series of short essays on various topics, well illustrated in colour. Zelanski & Fisher's (1988) *The art of seeing* is an excellent book, dealing with many aspects of composition and design, well illustrated in colour.

Part II

Microscopy

This part deals with the microscope optical system in detail, using transmitted light only. Details of other techniques of microscopy are given in Part III.

- Aims: to describe the optical system of the microscope.
- Prerequisite knowledge: Chapter 2.
- Exercises: see Appendix A3.
- Further information: Specialised forms of microscopy are described in Part III. See also sections entitled Further reading, at ends of chapters.

6
The optical magnifying system

A brief overview of the optical system of microscopes was given in Chapter 2. The present chapter deals with the magnifying system in detail.

The magnifying or viewing system of a microscope is that part of the optical system that produces a magnified image of the object. The magnifying system includes the objective, eyepiece (ocular), intermediate magnifying system (if any), and the camera. It may include accessories such as a filter.

The objective produces a real, magnified image (the intermediate image) in the plane of the diaphragm of the eyepiece (Fig 2.9). The eyepiece further magnifies this image, producing a virtual image at infinity, below the specimen. This virtual image is seen by the eye, the lens of the eye converting the virtual image to a real image on the retina. The virtual image produced by the eyepiece used to be regarded as being 250 mm in front of the eye, that being regarded as the nearest comfortable focusing distance of the eye; the magnification of the eyepiece is still calculated on the assumption that the image is in that position. In many microscopes, the intermediate image is situated about 150 mm above the objective (Fig 2.9, left); however, with infinity-corrected objectives, the objective produces a parallel beam of light, from which the intermediate image is produced by a tube lens (Telan lens), as shown in Fig 2.9 (right).

In a photomicrographic camera, either the camera has a lens corresponding to the lens of the eye, projecting an image onto the film (instead of the retina of the eye); or the eyepiece is replaced by a similar device called a projective that directly projects a magnified image of the intermediate image onto the film (see Chapter 14).

Refraction

The functions of lenses depend upon the phenomenon of refraction, in which light rays are bent when passing from one medium to another, such as from air to glass, or from glass to air. The angle through which light is bent depends upon the angle at which the light hits the interface between the media, and the refractive indices of the two media. Refractive index is defined in Fig 6.1, and a list of refractive indices of some fluids is given in Table 6.2.

Lens aberrations and corrections

All lenses are subject to imaging faults, known as aberrations (see Table 6.1). It is the skill and art of the optician to design systems of lenses to minimise these inherent defects. The higher the degree of correction, the higher is the cost; for this and other reasons, objectives are commonly sold with varying degrees of correction. It is useful for the microscopist to have at least a general understanding of these aberrations, so as to be able to choose the most appropriate equipment for a particular purpose, or to obtain the best possible result from a given set of optical equipment. Specifically, one needs to know about chromatic aberration and curvature of field, because objectives

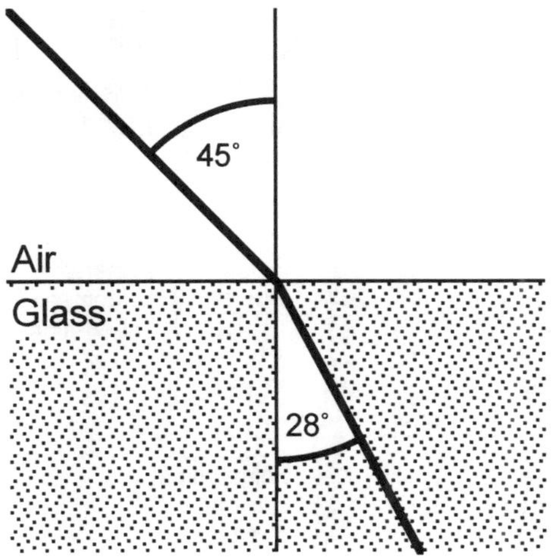

Fig 6.1. Definition of refractive index. The refractive index n is defined as the ratio of the sine of the angle of incidence to the sine of the angle of refraction. In this example, a light ray (represented by the thick line) incident on a glass–air interface, with an angle of incidence of 45°, is refracted to an angle of 28°. The refractive index of the glass is given by sin 45° / sin 28° = 1·51. A light ray travelling from glass to air with an angle of incidence of 28° follows the same path.

are classified according to their degree of correction for these aberrations. One also needs to know about spherical aberration, and how to avoid and control it, because the photomicrographer may inadvertently increase this aberration. Some aberrations can be minimised by reducing the numerical aperture (NA) of the system, or by using monochromatic light. Readers interested in taking the subject of aberrations beyond the coverage of this book should consult the book by Ray (1994a) or other textbooks of optics.

Table 6.1. Effects of lens aberrations

Aberration	Effect produced	Effect reduced by	
		Smaller aperture	Monochromatic light
Chromatic aberration			
Longitudinal	Colour fringes as focus changed	No	Yes
Lateral	Colour fringes in one focus plane	No	Yes
Spherical aberration	Unsharp, low-contrast image	Yes	No
Field curvature	Centre and periphery not sharp simultaneously	No (yes)	No
Coma	Low-contrast image	Yes	No
Distortion	Distorted shapes	No	No
Astigmatism	Unsharp image	Yes	No

Chromatic aberration

The refractive index of a substance varies according to the wavelength of light passing through it. White light is therefore dispersed by all simple lenses into its spectral colours, and for any object, there will be a separate image for each wavelength of the light source, resulting in coloured fringes around objects (Plate 1c).

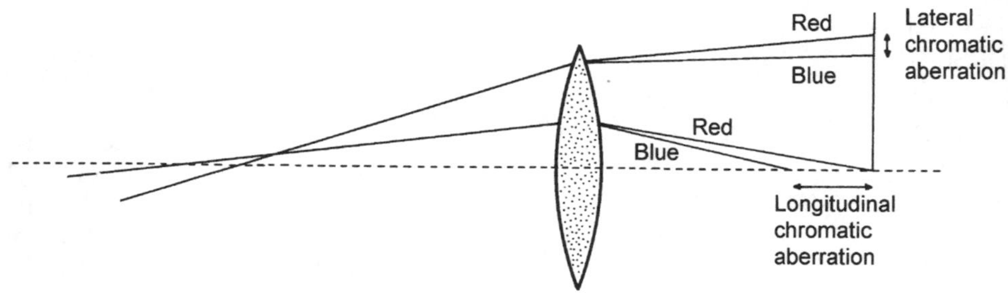

Fig 6.2. Chromatic aberration. Blue and red rays are focused to different points.

Two types of chromatic aberration are shown in Fig 6.2. *Longitudinal chromatic aberration* is detected as a coloured fringe around colourless objects: blue at a focus nearer to the lens, red at a focus further from the lens, with the other spectral colours lying at intermediate points of focus. With *lateral chromatic aberration*, an off-axis object point is reproduced as a line, coloured blue towards the axis, red away from the axis. The result is that the size of the image of an object will vary according to the wavelength of the illumination. This phenomenon is called *chromatic difference of magnification*.

Chromatic aberration can be reduced by designing lens systems using a combination of two or more glasses with different dispersive powers, a process known as achromatisation. Both lateral and longitudinal chromatic aberration may appear with a reversal of the colour positions if the design of a lens is such as to overcorrect for the aberration.

Chromatic aberration occurs for all light rays, and is therefore not reduced by decreasing the numerical aperture (NA). However, if the illumination is monochromatic, or at least confined to a narrow band of the spectrum, chromatic aberration cannot occur. This is one very good reason for the employment of coloured filters for black-and-white (B&W) photomicrography. It is also of practical interest that reflecting (mirror) lens systems do not have chromatic aberration.

Spherical aberration

This, and the other aberrations described below, occur even if monochromatic light is employed.

For technical reasons, lenses are normally manufactured with surfaces which are portions of a sphere. This is not the ideal shape, and results in *spherical aberration* (Fig 6.3). Compared with the central portion of a lens, which is almost parallel-sided, the periphery of a lens is highly prismatic. Therefore axial rays are less refracted than marginal rays and will come to focus at a greater distance from the lens. In consequence, in any plane perpendicular to the lens axis, a point object is imaged as a disc, called the *circle of confusion*.

The plane of the best image, at which the diameter of the circle of confusion is least, will not coincide with the plane of the axial image. In consequence, reducing the aperture of the lens will result in a shift of the plane of best focus.

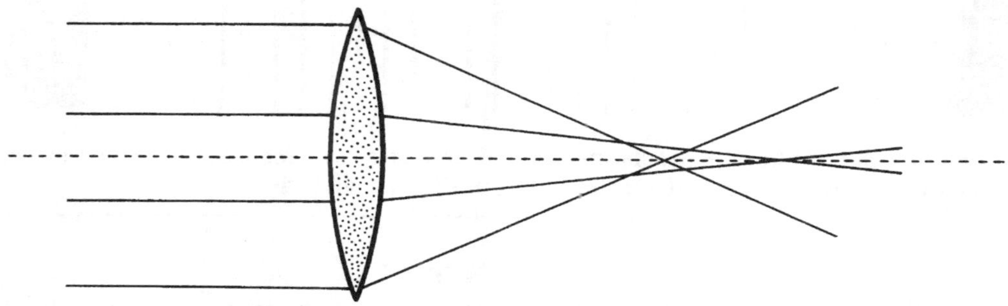

Fig 6.3. Spherical aberration. Marginal and axial rays are focused to different positions.

Spherical aberration may be introduced, particularly with objectives of high NA, by a coverslip of incorrect thickness or refractive index, and also by use of immersion fluid of incorrect refractive index. An example of a coverslip of incorrect refractive index is a plastic slip used for growing cells, which are examined through the plastic. An example of incorrect medium is the use of an oil-immersion objective in air (without oil), or a dry objective in oil. 'High-dry' objectives (with high NA and magnification, and for use in air) are particularly subject to this problem, and may have movable elements controlled by a ring that can be used to correct for variations in coverslip thickness. In conventional transmitted-light systems, spherical aberration can be reduced (at the expense of resolution) by decreasing the NA of the system, eg by partially closing the condenser aperture.

Curvature of field

A simple lens will form a curved image from a flat object (Fig 6.4). When you look through the microscope at a very thin, flat specimen (such as a blood smear, or the surface of a computer chip), curvature of field prevents the central portion of the field and the edges of the field being focused simultaneously. This is a very common fault in microscope objectives, except those specifically designed for a flat field. For visual observation, curvature of field is not a serious lens fault, since anything in the field can be brought into focus by slight adjustment of the fine-focus control. Curvature of field is very serious in a system used for photography, causing the picture to be unsharp either at the corners or in the centre.

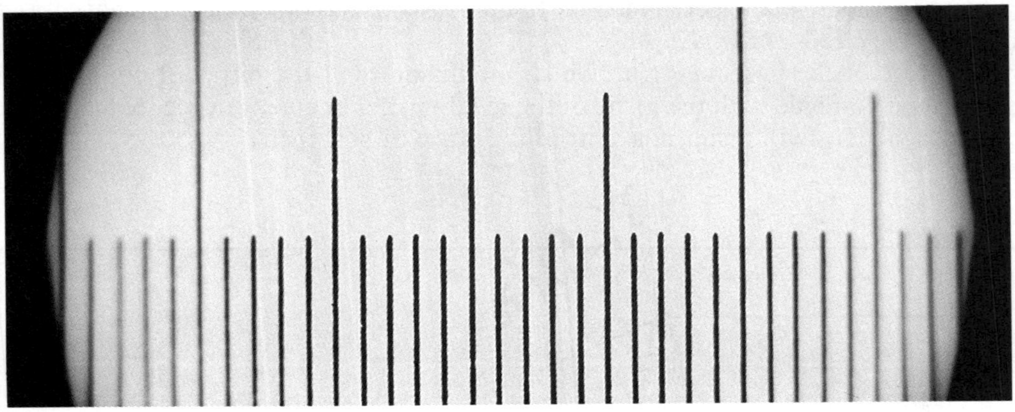

Fig 6.4. Curvature of field. A flat object (a stage micrometer) is reproduced as a curved image, which can be focused either at the centre, or at the edge, but not both.

The objective

Objectives were described briefly in Chapter 2. The prime purposes of the objective are to provide resolution of the object and initial magnification. The brightness of the final image is also determined in part by the objective.

Magnification

The magnification of an objective is determined by the focal length of the lens; the shorter the focal length, the greater is the magnification.

Numerical aperture

Numerical aperture (NA) is (roughly speaking) a measure of the diameter of a lens, such as an objective or condenser, compared to its focal length. NA is defined by the equation NA = $n \sin \alpha$ (see Fig 6.5), where α is half the angle subtended by the lens as seen from the specimen, and n is the refractive index of the medium (air, oil, water) between the lens and the specimen (see next section, Immersion). NA is related to the *f*-number of a camera lens, which is equal to $1/(2 \tan \alpha)$. For small NAs, in air, the NA is approximately equal to half the reciprocal of the *f*-number.

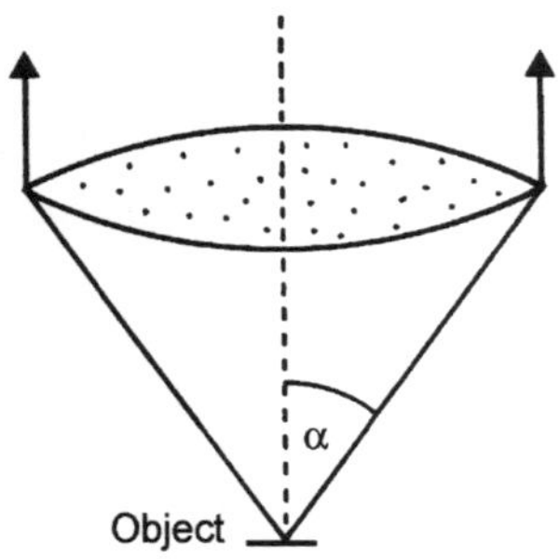

Fig 6.5. Explanation of numerical aperture. NA = $n \sin \alpha$, where n is the refractive index of the immersion medium (n = 1·00 for air), and α is half the angle subtended by the lens at the object.

The numerical aperture affects the resolution (minimum resolved distance, see next page) of the objective, and also the amount of light gathered by it. The brightness of the intermediate image varies as the square of the objective's NA and inversely as the square of its magnification.

Immersion

Objectives with an NA greater than about 0·9 require that the space between the object and the objective be filled with a liquid medium, such as immersion oil or water. Objectives used this way are commonly referred to as 'immersion' objectives, while those designed for use in air are called 'dry' objectives. The reason for immersion is that the refractive index of air is 1·0, and the maximum value for the sine of an angle is 1, so that a lens that has a NA greater than 1·0 must be an immersion lens. In addition, the use of an immersion medium with a refractive index greater than 1 gives increased depth of field (see below, Depth of field). Objectives with a lesser NA can also be designed for immersion, usually as a matter of convenience in having high and medium powers available when the specimen is immersed. The refractive indices of the common media are: air, 1·000; water, 1·33; standard immersion oil, 1·5180 (see Table 6.2).

When the glass slide, the mounting medium, the coverslip, the immersion medium and the glass of the front lens of the objective all have the same refractive index and dispersion, the objective is said to be *homogeneously immersed*. Under these conditions, geometrical optics predicts that it should be possible to achieve an image that is free from spherical aberration and coma. These advantages are lost if the wrong immersion fluid is used; each immersion objective must be used with immersion fluid of the refractive index and dispersion for which it was designed.

Immersion objectives are of two main types: those intended for use with standard immersion oil, and water-immersion objectives intended for examining specimens under water. However, the immersion medium may alternatively be silicone oil, glycerol, or indeed almost any liquid. Various media are listed in Table 6.2. Conventional immersion fluid, according to international standards DIN 58 884 and ISO 80 36/1, should have a refractive index of 1·5180 for the spectral E-line (green, 527·0 nm) at 23 °C, and dispersion v_E = 44. Formerly, the standard refractive index

Table 6.2. Immersion fluids for objectives

Fluids are listed in order of refractive index (n) for the sodium D line (589·3 nm, yellow), at the temperature specified. The DIN standard relates to the E line (527·0 nm, green). (For more data see Rost, 1992.)

Type	Refractive index	
	n_E	n_D
Air	1.000	1·0003
Water		1·3330 @ 20 °C
Olympus silicone		1.404 @ 25 °C
Glycerol		1·4730 @ 20 °C
Immersion oil (DIN standard)	1·5180 @ 23 °C	1·515
Cedarwood oil		1·516

was 1·515 for the sodium D line (589·3 nm, yellow). Special oils are available with high or low viscosity, or for fluorescence microscopy, or for use at 37 °C. Water-immersion objectives are useful for studying objects under water in a vessel without a lid. Some objectives are designed to be adjustable for use with various immersion fluids, such as oil, glycerine or water.

Contrast

The ratio of the intensities of dark and light areas in an object or image is known as the *contrast*. Lens aberrations and uncleanliness will always have the effect of lessening image contrast. In B&W photography, contrast can be controlled (ie increased or decreased) by choice of film and processing and printing procedures.

Resolution (minimum resolved distance)

The fineness of detail in the object that can be reproduced in the image by any lens system is always limited. The ability of a lens or lens system to reproduce fine detail is known as its *resolution* or *resolving power*. The closest distance apart at which two point objects can be distinguished as separate in the image is known as the *minimum resolved distance* (MRD) (Fig 6.6). The limitation on resolution arises from two causes: aberrations in the lens (which can be minimised by excellent design and manufacture), and diffraction effects (which are due to the wave nature of light and are therefore unavoidable).

The theoretical resolution depends primarily on the NA of the objective (see Fig 2.1), and on the contrast of the specimen (see above, Contrast). Contrast, and therefore resolution, are adversely affected by lens aberrations. In many optical systems, it is helpful to describe lens performance in terms of ability to *transfer* the fine detail and contrast of the object to the image. For this purpose, the test object can be considered as having square wave or sine wave characteristics of changing spatial frequency. The image quality is assessed across the range of frequencies. There is always a loss (modulation) of contrast in the imaging process, detected as a decrease in the amplitude of sine waves as produced in the image. The contrast loss is more severe at high frequencies, ie where the detail is finer and more closely spaced. A graph of contrast loss against spatial frequency is known as the *modulation transfer function*.

In practice, lenses are designed to minimise aberrations as much as possible, consistent with producing lenses at an affordable price. Optical designers have to arrive at a compromise according to the specific intended use of a lens. The terms of the compromise will also include NA, contrast, working distance, and magnification.

According to the Abbe formula (due to the German physicist Ernst Abbe, whose name is sometimes erroneously spelt Abbé) the MRD or resolution, using light of wavelength λ, is given by the formula

$$\text{MRD} = \frac{\lambda}{2\ \text{NA}}$$

Photographic technicians may be more accustomed to thinking of resolution in terms of *line pairs per millimetre* (LP/mm), the number of pairs of black/white lines in 1 mm which can be resolved in the microscope. The number of line pairs per millimetre (LP/mm) at the specimen is obtained by assuming that a certain number of resolved pairs can be accommodated in a distance of 1 mm.

For example, using a typical high-power dry objective with NA 0·65, for green light such that $\lambda = 500$ nm, ie $0{\cdot}5 \times 10^{-3}$ mm, the MRD is 0·38 μm or 0·00038 mm, corresponding to a resolution at the specimen of 1/0·00038 = 2600 LP/mm. If the magnifications used are those of a 40× objective and 3·3× projective, the magnification to the film is 132×, producing an image on the film with 2600/132 = 20 LP/mm. A further enlargement of 2× gives a total magnification of 264× and a resolution of 10 LP/mm, with detail just resolvable by the eye.

For a print, to be viewed satisfactorily at normal viewing (reading) distance, the total magnification (microscope and enlargement) should not exceed 1000 times the NA of the optical system. In the above case, the maximum total enlargement would be calculated as 1000 × 0·65 = 650. Of course, for a poster (to be viewed at a greater distance) the maximum total enlargement would be correspondingly greater.

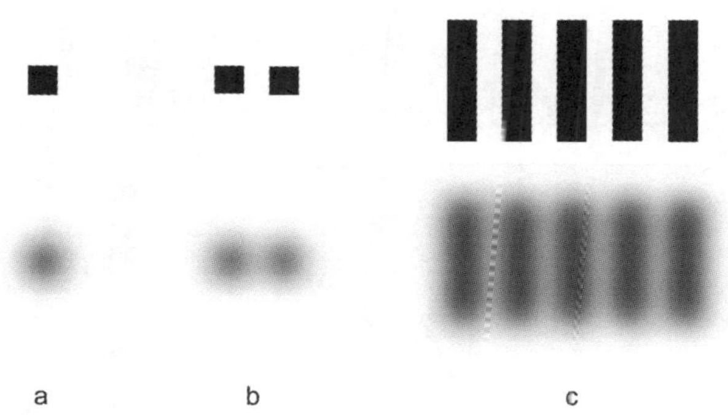

Fig 6.6 Illustrating circle of confusion, MRD, and LP/mm. The top row shows hypothetical objects, and the lower row shows images of them. (a) A point object is imaged as a hazy disc; its diameter is the *circle of confusion*. (b) Two point objects, when their images are only just seen to be separate, are separated by the *minimal resolved distance* (MRD). (c) Alternate black and white bars each the width of the MRD, constituting a line pair, define the number of *line pairs per millimetre* (LP/mm).

Reverberation

Objects seen or photographed in transmitted light with considerable empty magnification (ie using an NA much too small for the magnification) show an appearance known as *reverberation* (Fig 6.7). The image is of high contrast, poor resolution, and with characteristic bright and dark outlines (diffraction haloes) around structural areas of the specimen. This is due to the NA of the illumination being much less than that of the objective. This appearance normally indicates that there is something wrong, eg the aperture diaphragm has been closed down too much, or the condenser is too low.

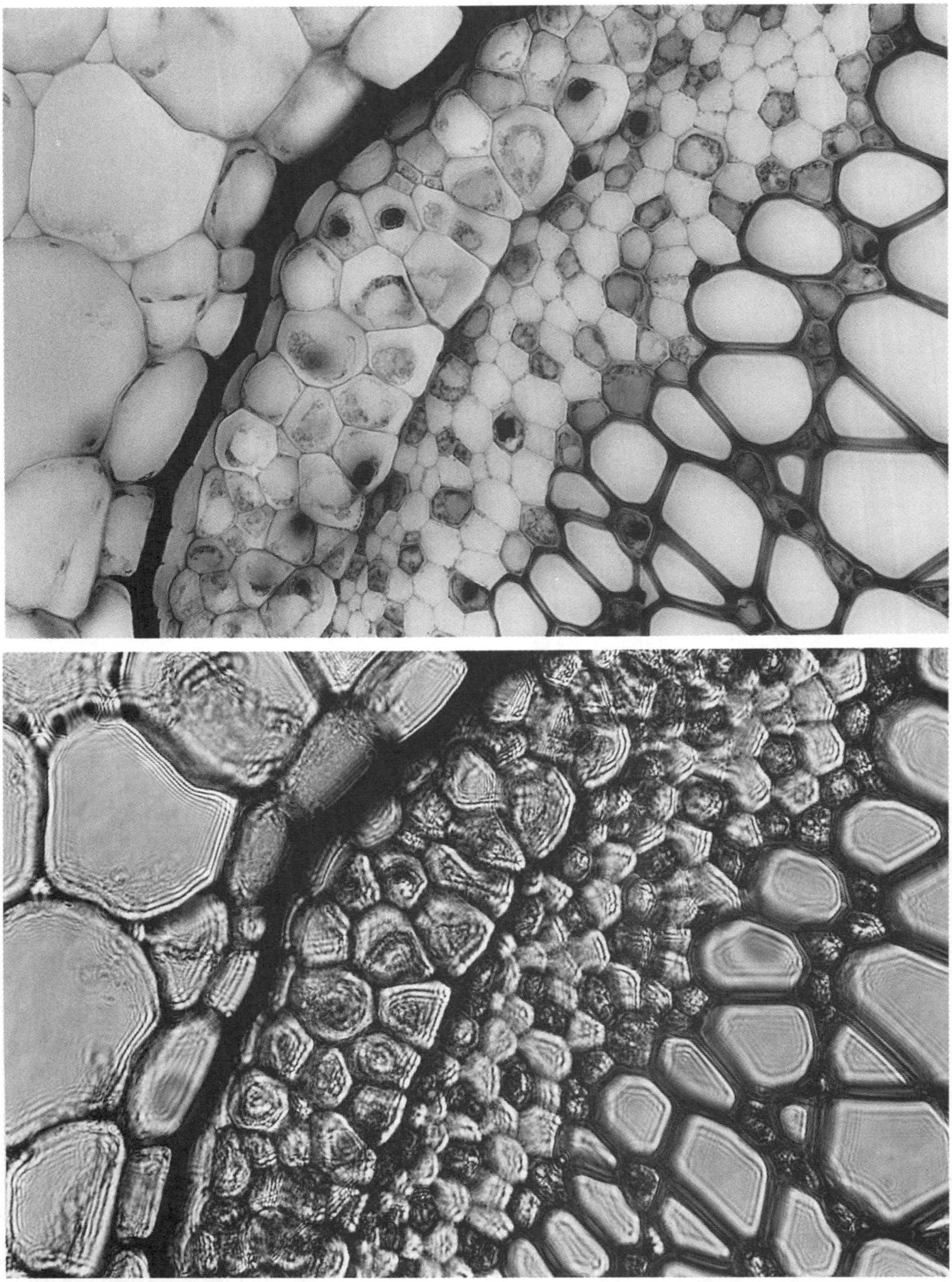

Fig 6.7. Reverberation (diffraction artefact) due to small-aperture illumination. Transverse section of fern rachis (stalk), field size 200 µm × 300 µm (0·2 mm × 0·3 mm). Above, normal image; below, with the condenser lowered and its aperture almost closed.

Types of objective

Objectives are available in great variety, differing in magnification, NA, chromatic correction, flat-field correction, other corrections, and the type of immersion fluid (if any). For photomicrography, a flat field and adequate resolution are essential.

Objectives varying in all of the above-mentioned characteristics are modified for specialised modes of microscopy, such as fluorescence (requiring a high NA in relation to the magnification, and non-fluorescent glass), polarisation (requiring strain-free glass), and phase contrast (requiring a built-in phase plate). High-NA objectives are made in two types, for use with or without a coverslip.

It is convenient to classify microscope objectives primarily according to the correction of chromatic aberration and field curvature (see Fig 6.8). The major types are: *achromats*, *semi-apochromats* (fluorite), and *apochromats*. In addition, those objectives that are particularly corrected for flatness of field are designated by the prefix *plan-* (eg *planachromat*).

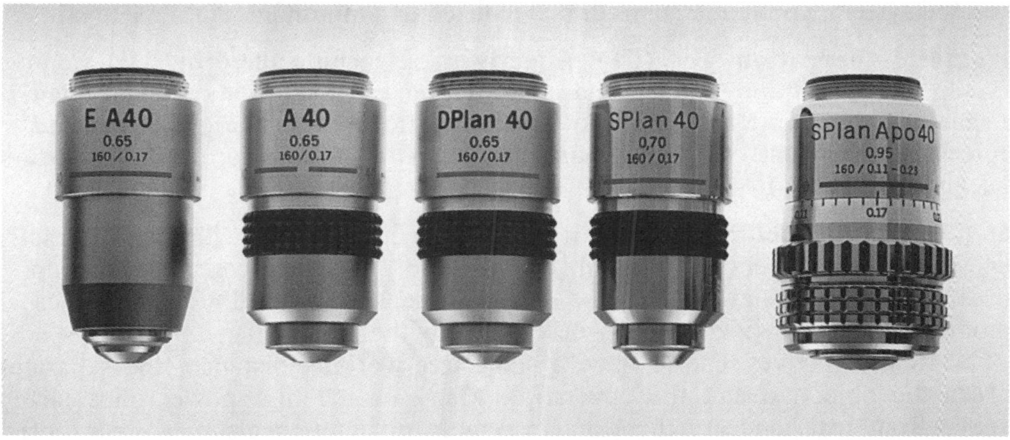

Fig 6.8. A group of objectives from Olympus (about 1990), with the same magnification and various degrees of correction. From left to right, *E* (economical) achromat, achromat, *D* planachromat, *S* (super) planachromat, *S* planapochromat. Improvement in optical correction is reflected in the price; the dearest is 10 times the price of the cheapest.

Achromatic systems. The most commonly used objectives in microscopy are achromatic ('colour-free') in design, in which glasses of different dispersion are used to recombine the spectral rays to produce an image much reduced in chromatic aberration.

An achromatic system is defined as being *corrected for chromatic aberration at two wavelengths* (normally 486 nm blue and 656 nm red), *and corrected for spherical aberration at one wavelength.* The correction of these lenses is best in the green region of the spectrum, and they give best results with monochromatic green light. Red and blue are brought to the same focus, and green to a different focus; since red and blue combine to appear magenta, this accounts for the observed magenta/green colour fringes (see Plate 1c).

Fluorite systems. Lenses of rather better performance than the achromats are known variously as fluorites or semi-apochromats. Their name is derived from the mineral fluorite, which is used in their construction, fluorite having a very low dispersion. Chromatic aberration is reduced and the image contrast very much improved in these lenses.

Apochromatic systems. Designed by Abbe in 1886, an apochromat is defined as being *corrected chromatically at three wavelengths, and corrected spherically at two wavelengths*. The lenses are characterised by a marked reduction in all aberrations (except curvature of field) and by rather higher NAs than the equivalent achromatic lenses. It is only for specialised microscopy that the very much higher costs of these objectives is warranted.

The design of conventional apochromatic systems is such that special 'compensating' eyepieces are required (see below, Eyepieces). An apochromatic objective and its *compensating eyepiece* used together produce an apochromatic system. Lateral chromatic aberration residual in the objective is eliminated by the eyepiece, which is designed to have chromatic aberration of opposite sign. In the combined system, chromatic aberration is reduced to a minimum.

Chromatic-aberration-free (*CF*) objectives are manufactured by Nikon and by Zeiss. In these, both longitudinal and lateral chromatic aberrations are corrected (to the specified degree, ie achromatic or apochromatic) in both the objectives and the eyepieces independently. This is characteristic of objectives corrected for infinite tubelength (see below).

Flat-field (plane-field) objectives. Some modern glasses with high refractive indices and low dispersion have made possible the commercial production of objectives with particularly flat image fields. These lenses find their greatest use in photomicrography. They are usually designated by the prefix 'plan-'.

Flat-field objectives tend to have a short free-working distance (the separation between the objective and the coverslip). Many of the high-power ones have a concave front lens, and are therefore extremely difficult to clean; a major effort should be made to avoid situations where dirt or liquids come into contact with the lens.

The achromatic and apochromatic corrections refer largely to correction for chromatic and spherical aberration, coma, and astigmatism; flat-field correction is for curvature of field. Therefore it is possible to purchase achromats, flat-field achromats, apochromats and flat-field apochromats. These last represent the most highly corrected microscope lenses available today, and their price reflects the extra design and care required for their manufacture.

Objectives for uncovered specimens are corrected for use without a coverslip. They are intended for use with uncovered preparations. They are sometimes referred to as metallurgical objectives, but are useful in biology also, for examining specimens without a coverslip (eg sections in process of staining).

Ultralow-power objectives have a magnification below 4×. Attention has recently been given to the design of new ultralow-power systems with more convenient usage, including parfocality with all other objectives and true Köhler illumination. A matching ultralow-power condenser is required for their proper use (see Chapter 7).

Infrared-transmitting objectives are available for photomicrography at infrared wavelengths (see Chapter 12).

Ultraviolet-transmitting objectives are required for photomicrography in ultraviolet light (see Chapter 12) and for fluorescence with epi-illumination using particularly short wavelengths (below 360 nm) for excitation (see Chapter 11).

The coating of lenses

In older lenses, there were annoying reflections from glass surfaces, that reduced the contrast of the image. These unwanted reflections can be reduced by coating the glass surfaces with one or more layers of a transparent material with a lower refractive index than that of the glass, as in modern camera and spectacle lenses.

The added contrast is a boon to the microscopist, but there is need for an awareness of the extreme vulnerability of these thin surface layers to damage, especially scratching, by fibres and grit in cleaning tissues. Internal surfaces may have a softer coating than external surfaces. If the film is scratched, to repair it the lens system has to be dismantled and the damaged surface re-polished and re-coated, seldom an economically viable proposition; the lens system may well have to be replaced rather than repaired.

Changing patterns in lens design

The advances in lens design during the past few decades are due mainly to the use of computers to carry out the laborious mathematical computations required for lens design. Also, more types of optical glasses of high refractive index and low dispersion are now available.

Manufacturers are claiming greater optical performance for their lenses (microscope and camera) and new phrases are being introduced in order to proclaim the wonders of advanced production technology. As seen above, apochromatic objectives required specially designed compensating eyepieces, in which chromatic aberration (perhaps better described as chromatic correction) was introduced into the eyepiece to compensate for residual chromatic aberration in the objectives. Strictly, when apochromats were being interchanged with achromatic objectives, it was necessary to change the eyepiece as well. Many manufacturers circumvented this inconvenience by introducing chromatic aberration into the achromats, just as it existed in the apochromats, so that compensating eyepieces served both systems.

For some of their lens combinations, Nikon (and now others) designed both objectives and eyepieces so that they were free from these introduced aberrations; that is, 'colour-free' (*CF*). These objectives are not literally 'colour-free', any more than achromats are 'a-chromatic'. They do show some chromatic aberration.

Other words which find their way into advertising pamphlets today reflect the need to make lenses of intermediate price (and performance). Some current examples are 'semi-flat', and 'economical'.

The testing of objectives

Lens testing, by the microscopist rather than by the trained optician, tends to be a subjective affair; a general impression is formed, a judgement based on past experience as to whether a lens is good, bad or indifferent (see Fig 6.9). Therefore, strictly comparable techniques of testing should be employed, such as uniformly produced test specimens and accurate setting of the microscope illumination. For detailed procedures for testing of microscope optical systems, see Oldfield (1994).

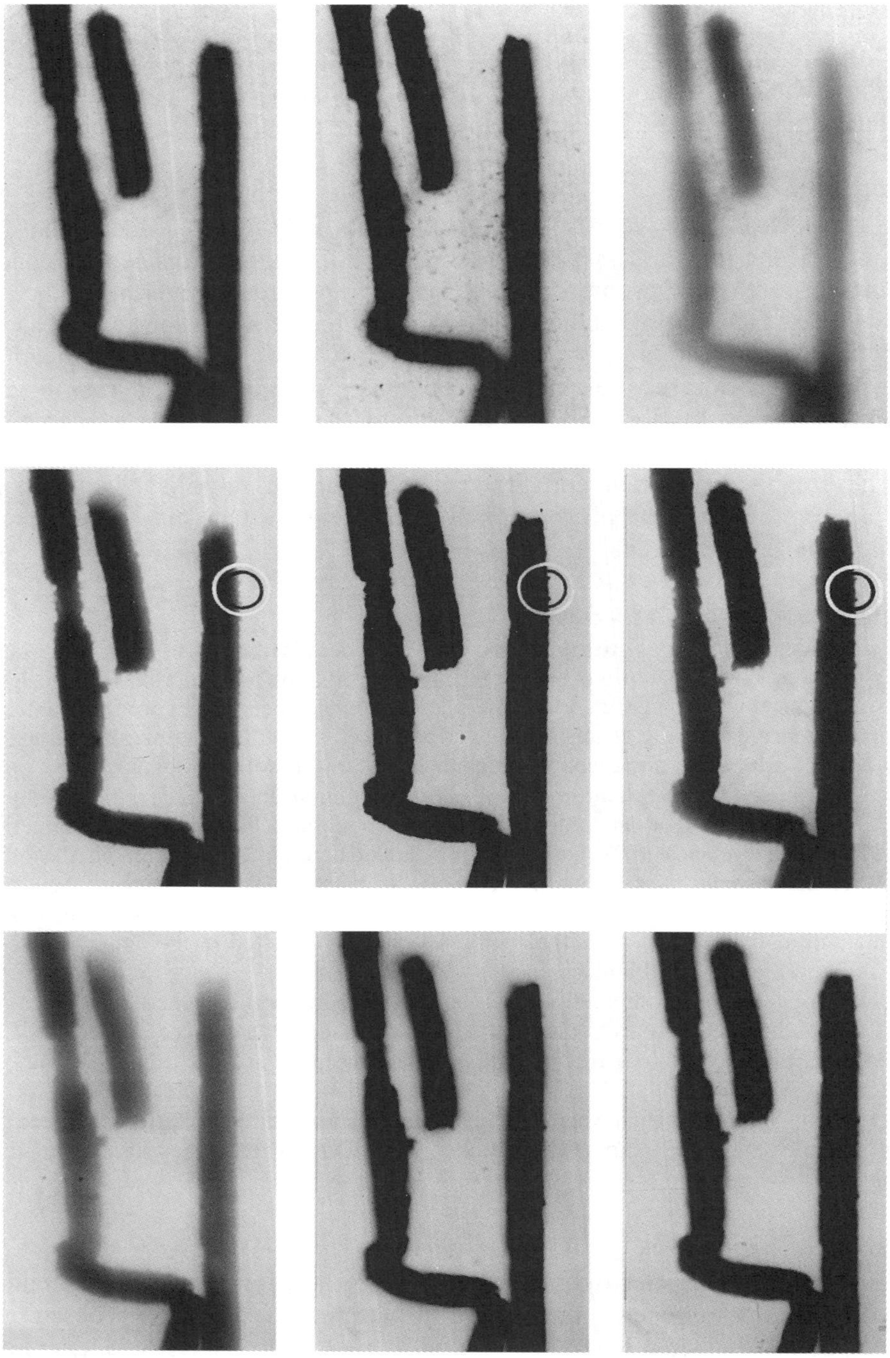

Fig 6.9. Testing for spherical aberration. Carbon particles, field size 130 mm × 200 mm. Objective 45×, 0·65 NA, dry. Top row, above focus; middle row, in focus; bottom row, below focus. Left column, no coverslip; middle column, correct thickness (No. $1^1/_2$) of coverslip; right column, too-thick coverslip (two No. $1^1/_2$ coverslips).

The coverslip

Coverslips (coverglasses) are made in a variety of thicknesses, as listed in Table 6.3. For nearly all biological work, the manufacturer has designed the microscope lens for use with a particular thickness of coverslip, usually 0·17 mm. The coverslip is an integral part of the optical system. If the wrong thickness of coverslip is used, spherical aberration is introduced into the system, with consequent loss of contrast in the image (see Fig 6.9). Some lenses, such as those used for metallurgical work, are designed for use with preparations without coverslips. Some examples of objectives with differing requirements are shown in Fig 6.10.

Table 6.3. Coverslip specifications

Grade number	Thickness (± tolerance) (mm)	Application
The 1986 ISO standard: (ISO 8255/1–1986)		
	Principal refractive index	$n_e = 1{\cdot}5255 \pm 0{\cdot}0015$
	Abbe number	$v_e = 56 \pm 2$
1	0·17 (+0·00, –0·04)	General purpose
1H	0·17 (+0·00, –0·02)	High performance
Currently available		
0	~ 0·08	Useful for oil-immersion work
1	~ 0·14	First choice for most purposes, allows for mountant thickness
$1^1/_2$	~ 0·17	For those fastidious with their preparations
2	~ 0·19	For low-power work only

With wet preparations and with mounted preparations, the fluid or mounting medium lying above the specimen adds to the effective thickness of the coverslip. Obviously, control of this total thickness to a hundredth of a millimetre is just not a practical proposition in the biological laboratory and it becomes useful to know the conditions under which coverslip thickness is optically significant.

For oil-immersion systems, there can be mechanical difficulties of focusing if the glass is too thick. But quite apart from this problem, as the oil and the glass are very nearly optically homogeneous, the relative thickness of glass and immersion oil is unimportant as far as spherical aberration is concerned. Even the absence of a coverslip is consistent with good imaging; for example, in haematology, blood smears are routinely examined without a coverslip, using an oil-immersion objective.

For dry (non-immersion) systems of NA less than 0·4, the effect of coverslip thickness errors is slight, and generally unimportant, but when the NA reaches 0·65 the coverslip thickness is important, and significant to within 0·01 mm. It is the high-power dry lenses that need special care with specimen preparation and choice of coverslip. The emphasis which was placed on the desirability of high aperture optics must be accepted cautiously. There is no doubt that a 60×, 0·8 NA objective has better resolving power than a 40×, 0·65 NA objective, but for general microscopy the practical demands of the 0·8 NA lens (for control of coverslip thickness) may well be too great!

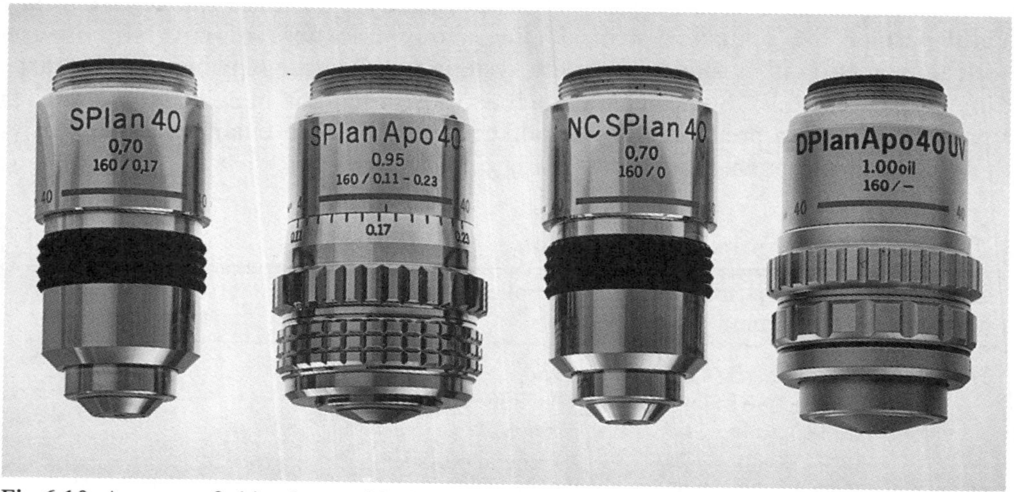

Fig 6.10. A group of objectives, with different corrections for thickness of coverslip, as shown in the bottom lines of engraving. The number '160' refers to the mechanical tubelength (160 mm). The symbols after the slash signify: '0.17', the correction for standard coverslips; '0.11–0.23'; a correction collar is fitted for compensating for coverslip thickness in the range 0·11 mm to 0·23 mm; '0', for use without a coverslip (zero thickness); '–', an oil-immersion objective, for which the coverslip's thickness, or presence or absence, is optically immaterial.

The correction collar

There may be occasions when the use of an oil-immersion system is undesirable, but high resolution is required. The best high-aperture dry objectives permit mechanical adjustment of the position of some of the internal lenses to compensate for different thicknesses of mountant and coverslip. The correction collar (Fig 6.10) is rotated so that the out-of-focus images appear identical on either side of focus (see centre column of Fig 6.9), indicating that spherical aberration has been eliminated. The range of coverslip thicknesses (including mountant thickness) for which correction is possible is from about 0·10 to 0·23 mm. Dry objectives of very long working distance and somewhat low NA, as used in inverted microscopes, may correct for thickness of a specimen chamber in the range 0–2 mm.

Dry apochromats, of aperture greater than about 0·7, if they are to be used with coverslips, have need of such a correction for spherical aberration. Unless this correction is attended to, or if excessively thick sections or layers of mounting medium are employed, the image produced by the apochromat will be inferior to that of the corresponding achromat, which could be purchased at one-tenth of the cost!

Depth of field and depth of focus

Depth of field is the thickness of the specimen that is acceptably sharp at a given setting of the focus control. The main factors involved are the NA of the system, the refractive index of the immersion medium, and the wavelength of the light. For monochromatic light of wavelength λ, with an immersion medium (air, oil, etc) of refractive index n, the depth of field T is given by

$$T = \frac{\lambda\left[n^2 - (\text{NA})^2\right]^{1/2}}{(\text{NA})^2}$$

Working with green light (λ = 527 nm) in air (n = 1·00) with an NA of 0·6, the depth of field is about 1·2 µm. Using immersion oil with a refractive index of 1·518, the depth of field is increased to 2·0 µm. Depth of field with various NA values, dry and immersed, is shown in Fig 6.11.

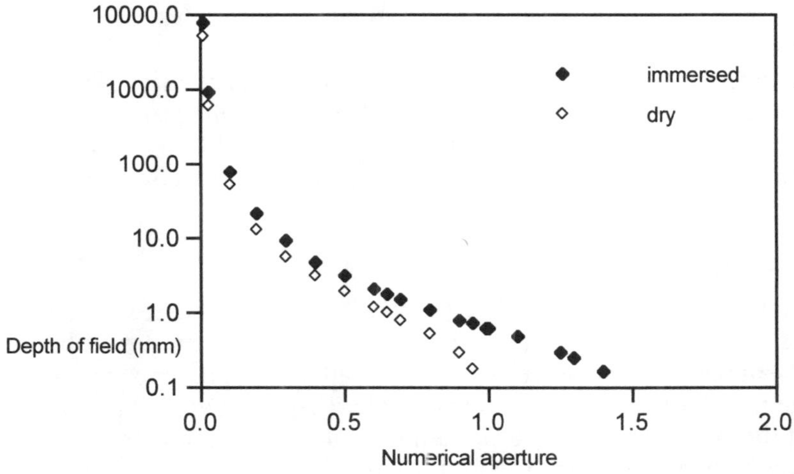

Fig 6.11. Graph of the depth of field at various NAs, dry (open diamonds) and immersed (solid diamonds). Horizontal axis: NA of system. Vertical axis: depth of field in micrometres (logarithmic scale). The bends at the right-hand ends of the curves are due to the NA tending to its maximum value, numerically equal to the refractive index of the medium (at which depth of field is zero).

Using objectives fitted with an iris diaphragm, depth of field is increased by closing down the iris. In transmitted-light and some other systems, the depth of field can also be increased by closing down the condenser diaphragm; this important topic is discussed in Chapter 15. In both cases, an increase of depth of field is obtained at the expense of resolving power. However, for photographic purposes this may occasionally be a legitimate trade-off. A very shallow depth of field is used to advantage with Nomarski differential interference-contrast (DIC) microscopy (see Chapter 10). An extremely shallow depth of field is obtained with confocal scanning microscopy (see Chapter 17). Depth of field is discussed in detail by Pluta (1988; Vol. 1, pp. 349–361), Ray (1994a) and Shillaber (1944).

Depth of focus is the range over which the image plane (eg film) can be moved while an acceptable sharpness of a specified object plane is maintained.

Limited depth of focus is not normally a problem in photomicrography, because, while there is normally only shallow depth of field, there is correspondingly great depth of focus. If there were a problem it might arise when a focusing graticule in the eyepiece is used for focusing, and the camera film plane is not correctly positioned in relation to the graticule; or if the eyepiece graticule is incorrectly used (as sometimes happens with low powers). Poor focusing technique in photomicrography is particularly serious with ultralow-power objectives.

Back focal plane

A lens focuses parallel rays to a point on the optical axis. The distance from the point to the lens centre is called the *focal length* of the lens; the point is at a principal focus; and the plane normal to the optical axis, through the principal focus, is called the *focal plane* of the lens. This focusing phenomenon occurs equally for light entering the lens from either side. Each lens therefore has two principal foci and two focal planes.

By convention, in an objective the focal plane nearer the light source is called the *front focal plane*, and the focal plane away from the light source is called the *back focal plane* (BFP). The physical position of this plane of an objective is inside the barrel of the objective; in low-power objectives, the back focal plane is fairly close to the level of the nosepiece.

Exit pupil of objective

The diameter of the objective's exit pupil is of importance in epi-illumination, because this is also the entrance pupil for illumination, and must be filled by an image of the light source. If this image is smaller than the pupil, uneven illumination will result; if the image of the light source is greater than the pupil, light is wasted and the intensity of the illumination correspondingly reduced. The diameter of the exit pupil of typical objectives varies from about 12 mm (low powers) to about 5 mm (high powers).

Working distance

The working distance of objectives is the mechanical distance between the specimen plane and the front of the objective. It is generally related to the NA, being usually least for objectives with highest NA. Some types of objective are designed with a particularly long working distance, and are useful for dealing with thick specimens or with specimens seen in thick-walled containers, such as the bottom of culture vessels examined with an inverted microscope.

Tubelength

The *mechanical tubelength* is the distance between the nosepiece surface and eyepiece flange. Early English microscopists established a tubelength of 250 mm (to coincide with the least distance of distinct vision of the human eye). However, the somewhat cumbersome length of these early instruments was superseded by the Continental standard tubelength of 160 mm (usually) or 170 mm (used by Leitz until comparatively recently). For engineering reasons, this mechanical tubelength cannot always be achieved, and we now talk of a corresponding *optical tubelength*, for which the current standards are 160 mm or infinity, and this optical tubelength is adjusted to the actual mechanical tubelength with additional lenses in the nosepiece or body tube.

The intermediate image is usually situated a short distance (eg 10 mm) below the top of the tube. The position of the intermediate image is important because correction for spherical aberration and coma can be effected for one object distance only, and by implication, one image distance.

Infinity correction

Many of the microscope techniques discussed in Chapters 10 and 11 require the insertion of optical devices between the objective and eyepiece. These devices may include vertical illuminators (for opaque objects and/or fluorescence), an analyser and compensation plates (polarisation), filters and a dichromatic mirror (fluorescence), beam combiners (interference contrast), as well as built-in telescopes and magnification changers or zoom systems.

In the classical optical systems described above, the introduction of these devices was at best inconvenient and at worst introduced spherical aberration. The modern solution is a system in which the light beam passing through these devices is composed of parallel rays. This means that the mechanical tubelength can be extended as far as necessary to accommodate the additional devices, and without introducing spherical aberration. For this purpose, the objectives are designed with *infinity correction*: the specimen is located at the focal plane of the objective which then produces parallel rays (ie the rays come to focus at infinity). A *tube lens* is required to bring these parallel rays to a focus in the intermediate image plane (Fig 2.9, right). Infinity-corrected lenses are usually marked with an '∞' sign, to distinguish them from the more common 160 mm tubelength objectives. Infinity correction is not a particularly new concept for microscope objective design; the advantage of parallel ray paths was recognised in the 1930s for metallurgical microscopes in which vertical illuminators were prone to imparting image ghosts.

Infinity-corrected objectives are now employed by all four of the major microscope manufacturers (Leica, Nikon, Olympus, Zeiss) except in some models designed for student use.

Infinity-corrected objectives cannot be used in a body tube designed for a finite (160 mm or 170 mm) optical tubelength, and objectives intended for a finite tubelength cannot be used in a microscope designed for infinity-corrected objectives.

Intermediate optical components

Particularly when using infinity-corrected objectives, a variety of optical components may be inserted into the body tube (ie between objective and eyepiece). These include filters (see Chapter 8), polarising devices (see Chapter 10), compensation plates (see Chapter 10), epi-illumination mirrors (see Chapters 7 and 11), and magnification changers.

Magnification-changing devices can be added as very desirable (but expensive) accessories to some types of microscope. They enable optimal magnifications to be obtained for photography. Magnification-changing devices consist either of a rotating turret with several lenses, any one of which can be turned into the optical pathway, or alternatively of a zoom system. They are convenient, but should be avoided in those forms of microscopy in which the image is dim and light loss should be minimised (particularly fluorescence microscopy).

Bertrand lenses are lenses used in conjunction with phase-contrast and polarisation systems (see Chapter 10). They enable the back focal plane of the objective to be examined through the eyepiece. Typically, they are incorporated into the turret of a magnification changer.

Eyepieces and projectives

Eyepieces (oculars) are of two main types: those intended for visual use, and projection 'eyepieces' (projectives) intended to project a real image of the object onto a photographic emulsion or a viewing screen. While the two types are often interchangeable in use, the magnifications marked on each type refer to the magnification actually obtained in the intended service.

Eyepieces magnify the intermediate image produced by the objective, and produce either a virtual image below it (for examination by the eye) or a real image above it (for photography). Optically, they contain two major components: a fixed diaphragm. which limits the field of view, and a lens system to provide the required magnification. In many microscope systems, the eyepiece lenses also help to correct aberrations introduced by the objective. The *entrance pupil* is formed by the diaphragm. The *exit pupil* is the image of the diaphragm formed by the lenses above it.

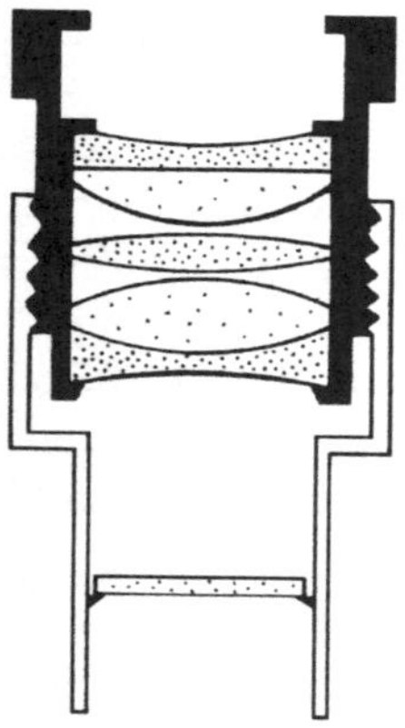

Fig 6.12. Positive eyepiece with graticule (near the bottom). A focusing movement in the eyepiece is required to focus on the graticule (the flat piece of glass near the bottom). A field diaphragm supports the graticule and limits the field of view.

Classical eyepieces have their lenses in two groups, one group (the field lens) at the lower end (assumed vertical), the other (the eye lens) at the top. In *positive eyepieces* (Fig 6.12), the diaphragm is situated at the bottom of the eyepiece, and the lenses are all above it. This is convenient for use with graticules (reticles). This kind of eyepiece can be used as a magnifier. In *negative eyepieces*, the diaphragm (and any graticule) is situated between the lenses, and is viewed through the eye-lens only, resulting in some chromatic aberration in its image.

The field of view is limited by the diameter of the entrance pupil, determined mainly or entirely by the diaphragm in the eyepiece, the diameter of the diaphragm being limited by the diameter of the body tube. Therefore, the full field of which any objective is capable can be visualised with an eyepiece with a magnification of about 10× (normal tube) or 6·3× (wide tube). Further reduction in magnification does not increase the field of view, and it is for this reason that lowest-power eyepieces are usually made only for fluorescence (where the brighter image is an advantage) or projection.

The *field number* of an eyepiece is the diameter of its entrance pupil, ie the effective diameter of the field stop (which may be affected by a *field lens* below it). The field number can be divided by the objective magnification to obtain the diameter of the field (in millimetres) in the specimen plane as seen through the eyepiece.

Compensation optics. Old achromatic and modern *CF* objectives are fully corrected for chromatic aberration at two or three wavelengths as described above. Other objectives (notably the old apochromats) are not fully corrected for lateral chromatic aberration. Instead, they are somewhat under-corrected, and this under-correction is intended to be balanced by compensating eyepieces which are over-corrected to an equal but opposite degree. Compensating eyepieces are sometimes designated with the letter K. The chromatic over-correction in the eyepiece results in an orange-coloured fringe around the edge of the field diaphragm and the edges of any graticule or scale. Moreover, these objectives cannot be used satisfactorily to produce images on their own, without an eyepiece.

Effects of optical parameters on the final image

The overall magnification is determined jointly by the objective, the intermediate magnifier (if any), the eyepiece or projective, and the camera lens (if any). Numerically, the overall magnification is equal to the product of the respective magnifications of the components named above. Any required overall magnification can often be achieved in more than one way, using different combinations of magnifications of the objective, intermediate lens, and eyepiece or projective. For example, given a 40× objective, 1·25× intermediate lens, and 10× eyepiece, one calculates the total magnification (M), as seen by the eye, to be

$$M = 40 \times 1{\cdot}25 \times 10 = 500$$

The resolution of the system depends on the NA of the objective and on the contrast of the image. The theoretical resolution in the image in the film plane can be calculated as follows. The minimum resolved distance (MRD) or resolution is given by the Abbe formula MRD = $\lambda/2$NA. The number of line pairs per unit distance (LP/mm) at the specimen is the reciprocal of the MRD in millimetres. Attention to specimen preparation and microscope usage should optimise the image. However, if specimen contrast is poor, the attainable resolution is impaired.

Empty magnification is the term used for magnification in excess of that required to make the MRD visible. Suppose that a photographic negative is made under optimal conditions, and a series of prints made at various magnifications, starting with quite small prints. As the magnification is increased there will be, at first, an increase in the amount of detail visible in the print. There will come a stage at which the smallest resolvable detail is enlarged big enough to be seen (about 0·1 mm for a print seen at normal close viewing distance). As a rule of thumb, this magnification is about 1000 times the NA of the objective. Further enlargement does not reveal any further detail in the object. Enlargement beyond that required to reveal the smallest resolvable detail is called *empty magnification*. For a poster, to be viewed at a greater distance, this magnification may be exceeded.

The brightness of the final image is determined in part by the objective, according to the square of its NA and inversely as the square of its magnification. The brightness of the final image (I) is also inversely proportional to the square of the total magnification.

$$I = \frac{\mathrm{NA}^2}{M^2}$$

In epi-illumination, the objective acts as both condenser and objective; as the condenser, the brilliance of the illumination of the specimen is proportional to the square of its NA and to the square of its magnification, since this produces a corresponding demagnification of the light source; as the objective, the brightness of the image is proportional directly to the square of its NA and inversely to the square of its magnification; and therefore in this case the brilliance of the final image is directly proportional to the fourth power of the NA of the objective, its magnification having no effect. The observable effect is that the image intensity increases when one changes from low to high powers (because of the increased NA). The brilliance of the image is affected by the square of the magnification taking place after the objective.

Closing the objective's aperture diaphragm (if it has one) or, in transmitted light, closing the condenser aperture diaphragm, reduces the NA of the system, thereby decreasing the resolving power, increasing the depth of field, and increasing the contrast of the image. Contrast of the image is also increased by reduction in flare (stray light). Spherical aberration is minimised; if the aberration was severe, the plane of focus is shifted slightly. Chromatic aberration is unchanged. Curvature of field is not changed, but its effects are reduced because of the increased depth of field. If the diaphragm is closed excessively, a diffraction artefact occurs (see above, Reverberation).

Further reading

The microscope optical system is described further by Oldfield (1994). For advanced discussions see the books by Pluta (1988, 1989) and Ray (1994a), and the article by Shimizu & Takenawa (1994).

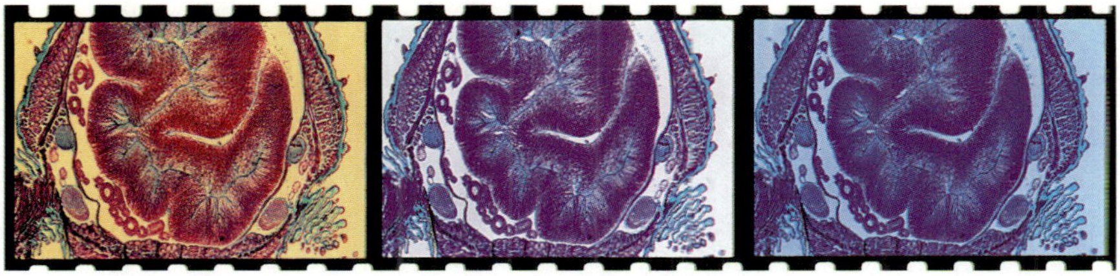

Plate 1a. The effects of colour temperature of the illumination. Transverse section through body of a peripatus, *Euperipatoides leuckartii*, stained with Milligan's trichrome, brightfield illumination. Zeiss *Universal* microscope, Olympus *PM-10ADS* photomicrographic unit. Illumination with 12 V 100 W lamp at full intensity (3200 K). Daylight-type colour film, Fuji *Velvia* exposed at speed rating 80. Left, without filter. Centre, with Olympus *LBD 2N* colour conversion (blue) filter. Right, with two *LBD 2N* blue filters. Field size 1·1 mm × 1·7 mm. See Colour temperature, Chapters 3 and 8.

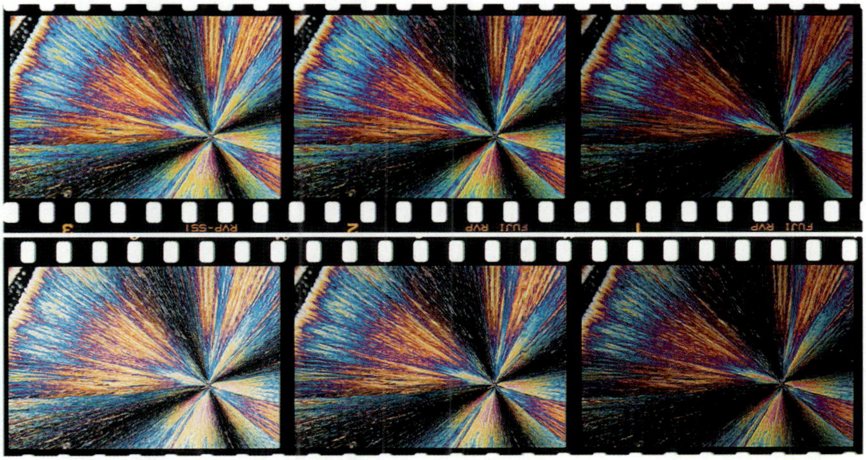

Plate 1b. Exposure latitude. Two sets of three frames of 35 mm film, with exposures of +1, 0, and –1 stops compared to the optimum. Fuji *Velvia* (50 ISO) and Kodak *Elite II ED* (200 ISO) films. Crystals of monosodium glutamate, transmitted-light polarisation microscopy with crossed polars. Field size 560 μm × 850 μm. See Chapters 10, 16 and 18.

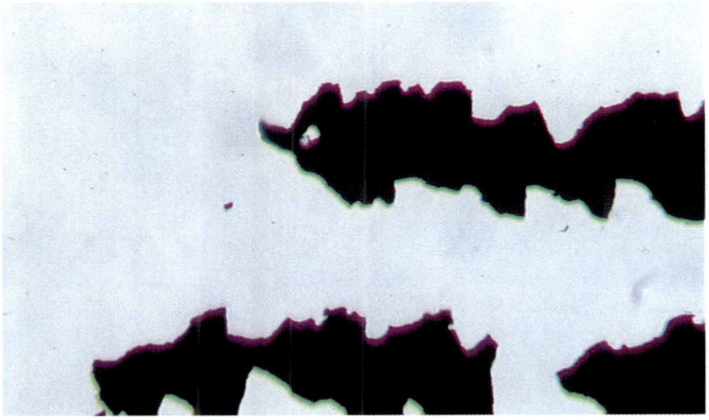

Plate 1c. Chromatic aberration (lateral), showing as green and magenta fringes. Wild Abbe test plate, with V-sector stop (in condenser filter holder) oriented at 90° to the test plate lines. Zeiss planachromat objective 40×, NA 0·65; immersed condenser. Fuji *Velvia* film. See Chapter 6.

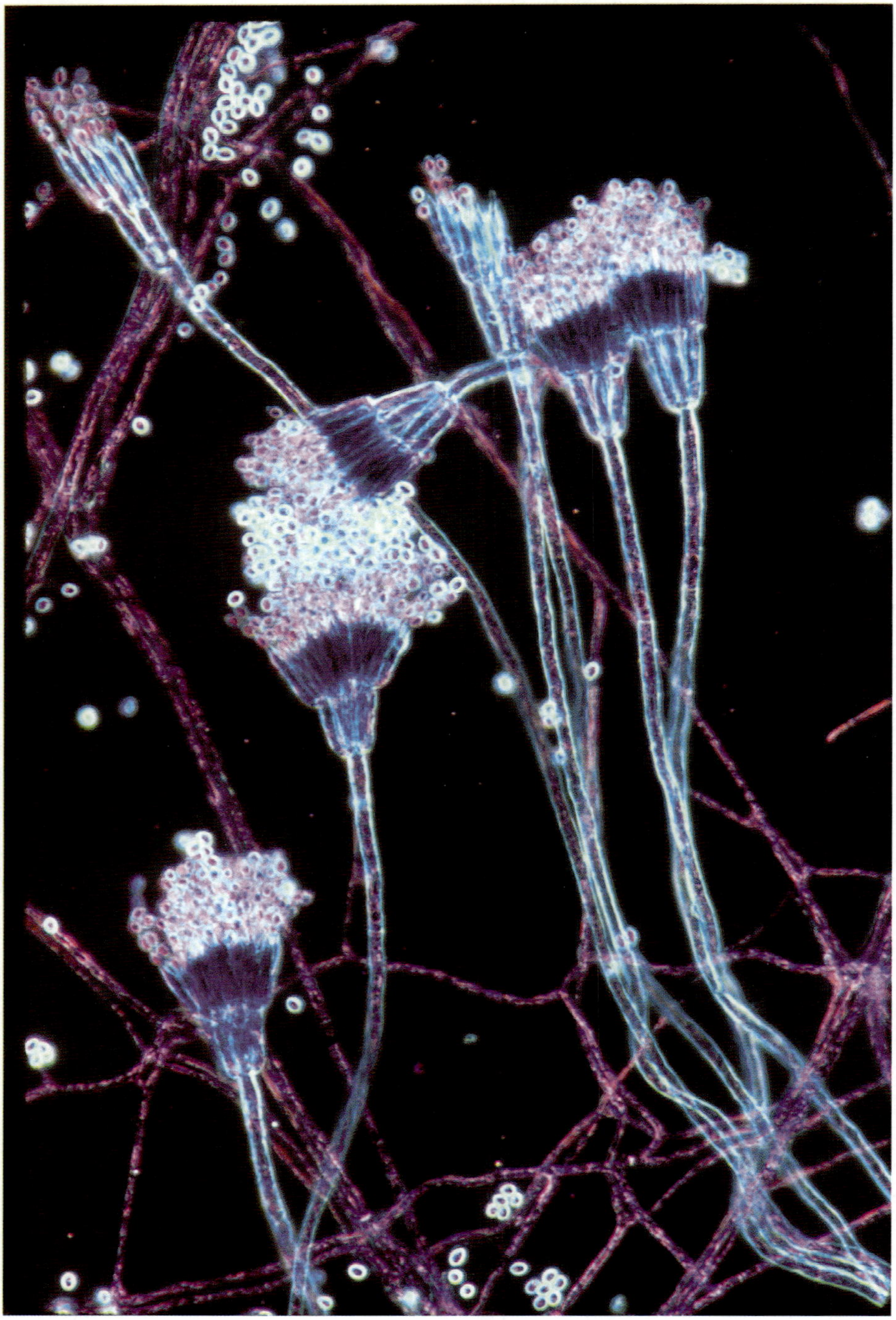

Plate 2. Darkground illumination with an immersion darkground condenser. The fungus (mould) *Penicillium funiculosum*. Field size 200 µm × 130 µm. Zeiss planapochromat immersion objective with iris, 40×, NA 1·0. Kodak *Kodachrome 25* film. See Chapter 9.

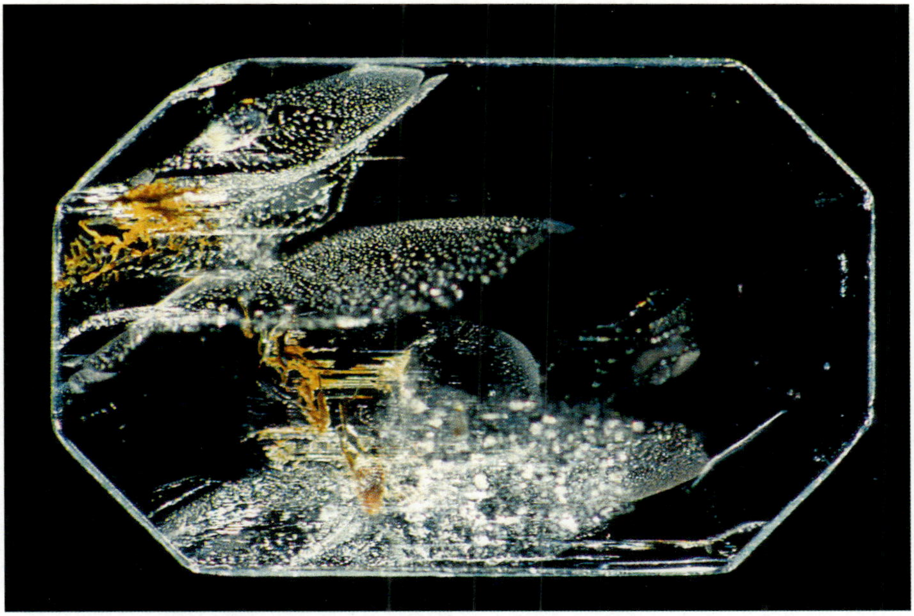

Plate 3a. Andalusite crystal, mounted in immersion oil to minimise edge refraction and reflection. Darkground illumination. This technique shows to perfection the inclusions which can be used to identify the gemstone. Andalusite is an aluminium silicate mineral found in small amounts in some metamorphic rocks. Field size 15 mm × 10 mm. Wild (Leica) *Photomakroskop*, darkground setting on illuminator, tungsten–halogen lamp at 3200 K, 80A blue filter; Kodak *Kodachrome 25* film. See Chapter 9.

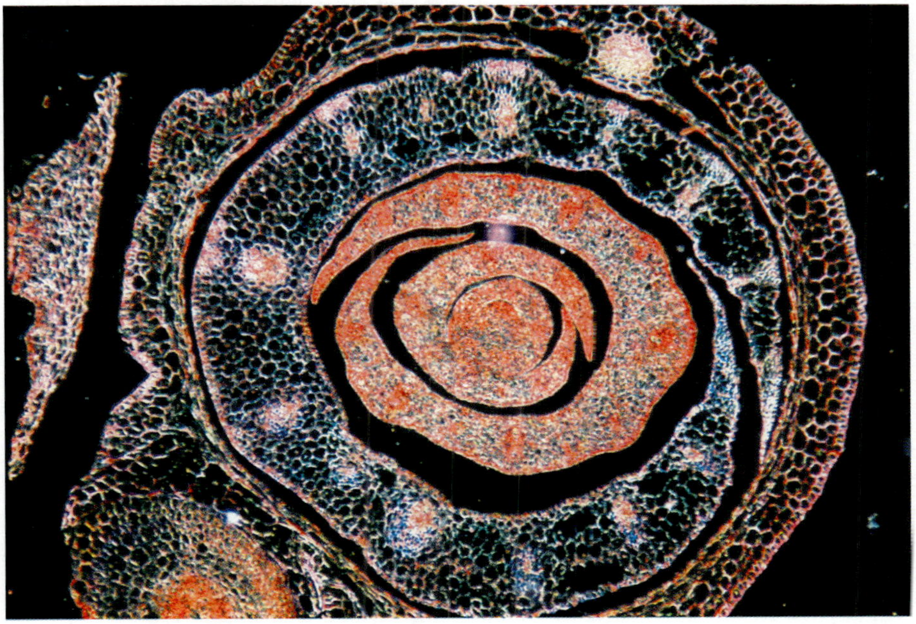

Plate 3b. Darkground illumination using, as a patch stop, the phase-contrast condenser annulus intended for the 100× objective. Section of apical shoot meristem of rice plant, *Oryza sativa*. Field size 530 μm × 800 μm. Zeiss planapochromat objective, 10×, NA 0·32. Kodak *Kodachrome 25* film. See Chapter 9.

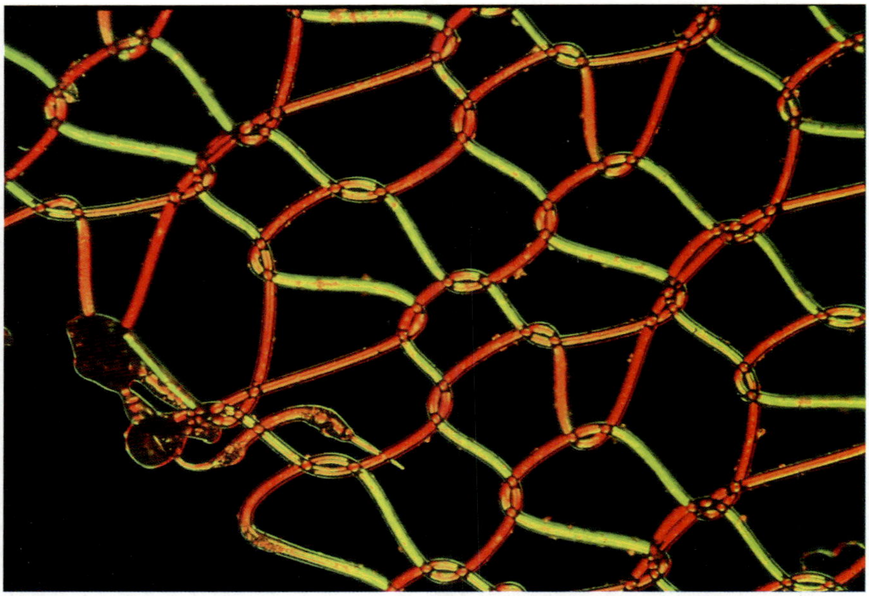

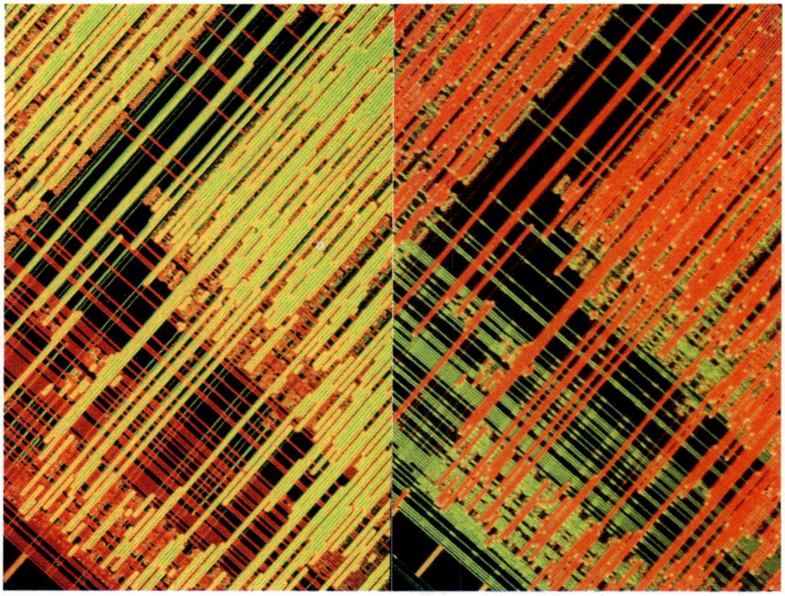

Plate 4. Rheinberg illumination (darkground illumination in colour), here using red and green filters in opposite sectors. See Chapter 9.

(Top) Edge of burn in nylon stocking. Field size 2·1 mm × 3·2 mm. Zeiss planachromatic objective, 2·5×, NA 0·08. Fuji *Velvia* film (50 ISO) rated at EI 200.

(Bottom) Epi-illumination. N71S integrated circuit. The two pictures show the same field, with the Rheinberg patch stop in different positions 90° apart. Field size 350 mm × 530 μm. Fuji *Velvia* film (50 ISO) rated at EI 250. We believe that this is the first published example of Rheinberg epi-illumination.

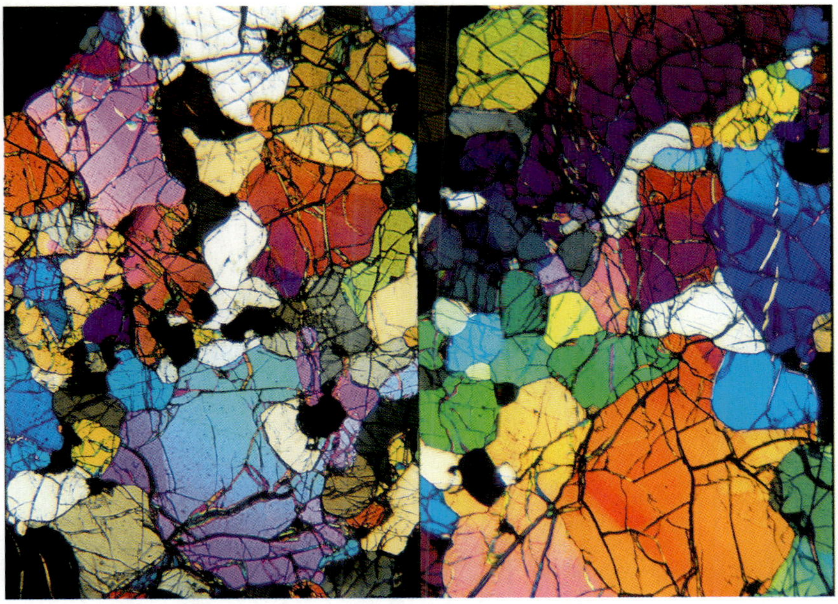

Plate 5a. Polarisation, transmitted light, crossed polars. Two sections of rock, mantle xenolith. Field size 5 mm × 8 mm in both cases. Xenoliths are fragments of rock embedded within an intrusive igneous rock, otherwise unrelated to the igneous rock. Wild *Photomakroskop* with polarisation attachments. Fuji *Velvia* film. See Chapter 10.

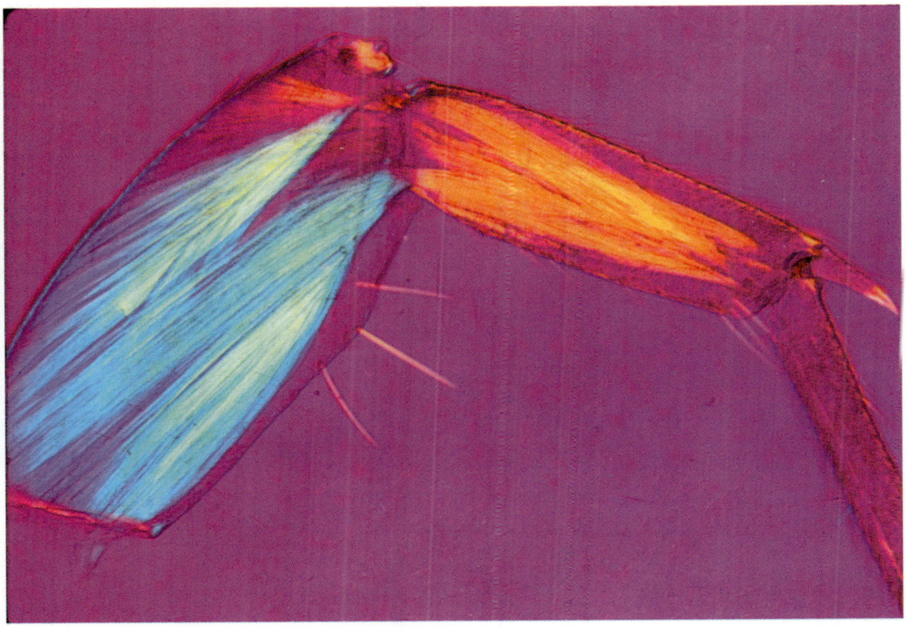

Plate 5b. Polarisation, transmitted light, crossed polars, with 1λ compensator. Leg of silverfish (*Lapisma saccharina*, Insecta), whole mount. Muscle fibres at 45° to the plane of polarisation. Field size 2 mm × 3 mm. Zeiss planachromat objective, 2·5×, NA 0·08. Kodak *Kodachrome 25* film. See Chapter 10.

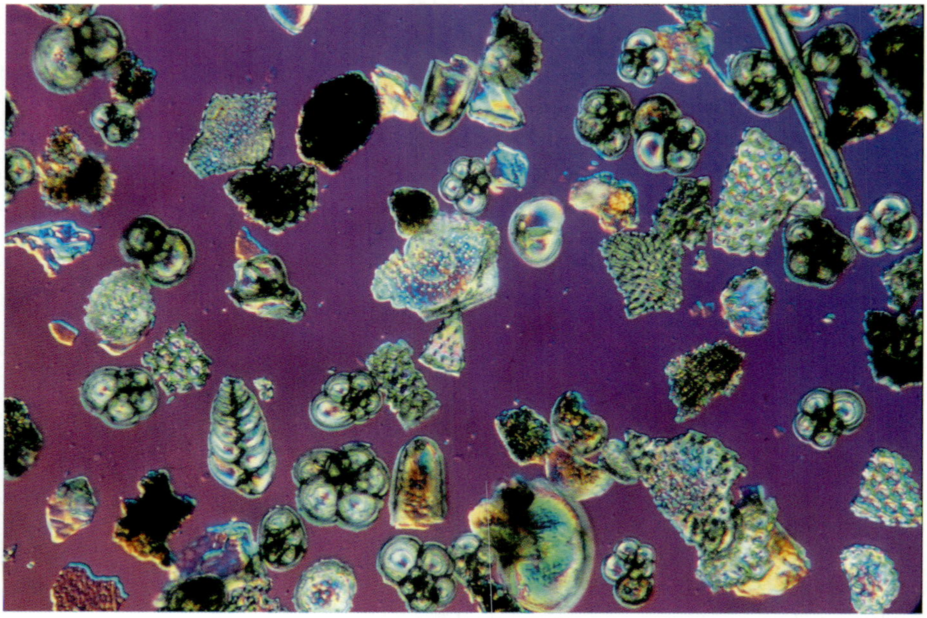

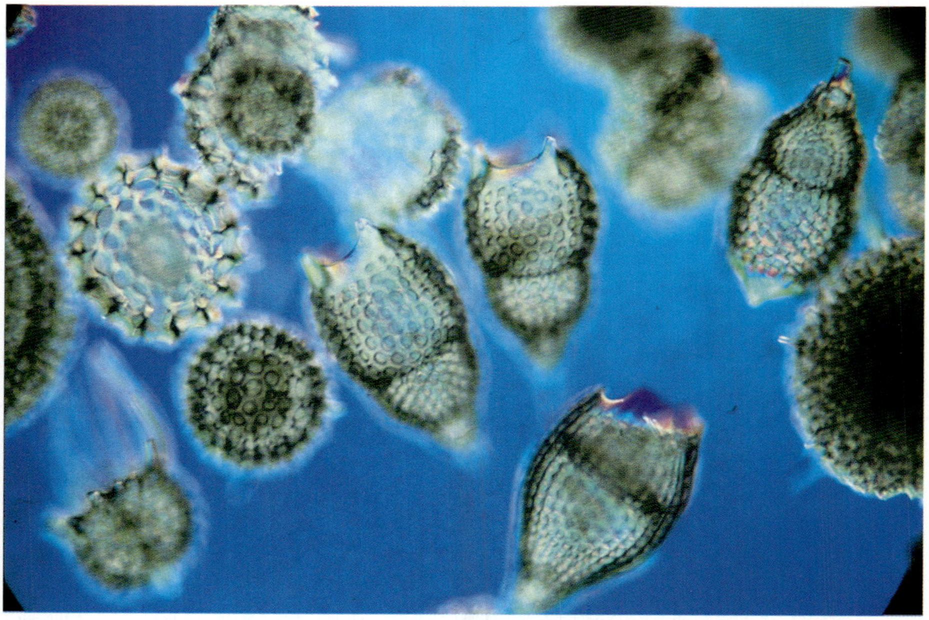

Plate 6. Differential interference contrast (DIC). Zeiss planachromat objective, 6·3×, NA 0·16. See Chapter 10.

(Top) Foraminifera. Transmitted-light DIC. Field size 0·7 mm × 1·05 mm (700 μm × 1050 μm). Kodak *Kodachrome 25* film.

(Bottom) Radiolaria. Transmitted-light DIC. Field size 0·4 mm × 0·7 mm (400 μm × 700 μm). Kodak *Kodachrome 25* film.

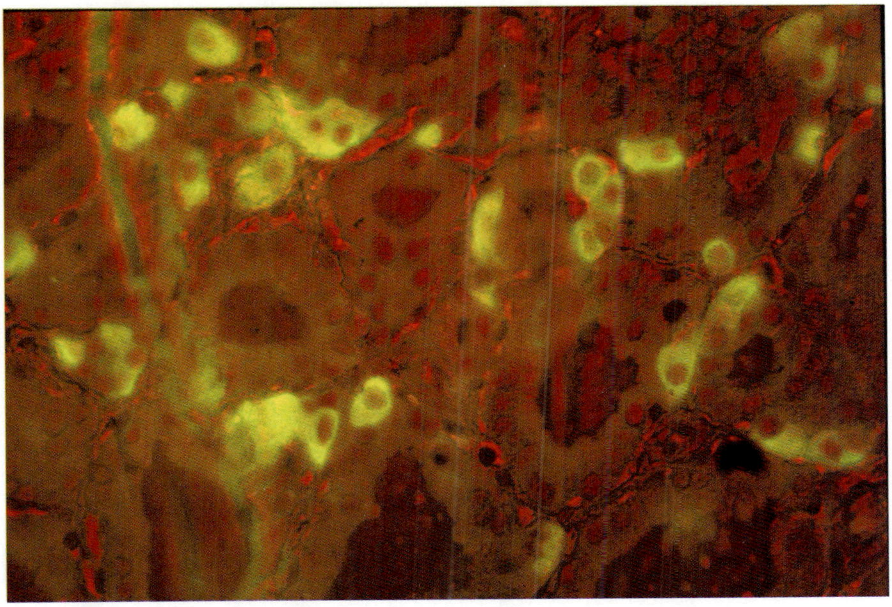

Plate 7a. Fluorescence and phase-contrast: immunofluorescence. Section of thyroid gland, stained with fluorescein isothiocyanate (FITC)-labelled anti-calcitonin, to show the location of cells producing the hormone calcitonin. Combined fluorescence epi-illumination (green) and phase-contrast transmitted-light illumination (red). See Chapter 11.

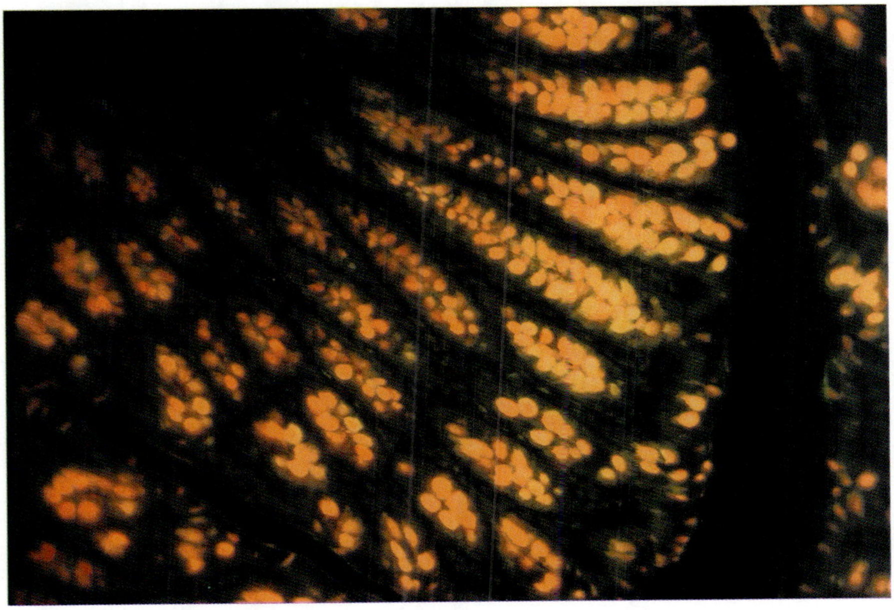

Plate 7b. Fluorescence. Mucin in rat colon, fluorochromed with Coriphosphine O after treatment with iron alum. The tissue was freeze-dried and fixed with formaldehyde vapour. Field size 0·7 mm × 1·0 mm. Zeiss *Universal* microscope, epi-illumination. Kodak *Kodachrome X* film. See Chapter 11.

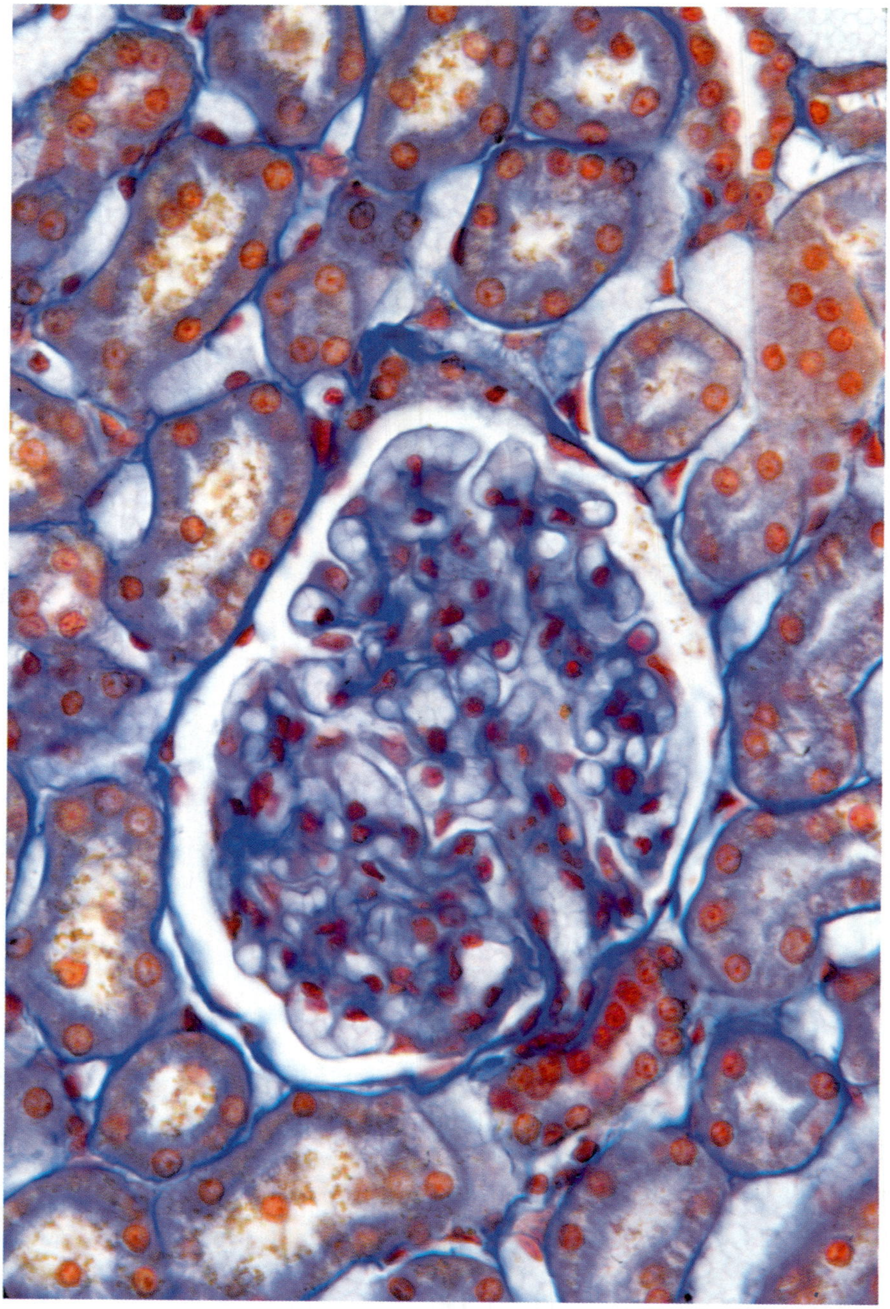

Plate 8. Transmitted-light illumination. Kidney of mouse (*Mus musculus*), stained with modified Masson's Trichrome stain (red, orange and blue). Field size 170 μm × 260 μm. Compare with the black-and-white photographs in Fig 15.2, which show the same preparation with various filters. Zeiss planapochromat objective, 25×, NA 0·65. Fuji *Velvia* film.

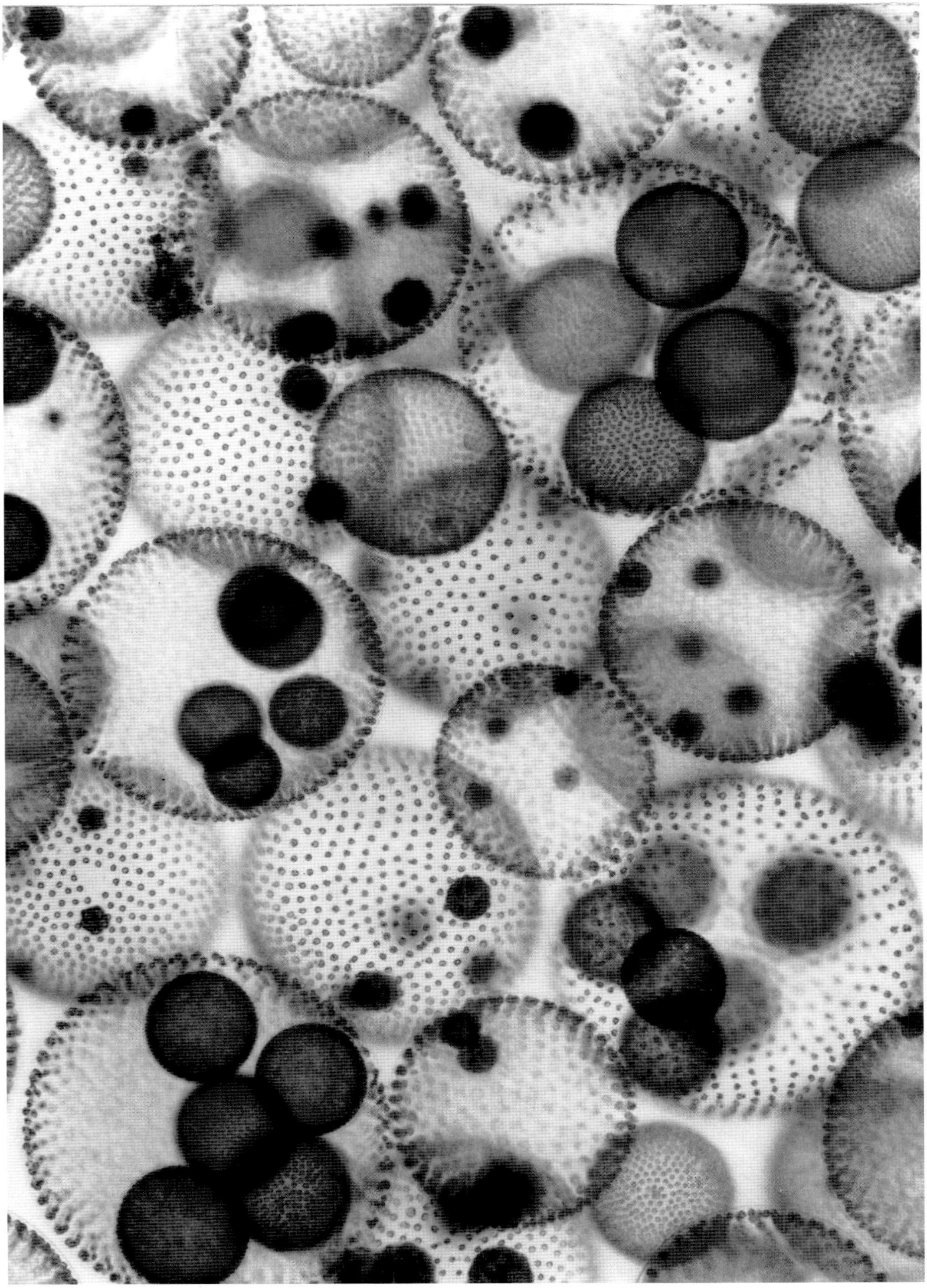

Plate 9. A first-class black-and-white photomicrograph, even if we say so ourselves as shouldn't! *Volvox* sp, field size 1·6 mm × 1·1 mm. *Volvox* is a small fresh-water green alga, consisting of cells surrounding a cavity, with daughter cells inside. Zeiss *Universal* microscope, planapochromat objective 4×, NA 0·14. Leitz *Aristophot* 4×5 inch camera (see Fig 4.6). Ilford *FP4* film.

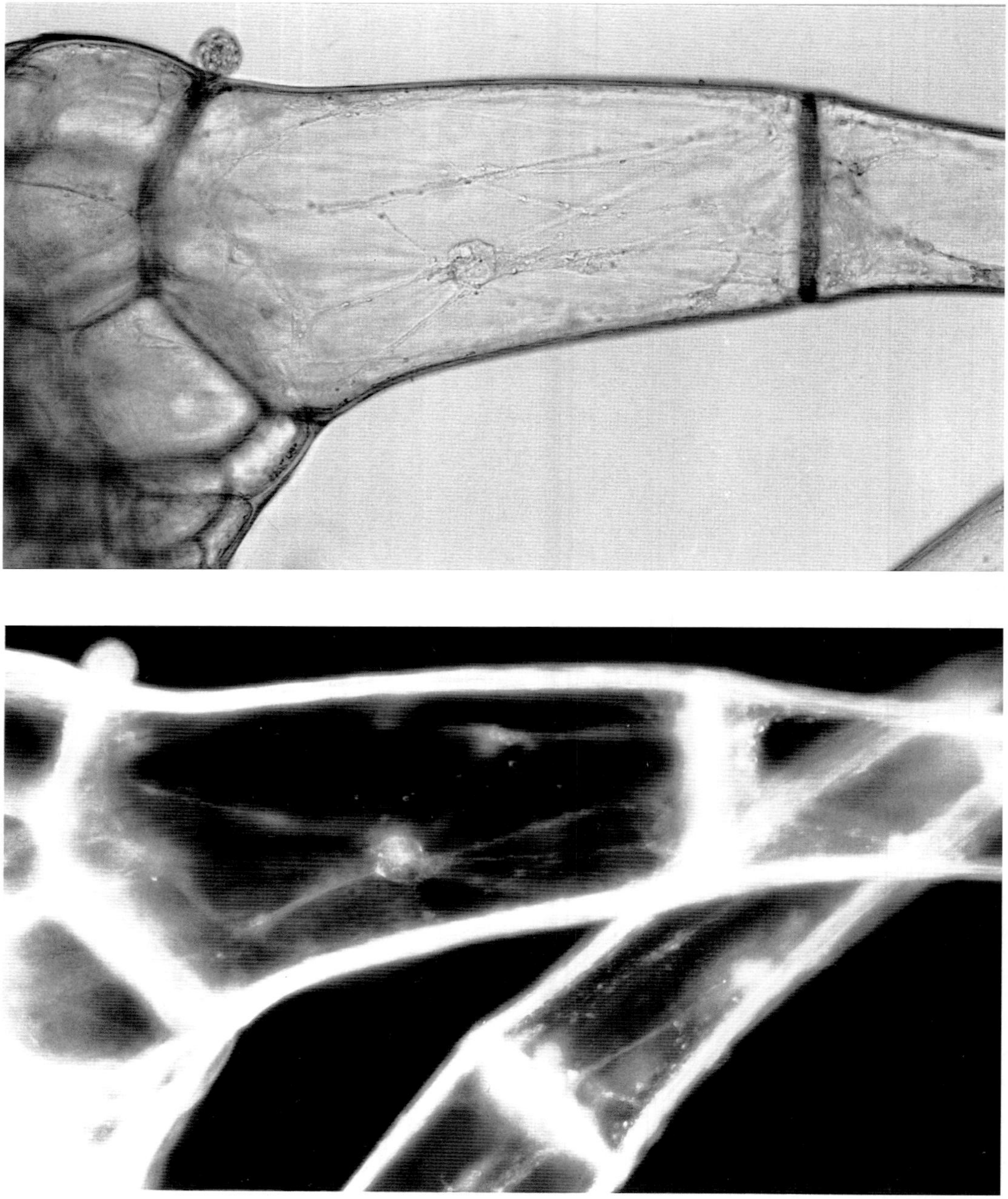

Plate 10. Comparison of brightfield, darkground, phase contrast, and DIC. Plates 10–12a show the same pumpkin (*Cucurbita* sp) hair cells, excised from a stem and mounted in water; the cells are living and unstained. Some specimen movement occurred after the first picture was taken. Olympus *BH2* microscope, with *PM-10ADS* photomicrographic system, Ilford *Pan F* film, Wratten 61 (green) filter. This plate, (top) brightfield, (bottom) patch-stop darkground. D-Plan objective, 10×, NA 0·25. Cf Plates 11 and 12a. See Chapter 10.

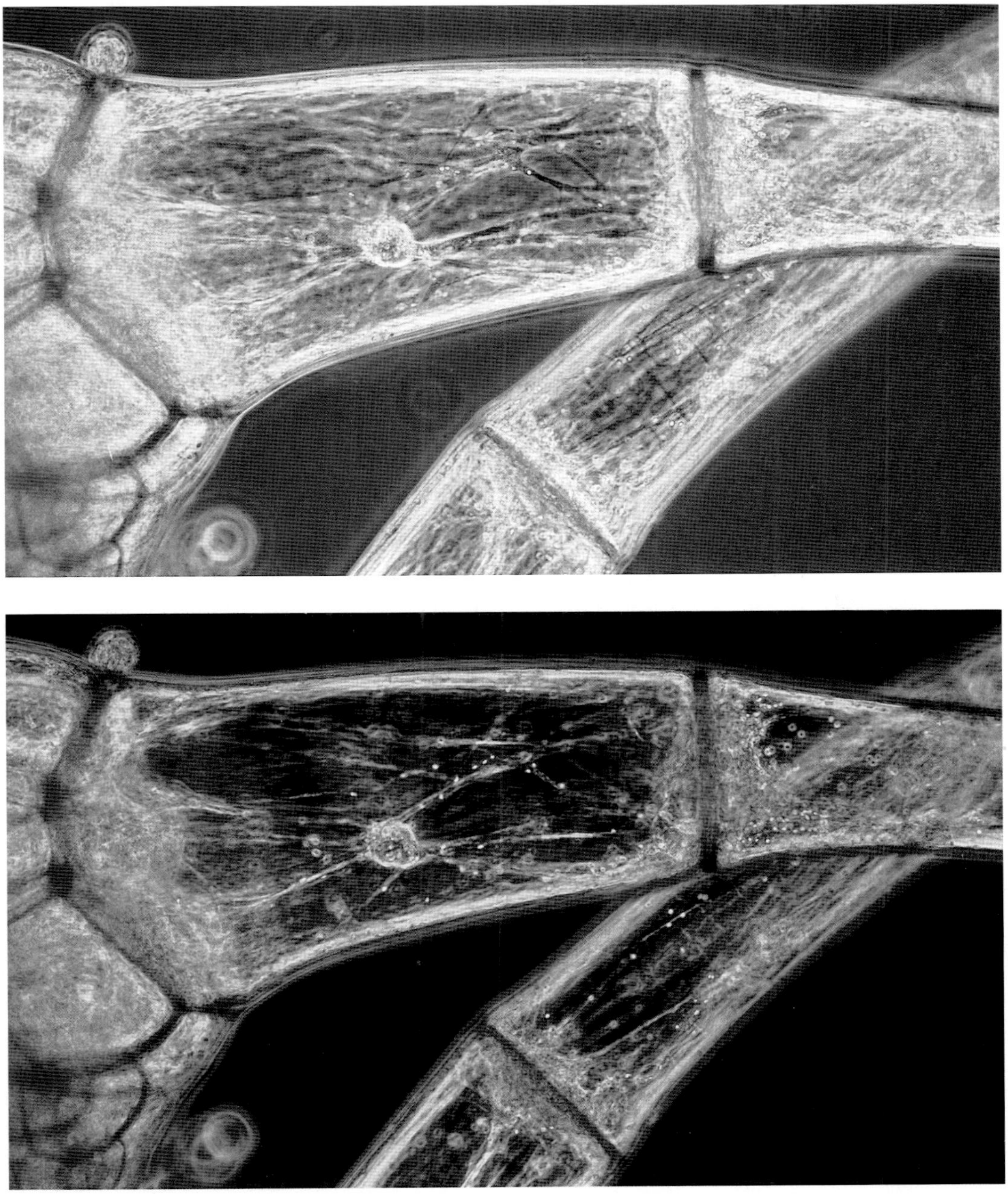

Plate 11. Pumpkin (*Cucurbita* sp) hair cells as in Plate 10, seen with positive phase-contrast microscopy (top) and negative phase-contrast microscopy (bottom). S-Plan objectives, 10×, NA 0·25. Cf Plates 10, 12a. See Chapter 10.

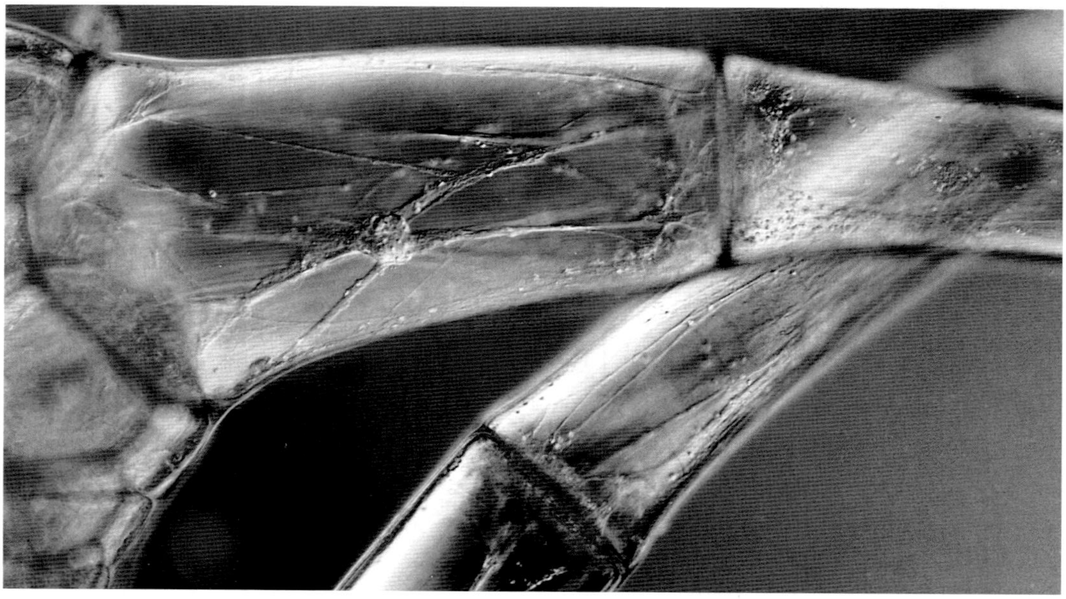

Plate 12a. Pumpkin (*Cucurbita* sp) hair cells as in Plates 10 and 11, differential interference contrast (DIC). S-Plan objective, 10×, NA 0·3. See Chapter 10.

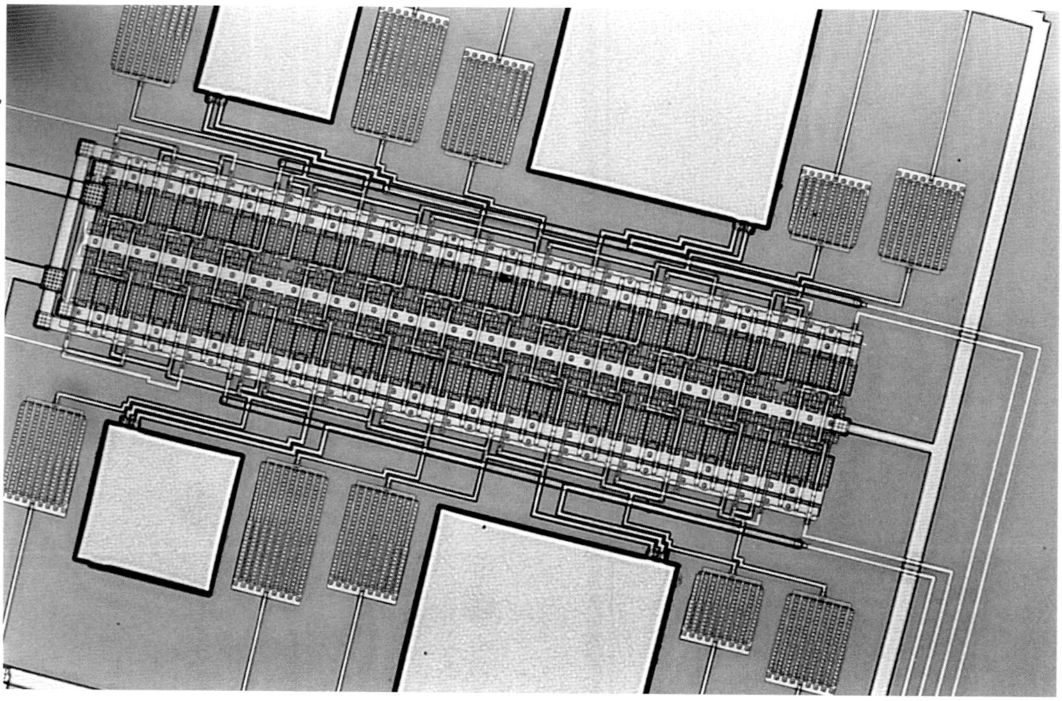

Plate 12b. Epi-illumination, brightfield. Microchip, field size 440 μm × 670 μm. Because of the sharp detail of the lines, vibration must be completely eliminated during photography! Zeiss *Universal* microscope, Zeiss objective *Epiplan HD*, 16×, NA 0·35. Olympus *PM-10ADS* photomicrographic system. Ilford *Pan F* film, light green filter. Cf Plate 13 (top, darkground illumination; bottom, polarisation, crossed polars). See Chapter 7.

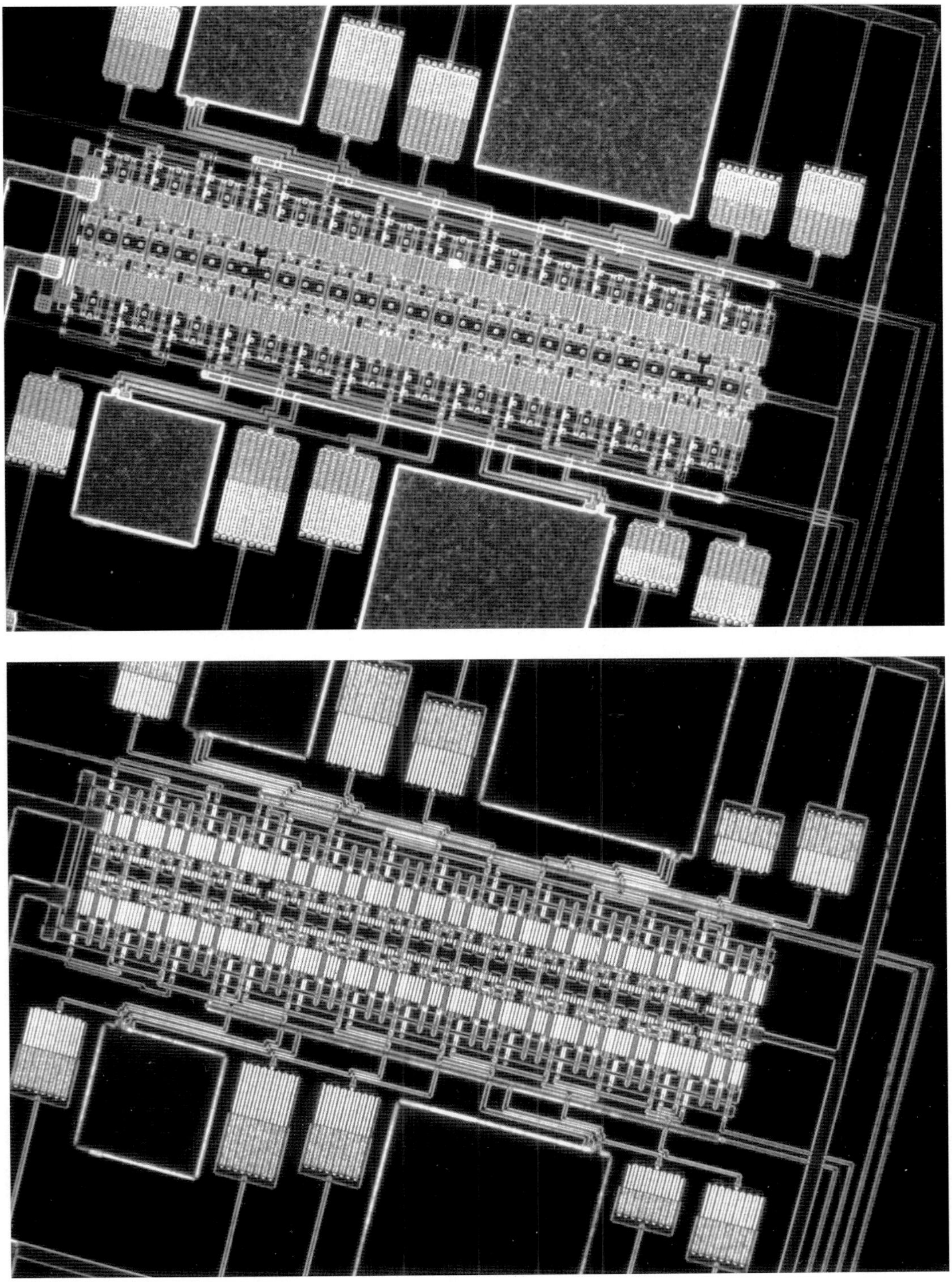

Plate 13. Epi-illumination. Microchip, field size 440 μm × 670 μm. Zeiss *Universal* microscope, with Olympus *PM-10ADS* photomicrographic system; Ilford *Pan F* film, light green filter. (Top) Darkground (darkfield) illumination. (Bottom) Polarisation, crossed polars. Cf Plate 12b. See Chapter 7.

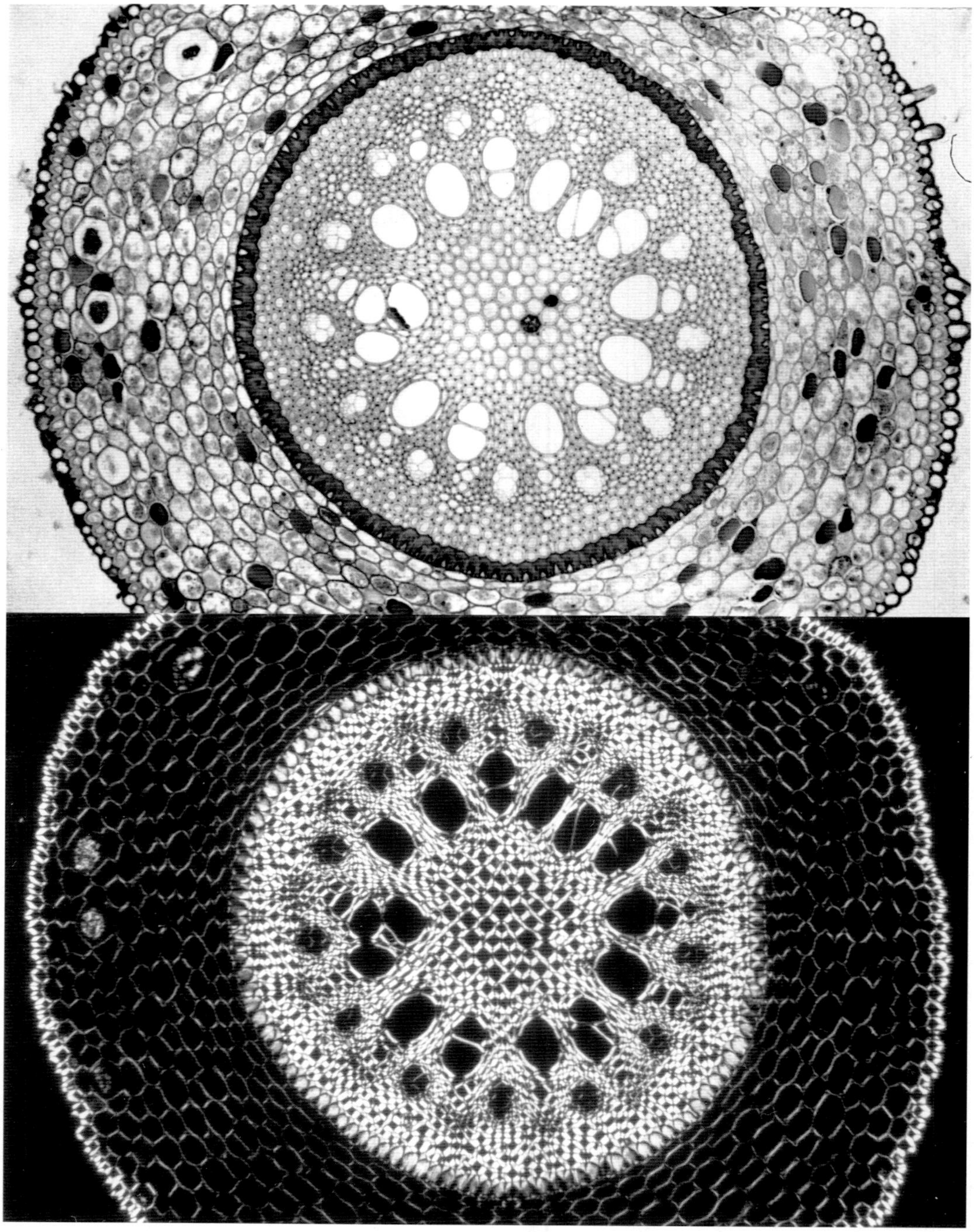

Plate 14. Comparison of normal transmitted light (brightfield, top) and polarisation with crossed polars (bottom). Transverse section of the root of the plant *Smilax* sp. Field size 0·9 mm × 1·4 mm. Zeiss planachromat objective 6·3×, NA 0·16. See Chapter 10.

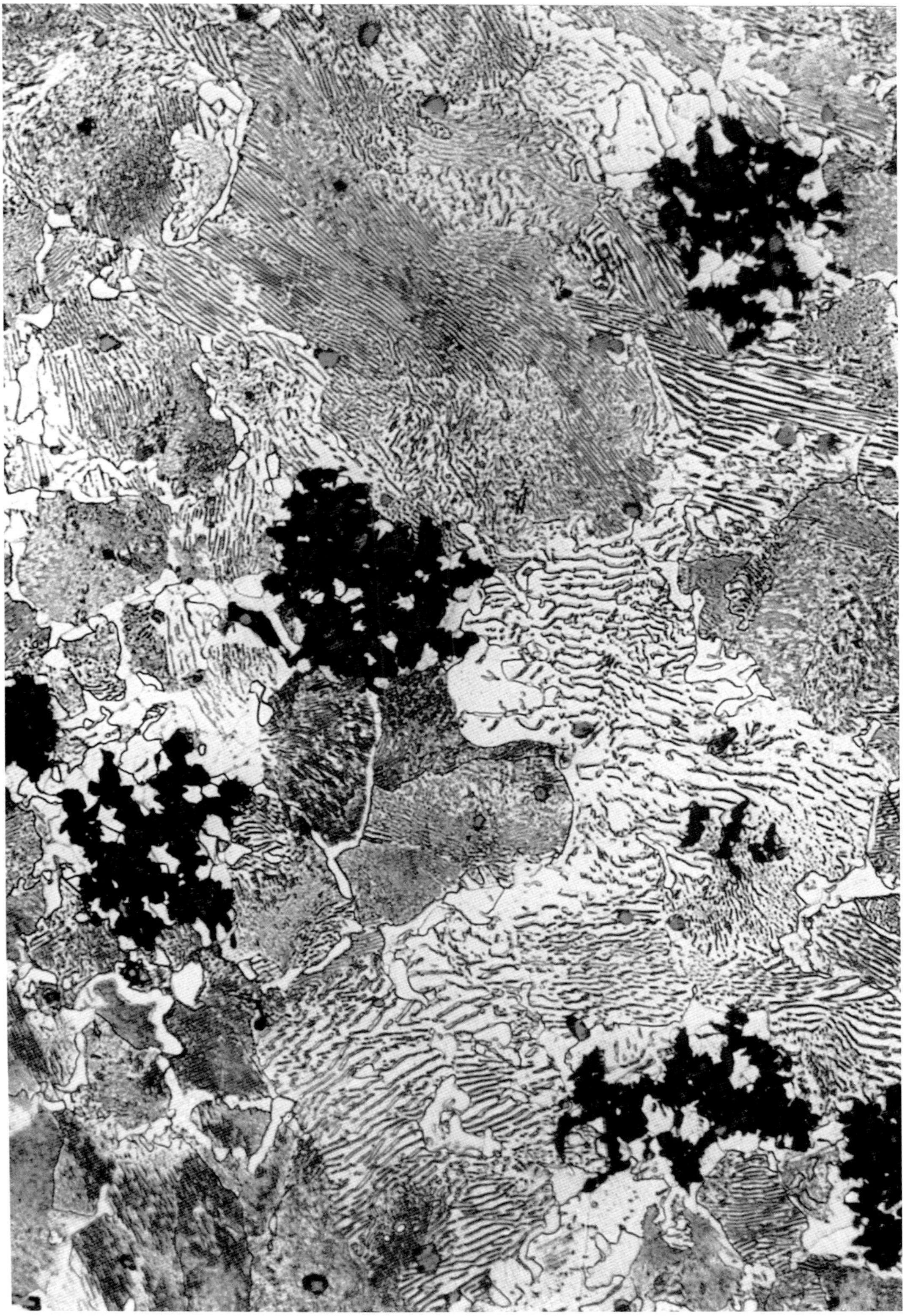

Plate 15. Malleable iron, polished surface. Epi-illumination, Zeiss *Universal* microscope, *Epiplan HD*, 16×, NA 0·35 objective, orange No 22 filter, Olympus *PM-10ADS* photomicrographic unit, Ilford *Pan F* film. Field 0·5 mm × 0·4 mm. Specimen courtesy John Budden, University of New South Wales. See Chapter 7.

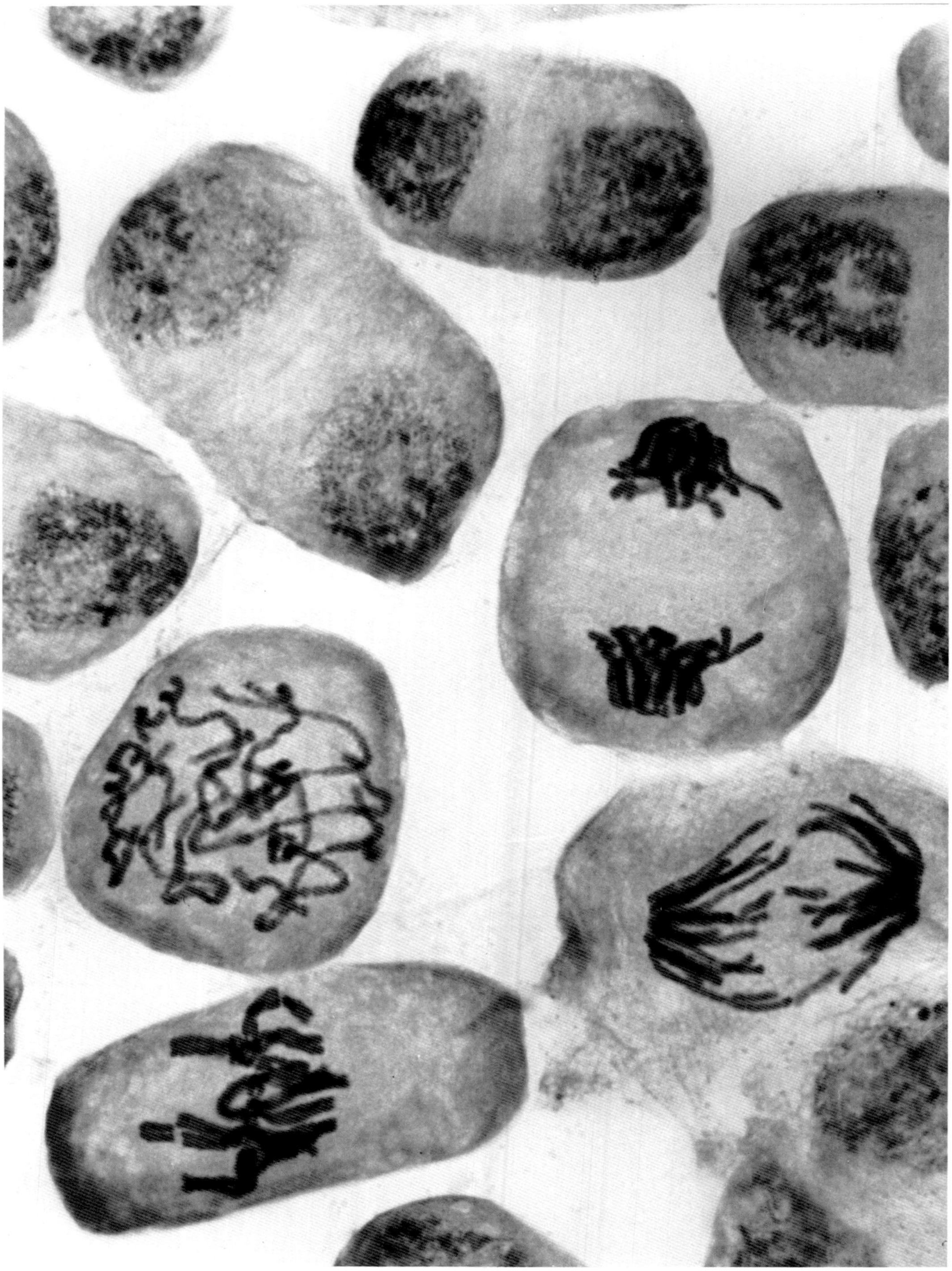

Plate 16. Mitotic figures, photographed in transmitted light. Root of bean (*Vicia faba*), squash preparation, after treatment with 5-aminouracil to synchronise cell division. The photomicrograph shows a unique grouping of mitotic phases. Anticlockwise from bottom left: prophase, metaphase, anaphase, telophase, and two nuclei in late telophase. Images of individual cells from this plate, assembled as a series, are shown in Fig 17.8. Field size 170 μm × 110 μm. Zeiss objective, oil-immersion apochromat 40×, NA 1·0. Ilford *FP4* 4×5 inch film. Photomicrography using transmitted-light techniques is described in Chapters 3 and 15.

7
The illumination system

The illumination system for conventional transmitted-light microscopy was described briefly in Chapter 2. The present chapter describes the system in more detail, and also describes illumination from above the specimen (epi-illumination).

The purpose of the illumination system is to illuminate the object with sufficiently intense light of an appropriate wavelength range, and to adequately fill the aperture of the objective. The illumination system may be required to provide this lighting in special ways for special techniques of microscopy such as darkground, phase contrast, or fluorescence (discussed in Chapters 9–13).

The classical method of illumination produces a beam of light that passes through the specimen into the objective (Figs 2.11, 7.7). This is known as *transmitted-light microscopy*, *transillumination* or (more rarely) *dia-illumination*. For opaque objects, and in some other circumstances, the light is directed downwards, around or through the objective onto the specimen. Illumination from the same side as the objective is usually referred to as *incident light* or *epi-illumination*. (Co-author Fred would prefer to refer to epi-illumination as *cis*illumination to match the term *trans*illumination, referring to the side of the object from which the illumination is directed.)

In conventional transmitted-light microscopy, the specimen is viewed as a dark or coloured object against a bright background. This is known as *brightfield* microscopy. If the aperture cone of the illumination has a hollow centre whose numerical aperture (NA) is greater than that of the objective, so that no light from the illumination enters the objective directly, the mode of illumination is said to be darkfield or *darkground*, because the background to the specimen appears dark. This method of illumination is discussed in Chapter 9.

Illumination for transmitted-light microscopy

A system of illumination acceptable for high-quality microscopy must fulfil a number of conditions:

- The specimen field should be fully and evenly illuminated.
- The intensity of the illuminated field should be variable within wide limits.
- The diameter of the illuminated field should be variable to match the field of view of the microscope, usually varying from about 0·2 mm to 4 mm.
- The numerical or angular aperture (NA, see Chapter 6) of the condenser should be variable to match the range of objective NAs (usually from about 0·1 to 1·3).

The illumination system will be discussed systematically, beginning with the light source and then tracing the optical path to the specimen. Lamps and filters are discussed separately in the next chapter (Chapter 8).

As explained in Chapter 2, light from the lamp is collected by a *collector lens* in the lamphouse and focused through a *field diaphragm* into the *condenser*, which focuses the light onto the specimen. Somewhere in the illumination system, a filter (see Chapter 8) may be inserted to select the appropriate wavelengths for illumination. The illumination and observation systems are similar, and symmetrical about the object. In principle, they are to some extent interchangeable – the objective can be used as a condenser, and vice versa. The basic transmitted-light illumination system will be described first, because it is the most widely used. However, the same principles apply to metallurgical microscopes.

There are two main types of illumination, generally known as *source-focused illumination* and *Köhler illumination,* respectively. Source-focused illumination (formerly called *critical illumination*) uses an image of the light source focused onto the specimen. This method was used in the early days of microscopy, but is no longer normally used for high-quality microscopy. A modified form is still sometimes used in inexpensive apparatus, and it is therefore described in Chapter 4. Köhler illumination uses a system of two lenses: a collector lens, which focuses an image of the light source into the aperture of the second lens (the condenser), which in turn focuses the aperture of the collector into the object plane. This gives a better and more controllable illumination, and is described in this chapter.

The condenser

To achieve its maximum resolution, the full NA of an objective must be used in image formation. To fill big objective apertures with light, a wide-angle cone of light for illumination is therefore essential, and a condenser is used for this purpose. Essentially, the condenser should fill the objective's aperture with light; more exactly, the condenser should image the light source across the whole of the back focal plane (BFP) of the objective. Only when this condition is met can the full NA (and therefore resolution) of the objective be realised.

For visual observation, it is not usually necessary for the condenser to be as highly corrected as the objective lenses, and a two-lens Abbe-type condenser is the general choice for routine microscopy. For the more exacting requirements of photomicrography, it is essential to employ achromatic-aplanatic or at least achromatic systems, with better lens corrections (Fig 7.1).

Condensers are also made with long working distances; condensers with flip-out tops may have special long working-distance tops available.

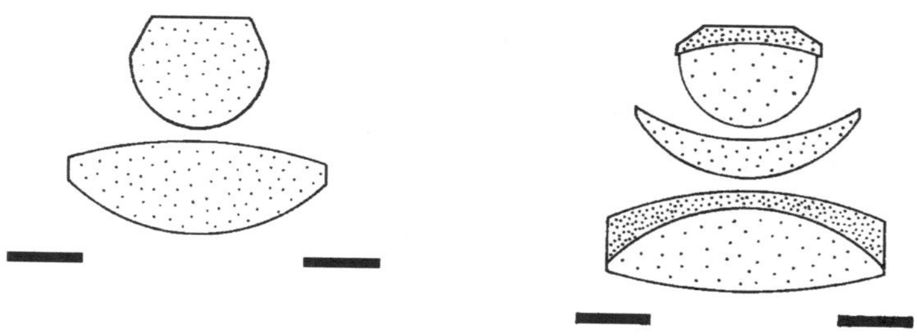

Fig 7.1. Cross-section diagrams of an Abbe two-lens condenser (left) and a highly corrected aplanatic-achromatic condenser (right) as preferred for photography.

Immersion of the condenser

Any condenser marked with an NA of 1·00 (or higher) is meant for immersion. Unless it is immersed it cannot reach its designed NA (see Chapter 6), and because of spherical aberration when the condenser is used dry, the effective NA is very much less – possibly no more than 0·7.

Whenever the microscope image needs to be the best possible, exploiting the full potential of a high-power objective, the oiling of the condenser is important, not only to achieve high numerical aperture, but also to eliminate the air–glass interfaces between the condenser and the slide, interfaces that are a source of undesirable reflection and flare. The circumstances that warrant the trouble of immersion of the condenser are:

- High resolution microscopy, NA exceeding 0·8.
- Photomicrography, NA exceeding about 0·6, to control one possible source of loss of contrast.
- Any situation where high intensities of light are preferred, eg for darkground or differential interference-contrast (DIC) microscopy.

On the other hand, condenser systems with an NA of 0·9 or less are not designed for oiling, and should not have immersion oil placed on them.

The condenser aperture (iris) diaphragm

It would appear that the full NA of a condenser should at least equal that of the highest NA objective, usually about 1·3. However, for most instruments, the condenser provided has an NA of 1·25 rather than 1·3. Only seldom is the high condenser aperture of 1·3 used in practical microscopy, and a slightly lower condenser aperture helps to increase image contrast. This condenser NA, 1·25, needs to be reduced further when using lower NA objectives, and for this function an iris diaphragm is located in the front focal plane of the condenser. The function of the condenser iris diaphragm is to control the NA of the condenser, to match the NA of the condenser to the NA of the objective (as described below).

Although the resolving power of a microscope is dependent primarily on the NA of the objective (see Chapter 6), the NA of the condenser is also a relevant factor in image formation. In the ideal case, the NA of the condenser should equal the NA of the objective (Fig 7.2, left).

If the condenser NA is less than the objective NA (Fig 7.2, centre), the effective NA of the system is approximately equal to the average (arithmetic mean) of the NA of the objective and the NA of the condenser, and the resolving power of the microscope system will be impaired accordingly. However, there will be a corresponding gain in contrast. In the extreme case, a very low condenser NA (relative to the objective's NA) results in an image with very high contrast and very poor resolution (see Reverberation, in Chapter 6).

The need to avoid having a condenser with an NA which is greater than that of the objective (Fig 7.2, right) is much less apparent. Under these conditions, the objective aperture is certainly fully illuminated. However, excessive condenser NA may lead to stray light, ie light not required for image formation, entering the objective. The effect of stray light is to reduce image contrast by flare introduced by reflection within the lenses and the specimen.

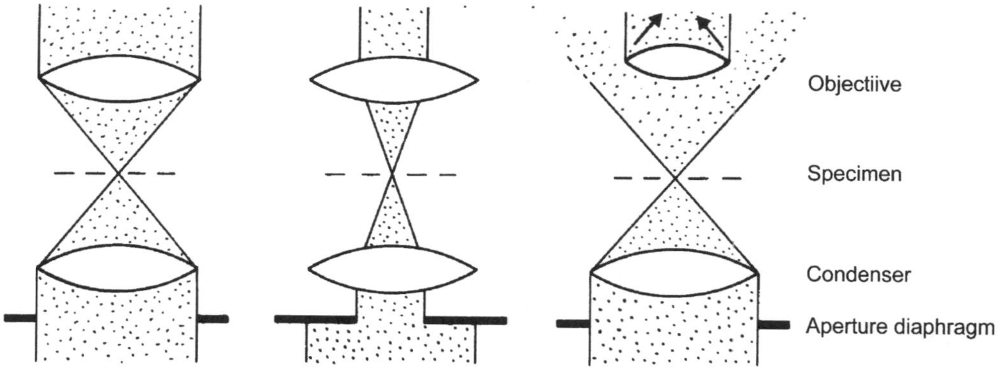

Fig 7.2. Diagram to show the effects of changing the condenser's numerical aperture (NA).

- When the NAs of condenser and objective are equal (left), the system is (theoretically) optimised.
- If the condenser's NA is less than that of the objective (centre), the resolution of the system is impaired because the effective NA of the objective is reduced.
- If the condenser's NA is greater than that of the objective (right) stray light may enter the objective.

Adjustment of the aperture diaphragm

How can it be known when the condenser NA has been adjusted to match the NA of a particular objective? By removing an eyepiece and looking down the microscope tube, one can see the back focal plane (BFP) of the objective (Fig 7.3). It is then possible to see the extent to which an objective aperture is illuminated, and in this way any effect on the objective aperture is detected. If the condenser iris is opened and closed while one is looking at the objective BFP, an image of the condenser iris is seen in the objective (Fig 7.3). When the iris is closed, the objective aperture is considerably restricted; as the condenser iris is opened, more of the objective aperture is illuminated, until a stage is reached where the image of the condenser iris just disappears outside the objective BFP. At this point, the NA of the condenser is set to match exactly the NA of the objective.

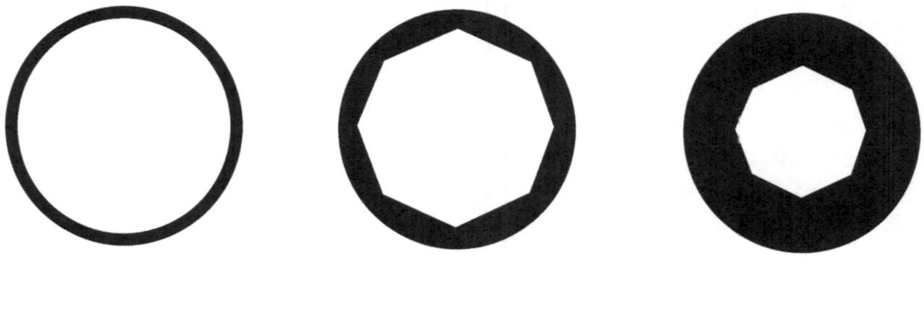

Fig 7.3. Appearance of the back focal plane of the objective, with various settings of condenser aperture. The optimal setting is usually as shown in the middle diagram.

In practical usage, the condenser NA is slightly reduced, below the point of matching apertures, until about $^7/_8$ to $^3/_4$ of the objective aperture is filled with light, as shown in the centre of Fig 7.3. The slight reduction in aperture is necessary in all but the most highly corrected of objectives to maintain image contrast. Closing the condenser iris further will reduce the effective NA of the objective. Opening the condenser iris beyond the $^7/_8$ths position will usually introduce loss of contrast, because of stray reflections.

There are two further important practical considerations in the setting of the condenser iris diaphragm: depth of field and contrast, which are dealt with below. In summary, although contrast and depth of field can both be increased by reducing the condenser NA, that same reduction in aperture must cause a loss in the objective resolving power. It is the effectiveness of the compromise made between these competing factors – resolving power, depth of field, contrast – that distinguishes a good image from a poor one.

Depth of field (defined and discussed in Chapter 6) is increased by reducing the effective NA of the optical system, because the depth of field is dependent on the NA. In transmitted light, depth of field can be increased by closing the condenser iris diaphragm (Fig 7.4).

Effect on intensity. If the intensity is proportional to the square of the NA, and if the condenser iris diaphragm controls the effective NA of the microscope system, it follows that the condenser iris (or any iris that is an aperture stop) will have the effect of changing image brightness. However, *the condenser iris diaphragm should never be used to control the intensity of the image*. The lamp rheostat, or neutral density filters (see Chapter 8) must be used for this purpose. There is complication enough in compromising the competing demands on the aperture iris of minimum resolved distance, depth of field and contrast.

Contrast in the image can be increased by partially closing the condenser iris diaphragm (Fig 7.4). This is caused as follows. The microscope image is a product of wave interference between the direct rays and the rays that are diffracted by the specimen, according to Abbe theory. If these interference phenomena are altered, the intensity distribution in the image plane will be altered and the contrast changed.

Lowering of the condenser

The following remarks refer to the full condenser, with its top lens in position. It is a common practice in classrooms and laboratories to lower the condenser, either to obtain a more even illumination for the 4× objective or to increase contrast with the 10× or 40× objectives. There is a difference of opinion as to the correctness or wisdom of such a displacement of the condenser. Most experienced microscopists are severely critical of the procedure, even making the judgement that lowering of the condenser is a certain sign of an absence of training in microscopy!

For the 40× and 100× objectives, or rather for objectives of NA higher than 0·4, the correct position for the condenser is almost fully raised. When the field diaphragm is correctly focused onto the specimen, the top lens of the condenser is usually about 1 mm below the level of the stage.

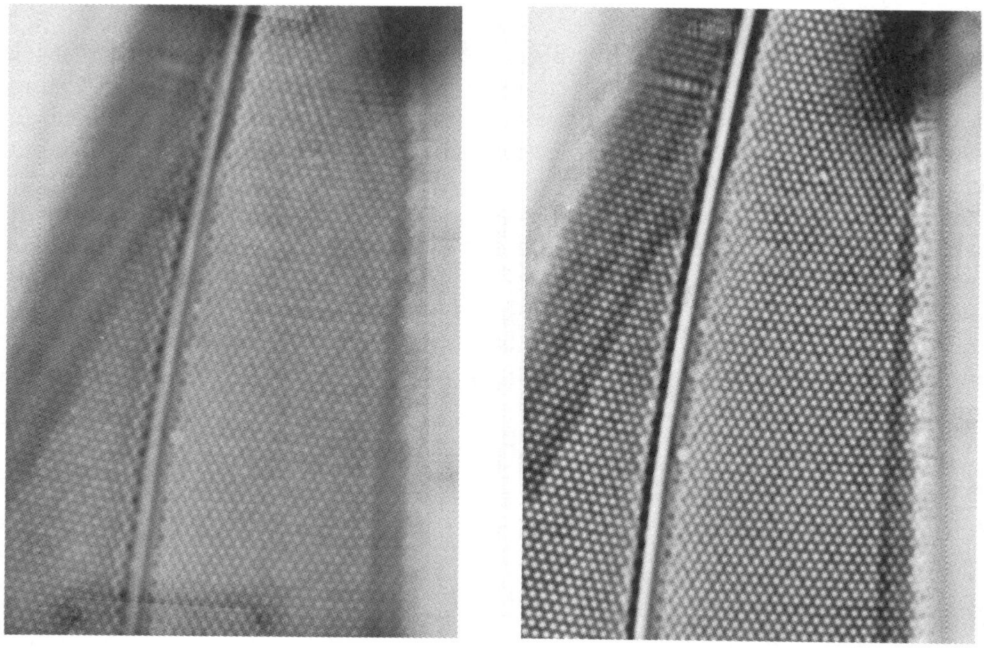

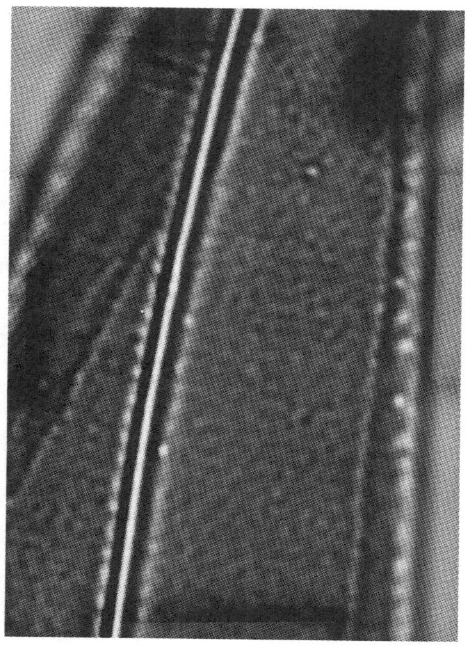

Fig 7.4. Photomicrographs showing increased depth of field and contrast obtained by use of the condenser aperture (iris) diaphragm. *Pleurosigma angulatum* (a diatom), field size 40 μm × 30 μm, objective 40×, NA 0·65. Top left, diaphragm fully open. Top right, diaphragm at its optimal setting. Lower left, diaphragm considerably closed down. The bottom photograph has been printed darker than usual to illustrate the reduction in light intensity. In the first picture, the diatom pattern is resolved, but with poor contrast. In the bottom picture, note the loss of resolving power, and increased contrast, due to reduced NA.

For low-power work, such as with the 4× objective, the difficulty of getting an evenly illuminated field is often overcome if the condenser is considerably lowered, by as much as 10 to 20 mm. In its lowered position, the aperture of the illumination system is much reduced, so that it is not possible to fill the NA of, for example, a 40×/0·65 NA objective. One objection to the practice of lowering the condenser is that once the condenser has been lowered, perhaps legitimately for the 4× objective, the condenser may be left lowered, and then all high-power work is effected at greatly reduced NA, which certainly is bad practice. The best practice is to avoid displacing the intact condenser. Increase in contrast is more properly obtained by partially closing the condenser iris diaphragm.

Adapting the illumination to the objective

A range of objectives will impose varying requirements on the condenser in terms of the diameter of the field to be illuminated, the appropriate NA of the condenser, and the intensity of illumination. These conflicting requirements are ideally met by using a separate condenser for each objective, but this is impractical (although microscopes have been made with such an arrangement). Most manufacturers provide a range of two or three condensers, from which the most appropriate is chosen for the job in hand.

High-magnification photomicrography requires relatively intense illumination of a small area in the object plane, by a light beam with a high NA. The condenser (Fig 7.5) needs to be highly corrected. For this purpose, manufacturers usually supply an expensive high-quality condenser, typically with an achromatic-aplanatic correction and an NA of about 1·4. To use such a condenser correctly requires immersion oil between its top surface and the slide; it is designed to give excellent results at high magnification, more strictly at NAs of 0·65 or greater, but the field of view of objectives below about 20× will not be covered.

Medium-magnification photomicrography, with objectives of 25×–10×, requires moderate illumination intensities covering a medium-sized area in the object plane, by a light beam with an NA of about 0·20–0·50. The condenser needs to be well corrected. The achromatic-aplanatic type is best, if it covers the field, but such a high correction is not strictly necessary. For this purpose, manufacturers normally supply a routine-quality condenser, typically with an achromatic correction and an NA of about 1·25. Used under the conditions stated, immersion oil between its top surface and the slide is not essential, but co-author Ron's practice is to oil all condensers designed for immersion, ie those with an NA greater than 1·0, whatever the objective magnification. Condensers of this type give adequate results at medium magnification, but will not cover the field of view of objectives below about 10×, and are unlikely to be good enough for photomicrography with the highest-power objectives, for which the achromatic-aplanatic type is preferred. An alternative approach for medium magnifications, currently fashionable and probably to be preferred, is to use a condenser of NA 0·9, with a swingout top lens (Fig 7.6). Such condensers do not have the highest optical correction, but because they will be used under the conditions for which they were designed, ie not immersed, will produce a more strictly controlled lighting system than the 1.25 NA condenser used without immersion.

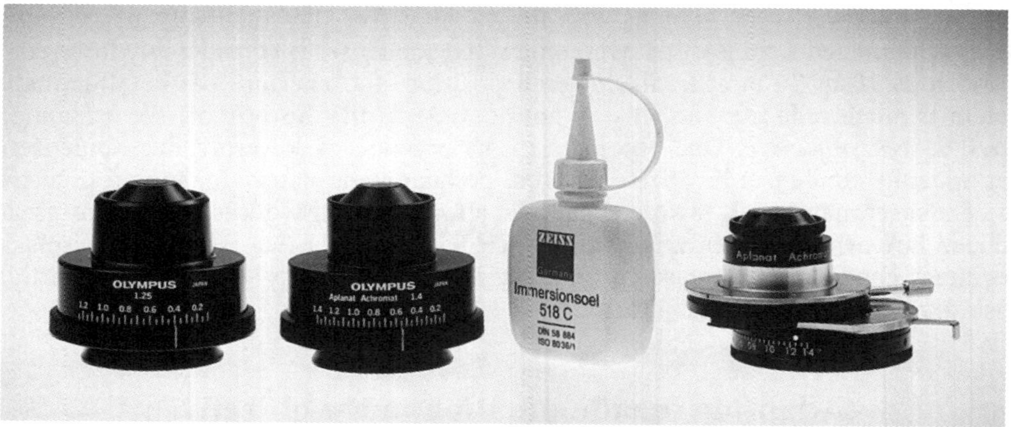

Fig 7.5. Types of brightfield condenser for high-magnification work. Left to right: Olympus achromatic-aplanatic condenser NA 1·4, Olympus achromatic condenser NA 1·25, a bottle of Zeiss immersion oil with DIN specifications, and an earlier model Olympus condenser NA 1·4 with shifting aperture diaphragm. In the latter, sideways displacement of the diaphragm effectively increases the NA and permits greater resolving power of structures at right angles to the direction of displacement.

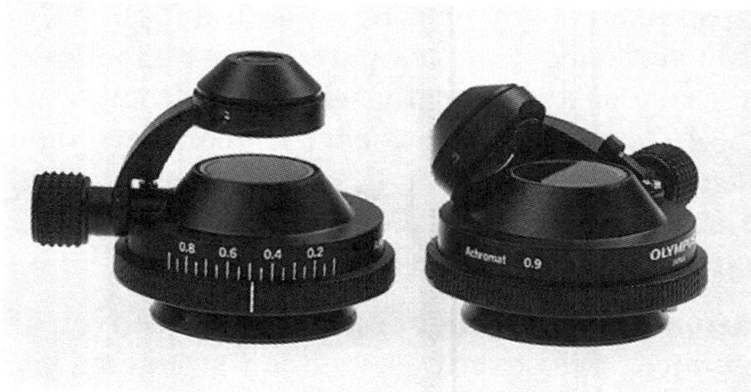

Fig 7.6. A brightfield condenser for medium-magnification work. Olympus, NA 0·9, with swing-out top for low and medium magnifications.

Low-magnification photomicrography, with objectives of 10×–4×, requires illumination of less intensity but of a largish area in the object plane, by a light beam with an NA of about 0·10–0·20. When using low power merely for the finding of a particular feature or suitable part of the specimen for more detailed examination under higher magnification, it is unnecessary to fuss unduly over the quality of an image; but for those instances where low-power images should have the best possible quality (eg for photography) it may come as a surprise that correct and even illumination is much more difficult with the lowest powers than with the high powers. As the magnification decreases, the field diameter increases, leading to difficulties in obtaining uniform illumination of the larger fields.

Typically, manufacturers provide a routine condenser with an NA of about 0·9–1·25 (as described above), of which the top lens can be swung aside by a lever for use at low powers. Otherwise, the top lens needs to be unscrewed. In either case, the condenser will need to be re-focused to maintain Köhler illumination; or the manufacturer may incorporate auxiliary condenser lenses, operated by a lever movement, to perform this re-focusing. In some models, the condenser without its top lens will not produce Köhler illumination (to save cost). The instructions of the manufacturer need to be consulted for the particular design of illumination system. One problem with any 'swingout' attachment is that it will not maintain its centration forever.

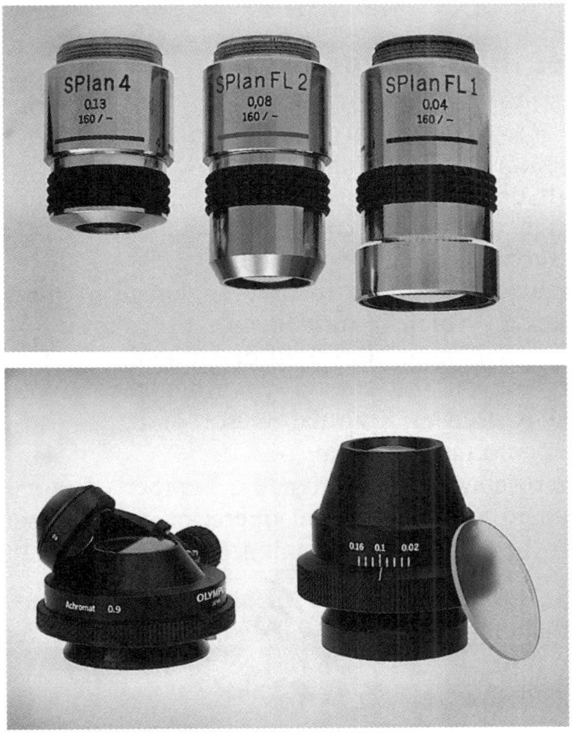

Fig 7.7. Olympus objectives and condensers for low and ultralow-power magnifications.

Top, left to right, Olympus objectives for low-power (4×) and ultralow-power (2×, 1×) work.

Bottom, left, standard Olympus condenser with the top lens swung out, giving adequate illumination for the 4× objective. Right, Olympus ultralow-power condenser specifically designed for the three low-power objectives (4×, 2×, 1×), and a ground-glass diffusing screen ('filter') to assist in producing even illumination.

With low-power objectives it is difficult to maintain even illumination to the edges of the field. The edges of the field tend to be dark – this is described as *vignetting* of the field. Some manufacturers incorporate removable ground-glass filters in the illumination path, or orange-peel finishes to the collector lens. The ground-glass filter is usually placed near to the lamp filament, and this is an acceptable compromise, giving minimum loss of light control; the unwelcome effect of contrast loss due to scattering of light rays is minimised.

Ultralow-power condensers

The wide field of objectives with a magnification 6× or lower creates some special problems. An ordinary condenser gives adequate illumination only for the central area of the field, leaving the periphery of the field relatively dark. The correct solution is an ultralow-power condenser (Fig 7.7), but they are quite expensive. Such a condenser gives a wide, uniformly illuminated field, of appropriate NA for the lowest-power objectives, including 1×. Ideally, the ultralow-power condenser should be used with all objectives having a magnification of less than 10×. If an ultralow-power condenser is too expensive, or not available for the particular microscope, there are alternatives (a ground-glass diffuser, lowering of the condenser, or doing without a condenser altogether) described in Chapter 4.

Köhler illumination

Köhler illumination is named after its inventor, August Köhler (1866–1948), who devised the system specifically for photography through the microscope. For all aspects of microscopy, including routine observation, it is now regarded as the preferred form of illumination. Its only disadvantages are that its luminous efficiency may be poor under conditions of high microscope magnification, and that it adds considerably to the cost of the microscope.

In Köhler illumination (Fig 7.8), a collector lens focuses an image of the light source into the aperture of the condenser, which in turn focuses the aperture of the collector into the object plane. An iris diaphragm, the field diaphragm, is placed on the optical axis near the collector lens on the side away from the lamp; this diaphragm is evenly illuminated, and is used as a virtual source of light. The field diaphragm is imaged by the condenser onto the specimen.

The various manufacturers of microscopes have designed a number of modes in which the basic Köhler system is obtained with convenient operation for the user. In general, all the systems have the following features in common:

- An image of the light source is focused onto the plane of the aperture iris diaphragm (ie the condenser iris diaphragm) (see Fig 7.9). Focusing is effected by relative movement of a lens (the collector lens) with respect to the filament. The lamp collector lens is sometimes called the *Köhler lens*.
- An image of the field iris diaphragm is projected onto the specimen field, using the condenser focusing mechanism for this process (see Fig 7.10). When this is effected, opening of the field iris will cause more of the specimen field to be illuminated, closing of the field iris will cause less of the specimen field to be illuminated. This affords control over the area of illumination, ie a control over the illuminated field of view. If more of the specimen field is illuminated than is observed through the eyepiece or in the camera, the image will suffer from a lack of contrast.
- The NA of the condenser is matched to the NA of the objective in use (see Fig 7.11). This affords control over the angle of illumination, and therefore the effective NA of the objective. This is the specific function of the condenser iris diaphragm, and it is therefore regarded as the *aperture diaphragm* (also known as the *aperture stop*).

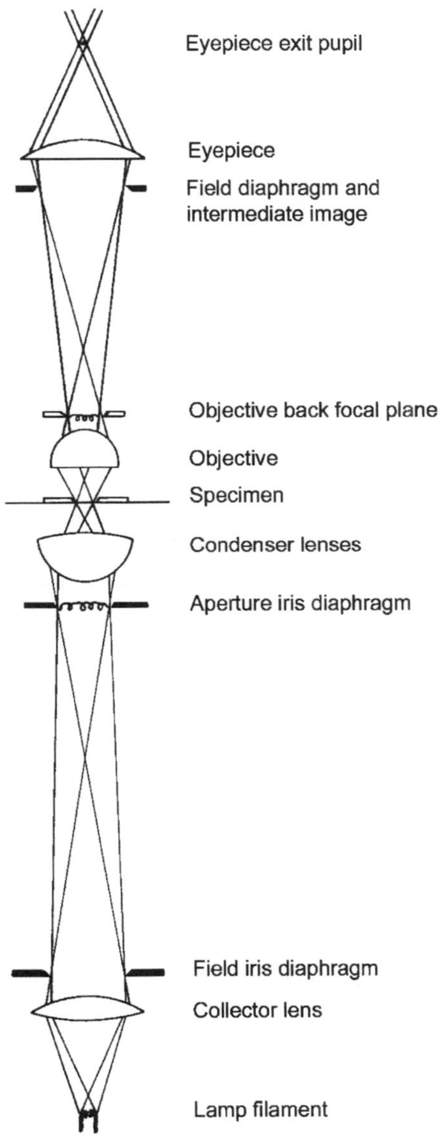

Fig 7.8. Köhler illumination: a schematic representation.

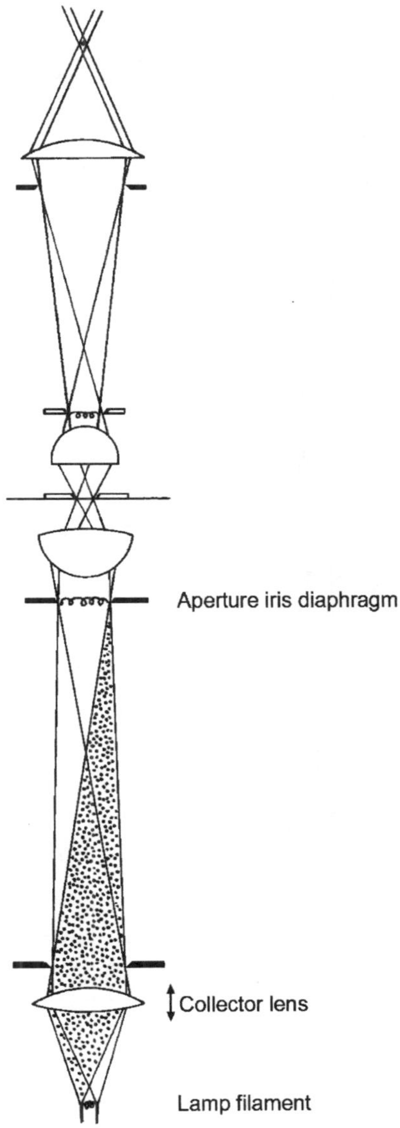

Fig 7.9. Köhler illumination, Stage I. The lamp filament is focused by the lamp collector lens onto the condenser iris diaphragm.

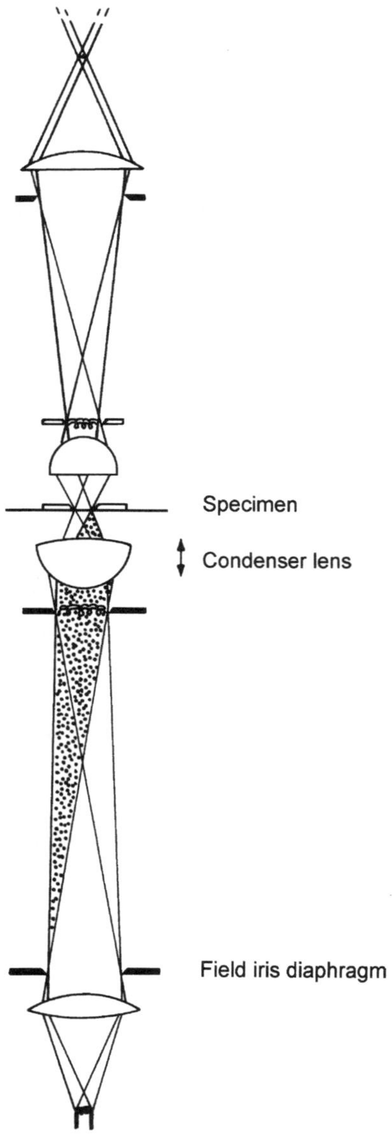

Fig 7.10. Köhler illumination, Stage II. The field diaphragm is focused by the condenser onto the specimen.

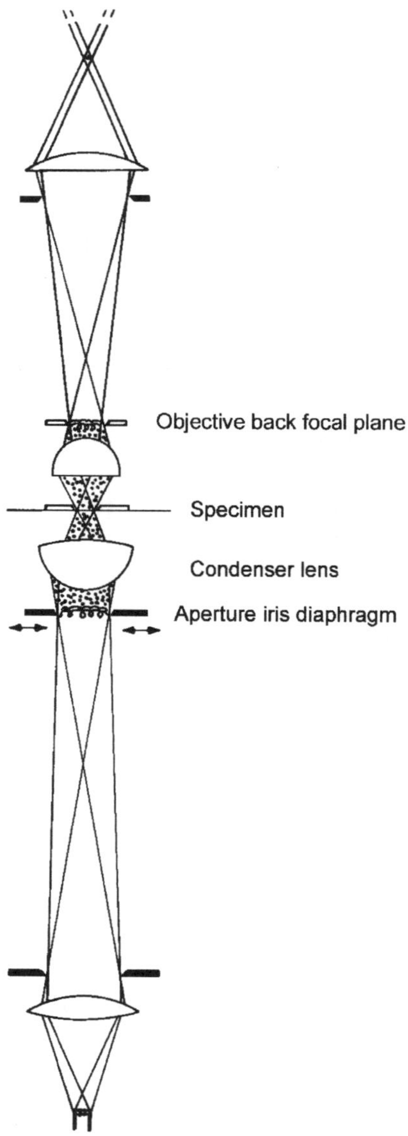

Fig 7.11. Köhler illumination, Stage III. The NA of the condenser is matched to that of the objective, using the condenser aperture diaphragm.

Conjugate planes in Köhler illumination

In a geometrical construction of lens systems, use is made of the concept of *object points* and *image points*. However, the positions of object and image are interchangeable, and the object point and image point are said to be conjugate. The planes that contain the points and which are at right angles to the axis of the optical system are called conjugate planes. In a microscope there are two sets of conjugate planes, namely *field planes* and *aperture planes*, listed in Table 7.1 and shown in Figs 7.12 and 7.13. It will be seen that there is a successive alternation of these planes from the filament of the light source to the final microscope image (Table 7.1).

Field planes (Fig 7.12 and Table 7.1) are associated with the specimen field and the images of that field. A pointer or graticule placed in any one of these planes will be superimposed on the image. A diaphragm placed in any one of these planes will limit the diameter of the image. Filters are best not placed in field planes, because dust on them can appear in the final image. The fact that the field diaphragm is in a field plane can be put to good use. Anything placed in the field diaphragm plane will appear in the image plane, and can be photographed. In practice, one can place a transparent object just above the field diaphragm, and re-focus the condenser slightly to bring it into focus. Photographic films can be identified by recording one's name and/or a serial number. Co-author Fred has used this arrangement with a CCTV (video) system used for teaching histology; a complete section, if not too big, can be demonstrated by placing it in this position, and 35 mm transparencies can be shown. The optical quality of the image is limited by that of the condenser.

Aperture planes (Fig 7.13 and Table 7.1) are the planes of the condenser iris diaphragm and of its conjugates. Collectively, these planes are known as aperture planes because the NA of the optical system can be controlled by fixed or iris diaphragms inserted in these positions.

Table 7.1. Field and aperture planes with Köhler illumination

Field planes	Aperture planes
Image (retina or film)	
	Eyepiece exit pupil
Intermediate image plane	
	Objective back focal plane
Specimen plane	
	Condenser iris (aperture stop)
Field stop (Köhler diaphragm)	
	Light source (lamp filament)

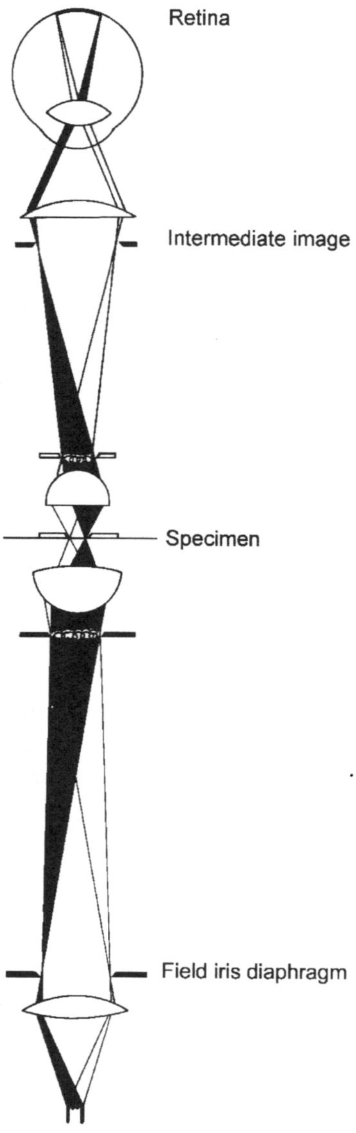

Fig 7.12. Conjugate planes of the specimen (field planes), in Köhler illumination.

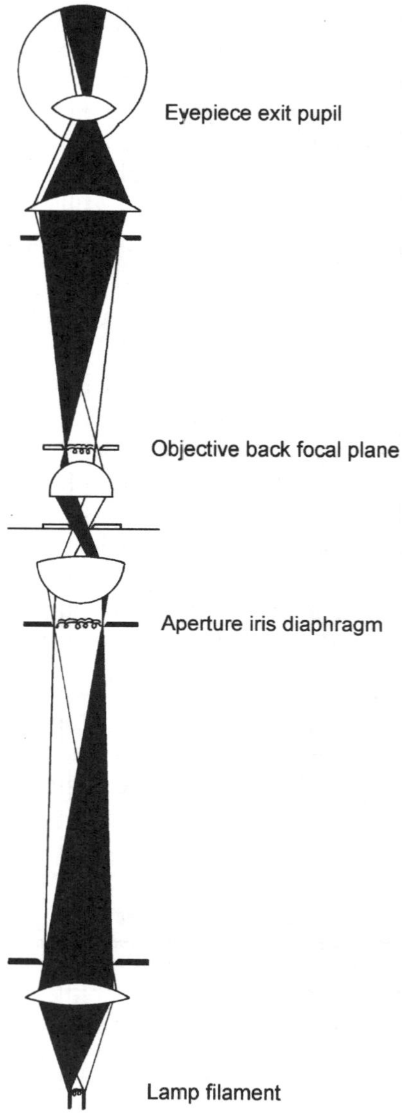

Fig 7.13. Conjugate planes of the light source (aperture planes), in Köhler illumination.

The field stop and the aperture stop

The two iris diaphragms, one which forms part of the substage condenser, the other which is usually but not always near the lamp, can lead to confusion in microscope operation. When the microscope is properly set for Köhler illumination, their differences are as outlined in Table 7.2.

More detailed instructions for Köhler illumination, found in manufacturers'' instruction books, will vary according to the ways in which the particular manufacturer chooses to meet the requirements stated above.

Table 7.2. The field stop and the aperture stop

Field stop	Aperture stop
Usually placed close to the collector lens	Placed at the condenser front focal plane
Controls area of illuminated field	Controls aperture of system
Will not affect NA of system	Will not affect area of illumination
Is imaged onto the specimen plane	Is imaged in the objective BFP
Does not affect image intensity	Affects image intensity (especially if reduced below two-thirds of the objective's NA)
Affects image contrast (stray light)	Affects image contrast and resolution

Checking Köhler illumination

There are two quick tests to check for the adequacy of the illumination, worth carrying out routinely and often.

Checking the field diaphragm. Slightly close the field iris diaphragm. When looking through the microscope, the field diaphragm should come into the field of view, be sharply superimposed on the specimen, and be centred to the objective field.

Looking at the objective's back focal plane (BFP). When the image quality is unsatisfactory, the experienced microscopist will usually start troubleshooting by checking the objective aperture. This is most easily done by removing an eyepiece, but some research microscopes may have a built-in lens system so that the BFP can be examined while one is looking through the eyepieces. In the BFP the following errors, if present, should make themselves evident:

- Uneven illumination, such as a poorly centred lamp filament.
- Failure to fill the objective aperture with light, thus reducing its effective NA. The condenser iris is set to about $^7/_8$ths of this aperture (Fig 7.3), unless there are special demands for depth of field or contrast.
- Any obstruction to the aperture, such as poorly centred lenses and auxiliary fittings, a condenser wrongly focused, or dirt within the lenses.
- The presence of air bubbles in immersion oil, either above or below the specimen. Air bubbles will appear as dark discs in the bright image of the light source.

Setting up Köhler illumination

To set up Köhler illumination, a sequence of operations similar to the following will usually be required.

1. It is essential to have a high-contrast specimen in the specimen plane, on which to focus the microscope and to define the specimen plane. The slide on which the specimen is supported must be thin enough to enable the condenser to be focused properly.
2. After rough alignment of the microscope, raise the condenser to its upper limit, and obtain an image of the specimen with a low-power (eg 10×) objective.
3. Project an image of the lamp filament onto the under surface of the condenser iris diaphragm. (Alas, not possible with some modern microscopes!)
4. Adjust the condenser focus so that a sharp image of the field diaphragm (field stop) is superimposed onto the specimen field. Centre the image of the field diaphragm. Open the field diaphragm until its image just disappears from the field of view when one is looking through the microscope – this controls the area of illumination. Since the condenser is not usually a highly corrected lens system, difficulty may be encountered in determining the position of the condenser focus when one is using high-power objectives. The outline of the field stop may appear hazy, and have a boundary which changes colour as the condenser is focused, due to chromatic aberration in the condenser. As a working rule, when in doubt, the upper focus of the condenser is the one to employ. The use of a green filter will eliminate the colour fringes.
5. Remove an eyepiece, and check that the objective's back focal plane (BFP) is uniformly filled with light. Stop down the aperture (condenser) iris until its image is seen in the objective's BFP. Then adjust the condenser iris until its image fills about $^{7}/_{8}$ths of the diameter of the objective's BFP. Replace the eyepiece and check the image.
6. Intensity control of the image is effected by controlling the lamp with a rheostat or filters, not by the condenser diaphragm.
7. Further adjustment of the condenser diaphragm may be needed, to obtain the desired contrast and depth of field.
8. With each change of objective lens, adjustments will need to be made to the field diaphragm (for the changed area of field), and the condenser diaphragm (for the changed requirements of numerical aperture (NA)).

Illumination with part of the condenser aperture

For various reasons, stops may be placed in the aperture plane of the condenser (Fig 7.13). The main types of illumination for which this is done are as follows.

Köhler illumination. An iris stop is used to limit the aperture of the condenser to that of the objective, or somewhat less, to control the NA of the system, as described above.

Darkground illumination. A central stop (Fig 14d), corresponding to the aperture of the objective, is used to block light from entering the objective directly; the specimen is illuminated by very oblique rays. This method is described in Chapter 9.

Rheinberg illumination. This is similar to darkground illumination, except that the central stop is coloured rather than opaque, and the peripheral part may be coloured in a contrasting colour (see Chapter 9 and Plate 4). The peripheral part may have more than one colour.

Phase contrast. A stop with an annular aperture (in effect, the combination of an outer stop and a central stop) produces a ring-shaped cone of light, used in conjunction with a special plate in the objective (see Chapter 10).

Oblique lighting. Interesting effects can be obtained if the cone of light used for illumination is incomplete (Fig 7.14a,b,c). This can be achieved in three ways. In one method, a quadrant (pieslice-shaped) stop blocks one-quarter (approximately) of the cone of illumination (Fig 7.14a). The result is a three-dimensional appearance (Fig 7.15). A similar effect can be obtained with an off-centre condenser (Fig 7.14b), or with a stop with an eccentric aperture (Fig 7.14c).

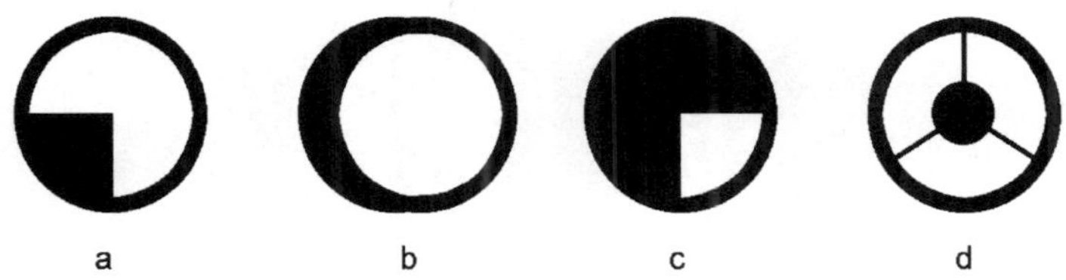

Fig 7.14. Aperture stops. (a), (b) and (c), oblique lighting; (d), darkground illumination.

Illumination of opaque objects

Epi-illumination

Light can be directed downwards onto the specimen through the objective (Fig 7.16) or by a built-in circular mirror surrounding the objective (Fig 9.4). This is usually called *epi-illumination*. As in transillumination, the illumination may be within the aperture cone of the objective (brightfield illumination) or outside it (darkground illumination). In brightfield epi-illumination, reflected light from the specimen is viewed, rather than transmitted light. All the other various modalities of optical microscopy (darkground, phase contrast, DIC, fluorescence) are equally possible using epi-illumination. Epi-illumination is necessary for opaque specimens; it is usually advantageous for fluorescence, whether the specimen is opaque or not (see Chapter 11). There are several methods by which epi-illumination can be achieved. The most common method uses a semi-transparent mirror placed above the objective. An alternative is by a prism placed above the objective (blocking part of its aperture). Some objectives are designed with an epi-illumination light path surrounding them. Epi-illumination is shown diagramatically in Figs 7.16, 7.17, 9.4 and 11.3; equipment is shown in Fig 11.2; and examples of photomicrographs obtained using epi-illumination are given in Figs 9.5, 9.6, and 11.1, and Plates 7, 12b, 13, and 15.

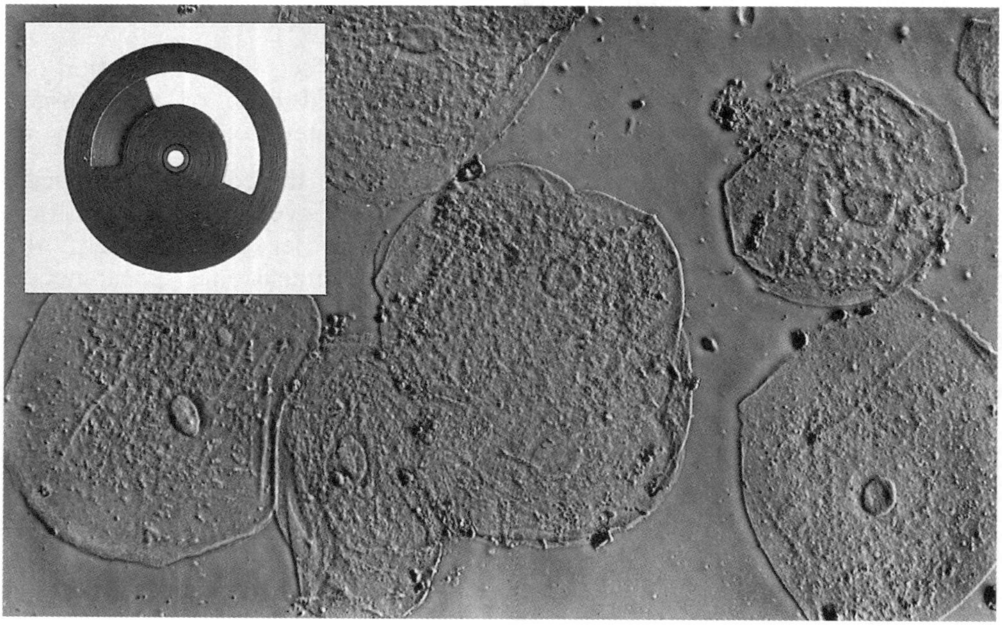

Fig 7.15. Photomicrograph showing the three-dimensional appearance obtained with oblique lighting. Human mouth epithelial cells, unstained. Field size 150 µm × 250 µm. Partial condenser aperture, as shown in the inset. Try the effect of turning the picture upside-down!

Semi-transparent mirror

In one form of epi-illumination, light is directed onto a semi-transparent mirror situated in the body tube of the microscope over the objective lens. Light is reflected by the mirror down through the objective onto the specimen. The objective thereby serves as the condenser, focusing the light onto the exact area being examined. The use of a semi-transparent mirror is the simplest to arrange, and has the advantage that the full NA of the objective is used for both illumination and for observation; on the other hand, it may suffer badly from flare, may give ghost images, and presents difficulties for polarisation studies. For fluorescence microscopy, because the excitation and emission are at different wavelengths, modern epi-illumination mirrors are *dichromatic*, designed to reflect preferentially at the excitation wavelength, and to transmit preferentially at the fluorescence wavelength (see Chapter 11).

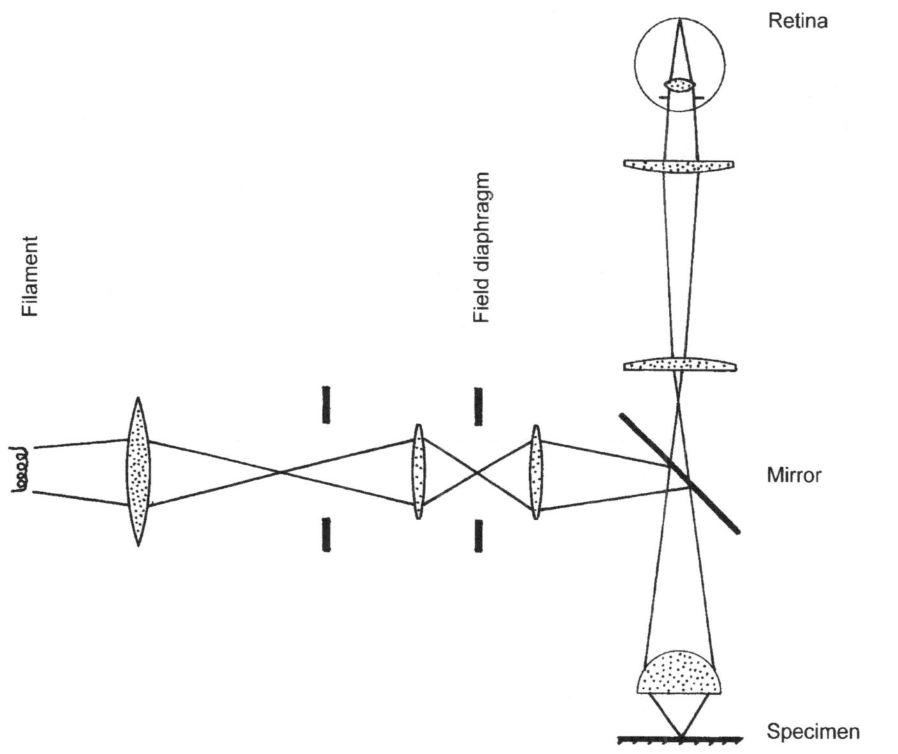

Fig 7.16. Epi-illumination. Conjugate planes of the specimen (field planes), in Köhler illumination.

Epi-illumination by prisms

For studies involving polarisation, a beamsplitter is not ideal because the amount of polarised light reflected or transmitted by a beamsplitter depends upon the orientation of the plane of polarisation. Therefore, for the more critical purposes, a prism is placed above the objective, occupying part of its aperture.

Darkground epi-illumination

Epi-illumination by a mirror surrounding the objective is described in Chapter 9 under the heading Epi-illumination darkground systems.

Field and aperture diaphragms in epi-illumination

The field diaphragm is focused onto the field of view (as in transmitted-light illumination) and is usually set so that its margins are just outside the field of view.

The field diaphragm is in a plane conjugate with that of the eyepiece diaphragm, because (on the one hand) the objective focuses an image of the field diaphragm onto the subject, and (on the other hand) the objective focuses an image of the subject onto the eyepiece diaphragm. When objectives are changed, the demagnification of the field diaphragm onto the specimen and the magnification of the object into the eyepiece are altered equally, so that the field diaphragm does not need to be re-set (in contrast to the arrangement with transillumination).

The aperture diaphragm has similar effects on resolution and contrast as in transillumination. For full discussion, see Chapter 15. Accordingly, the aperture diaphragm should be set for each objective. With opaque specimens of low contrast, reducing the *field* iris considerably increases image contrast. This unexpected effect is due to the minimising of reflections in the illumination system.

Objectives. The exit pupil of the objective serves as an entrance pupil for the epi-illumination system. Therefore, objectives with a large exit pupil are able to accept more light from the epi-illumination system, and give a brighter image.

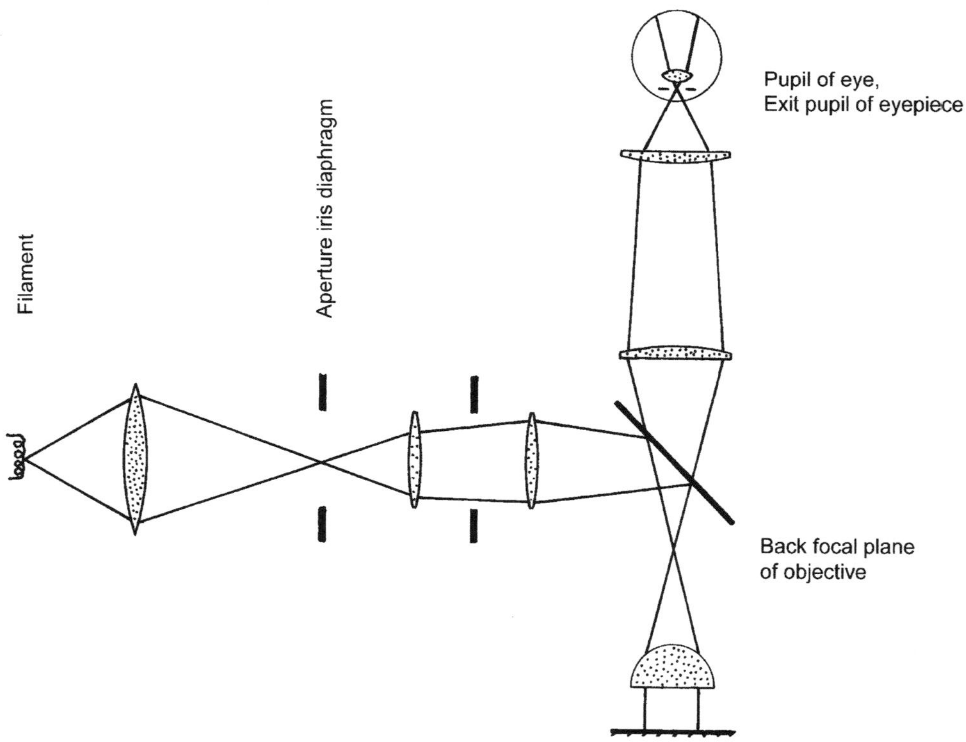

Fig 7.17. Epi-illumination. Conjugate planes of the light source (aperture planes), in Köhler epi-illumination.

Relationship of NA, magnification and intensity

Epi-illumination through the objective gives increasingly bright images as the magnification is increased, whereas the reverse is usually the case with transmitted light. Theoretically, the intensity of illumination depends upon two factors: (1) the square of the NA of the condenser, and (2) the square of the demagnification of the image of the light source (ie as the image of the field diaphragm is made smaller, it becomes brighter according to the square law). Similarly, the brilliance of the image of the specimen as it reaches the eyepiece is directly proportional to the square of the NA of the objective, and also inversely proportional to the square of the magnification. Hence, in transmitted light, changing the objective (without altering the condenser) results in changes to the brightness of the image according to the changes in NA and magnification of the objective. With epi-illumination, the same considerations apply, but because the objective acts as its own condenser, the intensity of illumination and therefore of the final image depend upon the squares of the NA and magnification of the objective. As the magnification of the objective increases, the image of the specimen is magnified more, but the image of the light source is demagnified by the same amount; these effects cancel out and therefore the brilliance of the final image is independent of the objective's magnification and depends only on the fourth power of its NA. In practice, the effect of changing objectives may be affected also by differences in the diameter of the rear of the objective and the matching of the illumination beam to that.

External illumination of opaque objects

Opaque objects can be illuminated by sources separate from the microscope. Possibilities include a spot lamp and fibre-optic illuminators (see Chapters 4 and 13).

Special modalities of illumination

The techiques described above are those generally applicable to all modalities of microscopy. For some puposes, particularly for increasing contrast, the standard illumination system requires modifications. Some of these are described in subsequent chapters, for darkground (including Rheinberg illumination) in Chapter 9, polarised light (Chapter 10), phase-contrast and interference-contrast microscopy (Chapter 10), fluorescence microscopy (Chapter 11) and infrared and ultraviolet light (Chapter 12). The uses of coloured or monochromatic light are discussed in Chapters 11 (fluorescence) and 15 (use of filters to increase contrast of coloured objects).

8
Lamps and filters

This chapter describes the main types of lamp and other sources of illumination suitable for microscopy, and also filters that may be used to modify the light.

Light sources

Daylight

Daylight and sunlight are now rarely used for microscopy, because they are unreliable, only available during daylight hours, and can be accessed only in the open or near a window. Also, sunlight is excessively bright, and should never be used for visual observation because of the risk of injury to the eye. White clouds and blue sky are useable; for photomicrography in colour, the blueness of blue sky needs to be corrected with a colour-correction filter (see below).

Artificial-light sources

The essential characteristic of an artificial-light source is a sufficiently intense output at the required wavelengths. Lamps can be compared objectively in terms of their total light output, spectral distribution of emitted light, intensity of light at a particular wavelength, the brilliance of the incandescent area, and their stability. The main types of lamp are incandescent (tungsten) filament lamps and gas-discharge (arc) lamps. Lasers are used in confocal microscopy.

Tungsten-filament lamps

Modern microscopes are most commonly equipped with incandescent tungsten–halogen lamps. Older microscopes used conventional tungsten-filament lamps, which deteriorate markedly with age, becoming blackened on the inside. The microscope lamp is powered by an electric current, which is regulated by a rheostat to adjust the intensity and colour of the light. There should be a meter (ammeter) to measure the current passing through the lamp, or a voltmeter to measure the voltage across the filament (measurement of current is said to be preferable, but we have no evidence about it). Some modern microscopes have, by way of a meter, an array of luminous diodes; these are more robust and cheaper than a meter, but if there are only a few diodes in the array, the current can only be set to a limited number of values, corresponding to the values at which the next diode is not quite lit.

Conventional tungsten-filament lamps (Fig 8.1) contain, as the name suggests, a tungsten filament in a transparent bulb; the filament is heated to incandescence by an electric current. The envelope may be of glass or of silica (quartz); the latter is better able to withstand high temperatures. The bulb contains an inert gas (such as argon) which does not react with the filament even at high temperatures. Because of the high temperature of the filament, some of the tungsten evaporates and deposits on the inside of the envelope, which is cooler; this has two deleterious effects, namely a gradual blackening of the bulb (reducing the lamp output) and a corresponding diminution of the substance of the filament, which ultimately fuses.

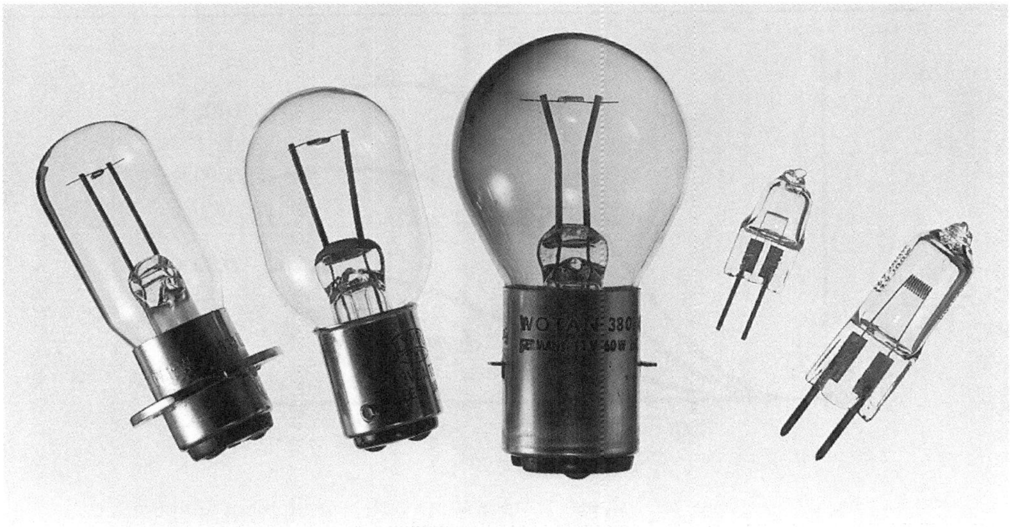

Fig 8.1. Lamps for microscopy. The three on the left are conventional low-voltage lamps; note the blackening of the big lamp. The two tungsten–halogen lamps on the right are much smaller, and also have more blue emission because they run hotter.

Tungsten–halogen lamps (Fig 8.1), also known as quartz–iodine (QI) lamps, are modern versions of tungsten-filament lamps, and are the preferred light source for most microscopy. Iodine vapour inside the bulb has the effect of causing any vaporised tungsten to be re-deposited on the filament. Also, these lamps have a small quartz envelope that runs at a high temperature (over 260 °C, or over 530 K), which further reduces deposition of metal. In consequence, the filament of these lamps can be run at a much higher temperature. It is important not to touch the envelope when installing one of these lamps, because even the small amount of grease on one's fingers, when baked onto the envelope, darkens and may weaken it. Because of the higher filament temperature, the lamps are more efficient, and emit a greater proportion of short-wavelength (blue) light. The necessity to run the filament at a specific temperature for colour work (see Fig 8.2) is discussed in Chapter 3 (under Colour photomicrography) and below (under Colour-compensation filters).

Gas-discharge lamps

Gas-discharge lamps consist of two electrodes surrounded by an appropriate gas in a quartz (silica) envelope. On application of a high enough voltage to start an arc, a small number of electrons present in the gas are accelerated by the electrostatic field until their energies become large enough to ionise the gas by collisions with neutral particles. The ions act as new current carriers, and the ionisation rate increases in a cascade effect. The electric current keeps the electrons, ions and neutral molecules in continuous motion. The gaseous molecules become excited and then radiate photons in returning to the ground state. It is a characteristic feature of arc lamps that they require a very high voltage to strike the arc, which can thereafter be maintained by a low voltage. In modern power supply units, the ignition voltage is applied automatically.

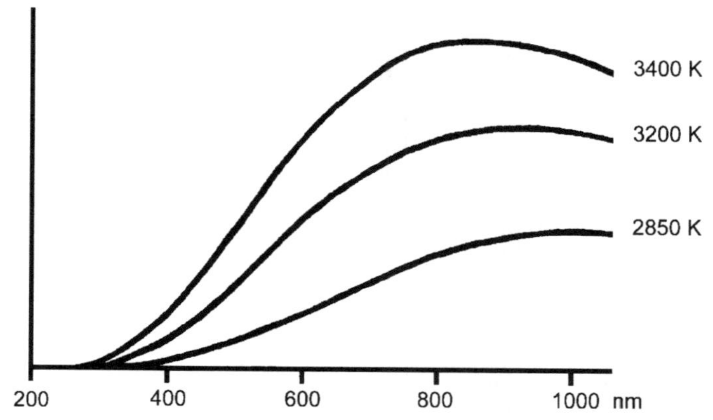

Fig 8.2. Spectra of tungsten–halogen lamp at three different filament temperatures.

Mercury arc lamps are widely used for fluorescence microscopy. Their suitability is based on their intense light emission, and the relative simplicity of the power supply required. The major part of the energy of the emitted light is concentrated in a few narrow bands, corresponding to mercury emission lines, with a much weaker broad spectrum radiation. The major bands are at wavelengths of about 365, 405, 436 and 546 nm (Fig 8.3). Each of these bands can be selected with a filter, and each one has specific applications for excitation in fluorescence microscopy. The disadvantages of these lamps are the need for an expensive power supply unit, the small arc size making it difficult to fill the aperture of the condenser for Köhler illumination, and a tendency to flicker due to positional instability. Some modern systems have an intensity control. Some advice on the maintenance of these lamps is given in Appendix A1.

Metal halide lamps are similar to mercury arc lamps, but have additional gases in the envelope, giving a more uniform spectrum. They are not used at present for microscopy.

Xenon arc lamps are similar in construction and operation to mercury arcs. However their spectral characteristics are quite different. There is a broad band of emission in the visible region, together with a substantial emission in the ultraviolet (UV). Because of the absence of prominent spectral lines, xenon arcs give a substantially 'white' light, which also makes them suitable for colour photography and for all forms of microscopy. The capital cost of xenon arcs is greater than that of mercury arcs. However, the life of individual lamps is proportionally greater, so that the actual running cost per hour may be less for xenon arcs. The disadvantages of these lamps are the need for an expensive power supply unit, and a small arc size, making it difficult to fill the aperture of the condenser for Köhler illumination.

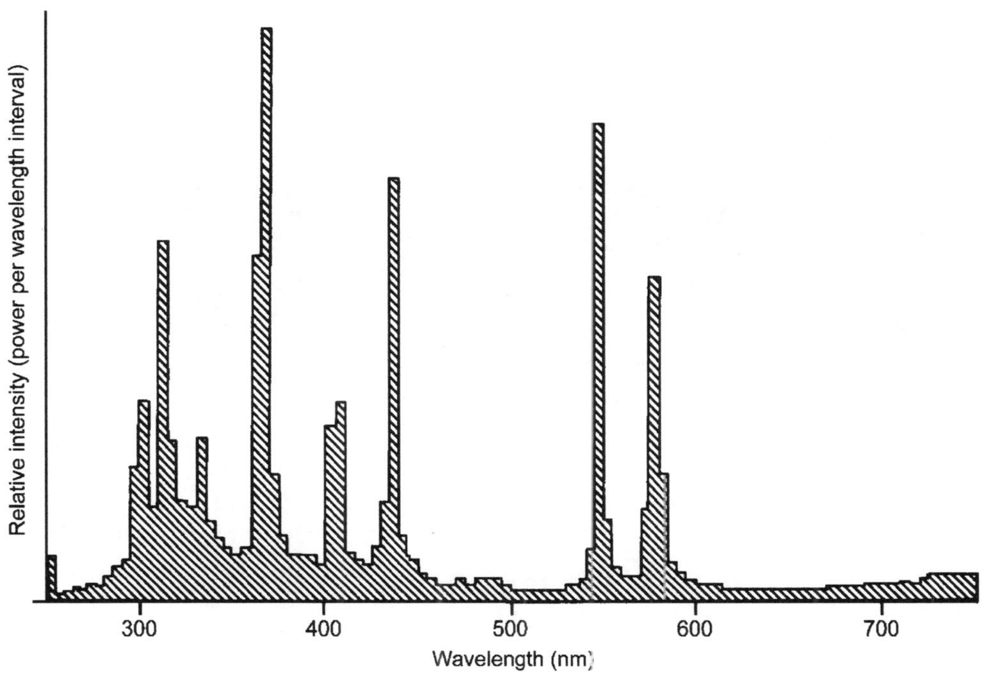

Fig 8.3. The spectral distribution of light emitted from a high-pressure mercury arc lamp. Data of a Philips CS 200W-2 lamp, redrawn after manufacturer's data, courtesy of Philips Lighting Industries.

Electronic flash

An electronic flash unit (Fig 8.4) is essentially a xenon arc, powered intermittently in single bursts. The length of a flash is typically about 0·1 ms to 1 ms (1/10 000 second to 1/1000 second). In principle, a flash can be used for all forms of optical photomicrography. An electronic flash has the same colour temperature as a xenon arc, namely about 6000 K. This means that it can be used with daylight film, either without a filter or with a warming filter to reduce the colour temperature to about 5400 K. For microscopy, the main advantage of flash is that it is possible to photograph moving objects. For static objects, if a single flash is insufficient for the exposure, two or more successive flashes can be combined on the same frame of film.

An ordinary lamp is required for composing and focusing the picture, and therefore it is usual to arrange either a beamsplitter device or a system whereby the flash is focused by a collector lens into the plane of the lamp filament, the normal illumination pathway being used from there on.

Lasers

A laser is a device for producing pure monochromatic light in a coherent beam. Lasers are not at present appropriate for general observational microscopy, but are ideal for quantification. They are used for confocal microscopy (see Chapter 17).

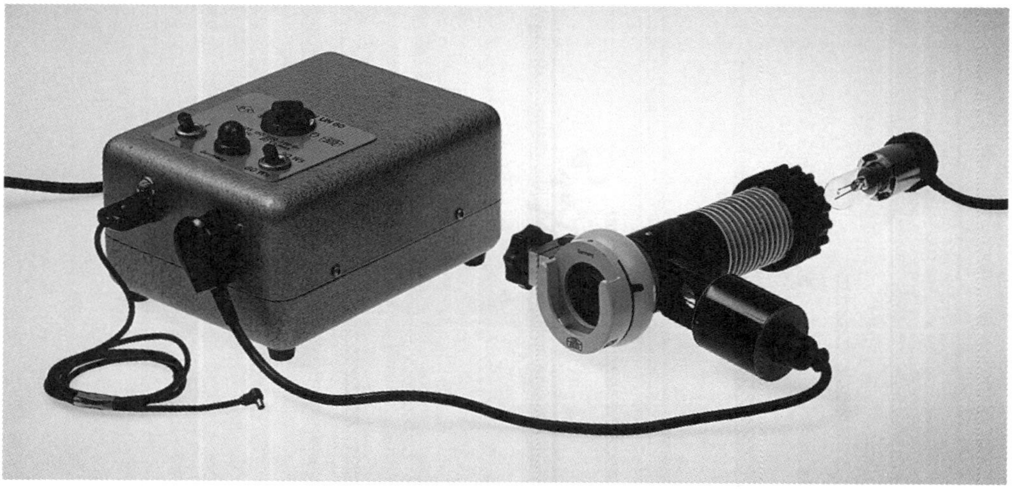

Fig 8.4. Zeiss electronic flash system for a microscope.

The lamphouse

The lamphouse is essentially a mechanical arrangement to hold the lamp and collector lens, sometimes with a reflector, heat filter and other filters.

The collector lens functions to collect as much as possible of the light emitted by the lamp, and to concentrate it into a beam directed at the condenser. The focal length of the collector lens must be appropriate for the particular lamp, so that an image of the lamp of appropriate size (ie completely filling the condenser aperture) is projected into the aperture of the condenser. For this reason, different collector lenses are required for different lamps, depending upon the dimensions of the filament or arc. Some collector lenses have one surface modified (as ground-glass or 'orange-peel') to act as a diffuser. This is not necessarily a good idea. For use in the UV range below about 360 nm, a quartz-glass collector lens is required, since optical glass does not transmit adequately. For the 365 nm mercury line, there is no need for quartz.

Filters

Filters are optical elements that selectively transmit or reflect light. Coloured filters preferentially absorb light of some wavelengths and preferentially transmit at other wavelengths, thereby colouring the light. Filters are used mainly for:

- Reducing the intensity of the light.
- Removing heat.
- Correcting the colour temperature of the light source.
- Changing the contrast of coloured areas, using black-and-white (B&W) film.
- Providing (relatively) monochromatic light to avoid chromatic aberration.
- Polarisation – selecting a preferred direction of vibration.
- Selecting excitation and observation wavelengths for fluorescence microscopy.
- Special effects of colour.
- Selecting short wavelengths for maximum resolution.

Nomenclature

The nomenclature of filters is, unfortunately, inconsistent and confusing. For example, a 'heat filter' is one which *absorbs* heat; whereas a 'green filter' is one which *transmits* green, absorbing every other colour! We ought really to refer to these as 'heat-absorbing' and 'green-transmitting', respectively.

Spectral characteristics of filters

Neutral density (grey) filters give a nearly constant transmission over a wide range of wavelengths (Fig 8.5a). There are employed to reduce the intensity of light.

Longpass (LP) filters preferentially transmit at long wavelengths, above a certain transition point, with minimal transmission at short wavelengths (see Fig 8.5b, c). Because they transmit at low frequencies, they are also known as *lowpass* filters. This type, with sharp cutoff (Fig 8.5c) is used for barrier filters in fluorescence microscopy.

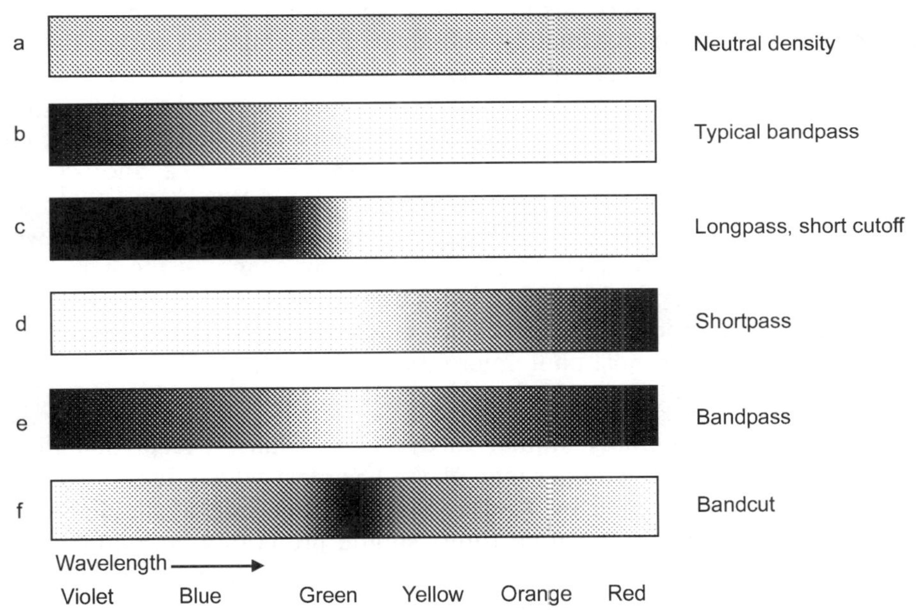

Fig 8.5. Transmission (light areas) and absorption (dark areas) of longpass, shortpass, bandpass and bandcut filters. The bandpass filter shown can be obtained by combining the longpass and shortpass filters. See also Rost, 1992, Fig. 3.9.

Shortpass (SP) filters preferentially transmit at short wavelengths, below a particular transition point, and transmit minimally at longer wavelengths (see Fig 8.5d). Because they transmit at high frequencies they can also be termed highpass filters. This type is required for use as excitation filters for fluorescence microscopy.

Bandpass (BP) filters have a bell-shaped transmission curve, transmitting maximally at a particular wavelength and less at shorter and longer wavelengths (see Fig 8.5e). A common example is a green filter.

Bandcut filters have characteristics inverse to those of bandpass filters: they transmit at all wavelengths except over a narrow range (Fig 8.5f). They are often referred to as *minus* filters, eg a 'minus-blue' filter transmits all wavelengths except blue.

Types of coloured filter

Several optical devices are available for monochromation (ie selective transmission of a specified wavelength band). These are: coloured glass, gelatine or liquid filters, interference filters and mirrors, and prism and grating monochromators.

Glass filters are of two basic classes. In the first, the colour is due to ions in true solution in the glass. In the second, known as temperature-coloured glasses, the colour is due to submicroscopic crystals, the optical effect of which depends on their composition and size. The final characteristics of the glass are obtained by heat treatment of an originally clear glass.

The transmission characteristics of the two types are quite different. Glasses with ionic coloration have an approximately bell-shaped transmission curve; that is, they transmit preferentially in a particular, relatively narrow region. This renders them suitable for use as excitation filters for fluorescence microscopy. The obtainable range of such curves is limited. On the other hand, temperature-coloured glasses are characterised by a long-wavelength region of high transmission and a short-wavelength region of lower transmission, which happily happens to be the characteristic required of a barrier filter for fluorescence microscopy. The cutoff wavelength, between the regions of high and low transmission, can be varied by changing the heat treatment; hence, a great variety of optical characteristics can be obtained.

Glass filters for a variety of purposes are made by Schott (Schott, nd). A more limited range, adequate for most photomicrography, is made by Hoya and sold widely and relatively inexpensively by photographic retailers. Many other brands exist.

Gelatine filters are essentially similar to dye-glass filters, except that the dye is dissolved in a sheet of gelatine rather than glass. The most widely used gelatine filters are the Wratten filters supplied by Kodak. Similar filters are available from other manufacturers. For protection, gelatine filters should preferably be mounted between two layers of optical glass. Projection slide mounts are convenient for this purpose: note that slide mounts are available in several sizes, eg 35 mm, Superslide (38 mm square), 7×7 (70 mm square, for 6×6 cm or 6×4·5 cm film), and the classical lantern slide size, 85 mm square (typically for 6×7 cm film).

Polycarbonate and acetate filters are widely used for colouring light sources in photographic studios. They are inexpensive, and can be used with very hot light sources without buckling or fading. Sample swatches of filters are available, probably adequate in size for microscopy. Lee filters are available in a very wide range, and their characteristics are well documented.

Interference filters function by selective reflection and transmission, instead of selective absorption and transmission as in the filters described above. They are comparatively expensive, but have the advantages of high transmission and the possibility of narrow bandwidths. Interference filters consist of two semi-transparent mirror surfaces separated by a thin layer of transparent material (the dielectric). In practice, they normally consist of a sheet of glass, coated on one side first with one thin semi-transparent coating of metal (eg silver), then the intermediate layer, followed by the second semi-transparent metallic coating. To protect the coatings, a second glass is cemented on. Light is successively reflected, bouncing between the coatings. Interference between light from successive reflections results in transmission of light of the desired wavelength, while other wavelengths are reflected back the way they came. The wavelength of light transmitted is dependent upon the spacing of the reflective coatings. On casual inspection, an interference filter therefore appears as a mirror. The thickness of the dielectric layer, and its refractive index, critically determine the wavelengths of the transmission bands, and the amount of background transmission. The same principles apply in interference mirrors, which are used mainly as dichromatic mirrors in lamphouses and for epi-illumination devices (see Chapters 7 and 11).

Interference filters transmit light also at wavelengths that are integral multiples of the primary (first-order) wavelength. Therefore, practical interference filters always require a supplementary filter to remove higher-order transmission bands and to decrease the background. The supplementary filter is usually a coloured-glass filter cemented to one side; such combination filters show one mirror surface and one coloured surface. Tilting an interference filter changes its transmission/reflection characteristics.

Applications of filters

Heat filters (ie infrared-absorbing filters) are used to absorb heat from strong illumination. They may give a greenish cast to the light. We strongly recommend that the illumination system include a heat filter (eg Schott KG1), to minimise heating of the specimen and to avoid erroneous exposure meter readings caused by infrared light.

Neutral density (grey) filters are used to decrease the intensity of the light, eg to keep the brightness within the exposure range of the camera, particularly for colour photography with tungsten–halogen lamps run at or near full brightness in order to obtain the correct colour temperature. Inexpensive neutral density filters can be made from partially fogged B&W negative film.

Colour-temperature conversion filters are of two types: blue ones to increase the colour temperature, and amber ones to decrease it. It is usual for all microscopes to incorporate a blue filter, to convert the yellowish light from a tungsten lamp to approximately the colour of daylight. These filters are described in detail below.

Colour-correction filters are supplied in series of varying intensities of blue, cyan (minus-red), green, magenta (minus-green), red, and yellow (minus-blue). Their use is described in Chapter 15. Blue filters are used also to select short wavelengths to increase resolution (see Chapter 6).

Bandpass filters to provide relatively monochromatic light for avoiding chromatic aberration, are usually green, this being the colour most easily seen by the eye and a colour for which optical systems are specifically corrected. Such filters can be used with B&W film, as well as for visual observation.

Colour contrast filters may be of any colour; they are chosen to be complementary in colour to whatever colour in the object is to appear dark on B&W film (see Chapter 15). They may be bandpass or bandcut filters.

Didymium filters are special filters to improve the reproduction of Eosin, a biological stain that is notoriously difficult to reproduce properly in a colour photograph (see Chapter 15).

Polarising filters have a preferred vibrational direction: they transmit preferentially light whose plane of polarisation is parallel to a particular axis of the filter, and progressively absorb light whose plane of polarisation approaches a right angle to that axis. Their use is described in Chapter 10.

Excitation (bandpass) and **barrier** (sharp-cutoff longpass) **filters** are used in fluorescence microscopy (see Chapter 11).

Diffusion 'filters' serve to diffuse the light rays, and are used especially in ultralow-power microscopy to achieve uniform intensity over large fields. There are usually made of clear glass, ie without selective transmission of wavelengths; blue frosted filters are also known.

Colour-temperature compensation filters

To a first approximation, it may be said that colour film records the amounts of red, green and blue light in the image. The light used for illumination must therefore contain red, green and blue light in the correct proportions. In an incandescent lamp, these proportions can be summarised as the colour temperature (defined in Chapter 3). The colour temperatures of some light sources are given in Table 8.1.

If necessary, the colour temperatures of a light source can be modified with a filter (Table 8.2) to render that illumination suitable for a particular type of colour film. To calculate the filters required to change one colour temperature to another (Table 8.3), it is necessary to use the reciprocal of the temperature. This gives rise to another system of colour temperature measurement, for which the common unit is a *mired*. Mired stands for *microreciprocal degrees*, and the mired value is obtained by dividing the colour temperature in kelvin into one million. The mired unit is now often replaced by *reciprocal megakelvin*, abbreviated MK^{-1}, which has the same numerical value (only the name of the unit is different). (Strictly, a better name would be *megareciprocal kelvin*.) Sometimes decamired values are used, as these are smaller numbers: one decamired equals ten mireds. MK^{-1} or mired values are used for filters because the same filter will produce the same numerical colour shift in mireds with any light source of any colour temperature, and the effect of two or more filters can be calculated simply by adding their mired values. Amber filters lower the colour temperature, raising the MK^{-1} value, and have positive MK^{-1} numbers. Blue filters raise the colour temperature, lowering the MK^{-1} value, and have negative MK^{-1} numbers.

Colour temperature meters operate by determining the ratio of red to blue light, from which the colour temperature can be calculated. Such meters are built-in to some photomicrographic cameras.

Table 8.1. Colour temperature and MK^{-1} (mired) values of light sources

Light source	Approximate colour temperature (K)	MK^{-1} (mired) value
Standard candle	1930	518
Dawn sunlight	2000	500
Tungsten lamp (vacuum)	2400	417
Tungsten lamp (gas-filled, general service)	2760–2960	362–338
Tungsten-halogen, 12 V 100 W, at 7·4 A	3100	323
'Photographic' lamp	3200	312
Projector lamp	3200	312
Photoflood lamp	3400	294
ANSI standard light source	5000	200
Mean noon sunlight	5400	185
Electronic flash	6000	167
Xenon arc	6000	167
Blue sky	12 000–18 000	83–56

Table 8.2. Colour temperature conversion filters

Amber series		Blue series	
Filter	MK^{-1} (mireds)	Filter	MK^{-1} (mireds)
85B	+131	80A	–131
85	+112	80B	–112
85C	+81	80C	–81
81EF	+52	80D	–56
81D	+42	82C	–45
81C	+35	82B	–32
81B	+27		
81A	+18	82A	–21
81	+9	82	–10

For detailed specifications, see Hanke (1979) and Anon (1990).

Table 8.3. Filters required to match light source and film type

Light source	Filters required for film			
	Daylight type	Artificial-light type		
Colour temperature	5500 K	Type A 3400 K	Type B 3200 K	Fuji 3100 K
Tungsten lamps				
2800 K	80A + 82C	82B + 82B	82C	82B
2900 K	80A + 82B	80D	82B	82A
3000 K	80A + 82A	82C	82A	82
3100 K	80A + 82	82B	82	none
3200 K	80A	82A	none	81
3300 K	80B + 81	82	81	81A
3400 K	80B	none	81A	81B
Xenon arc or electronic flash				
6000 K	81A	85B	85B + 81A	85B + 81

Some combinations of two filters can be replaced by equivalent combinations, eg 80A + 82 = 80B + 82B; see Table 8.2.

Part III

Special optical techniques

This part describes specialised optical techniques of microscopy, and the use of a stereomicroscope.

- Aims: to describe techniques by which optical contrast may be increased, the use of invisible wavelengths (infrared and ultraviolet), and three-dimensional optical microscopy (stereomicroscopy).

- Prerequisite knowledge: Chapters 1–3 and 6–8.

- Exercises: see Appendix A3.

- Further information: the techniques described in Chapters 9–11 typically involve dim images, for which see Chapter 16. Otherwise, see sections entitled Further reading, at the ends of Chapters 11 and 12.

9
Darkground microscopy

Darkground illumination (Fig 9.1) is a technique that greatly improves the contrast of many specimens and substantially changes the appearance of the image. (Darkground illumination is also known as *darkfield* illumination, a term that co-author Ron prefers.) The technique was referred to briefly in Chapter 4. When sunlight or a projector throws a beam of light into a darkened room, we can recognise dust particles in the air not by looking into the blinding light, but by looking at right angles to the path of the beam. The dust particles, although they may be well below a size that enables them to be resolved by the eye, are detected as bright objects against the dark background. The dust particles are detected, seen, or made visible, but are not resolved. Measurement may be made of the number of dust particles shown, of their speed and direction of movement, but a description of their size or shape is not so certain. Perhaps more important is the ability to determine readily the presence or absence of the particles, even though they are too small to be resolved.

Darkground microscopy is one of several optical techniques that can be used as alternatives to transmitted-light microscopy. Comparisons of results obtained by several optical techniques are shown in Figs 9.2, 9.5, 9.6, and Plates 10–13.

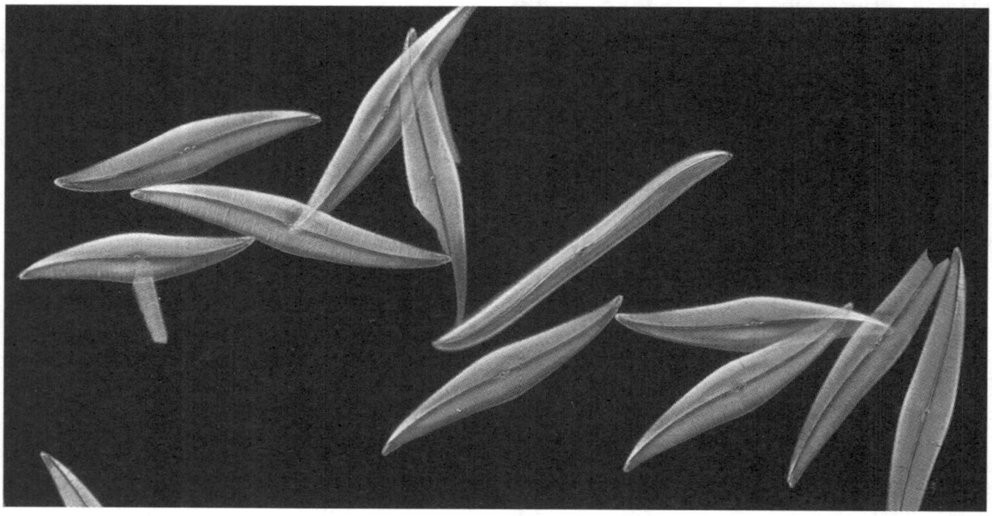

Fig 9.1. Photomicrograph using darkground microscopy (low magnification). Algal cells, *Pleurosigma angulatum* and *Gyrosigma* sp (diatoms), scarcely detectable in brightfield, are shown clearly in darkground illumination. Field size 0·45 mm × 0·9 mm (450 μm × 900 μm). Zeiss *Universal* microscope, patch stop in condenser, objective 4× planapo, Ilford *Pan F film*, *ID11* developer.

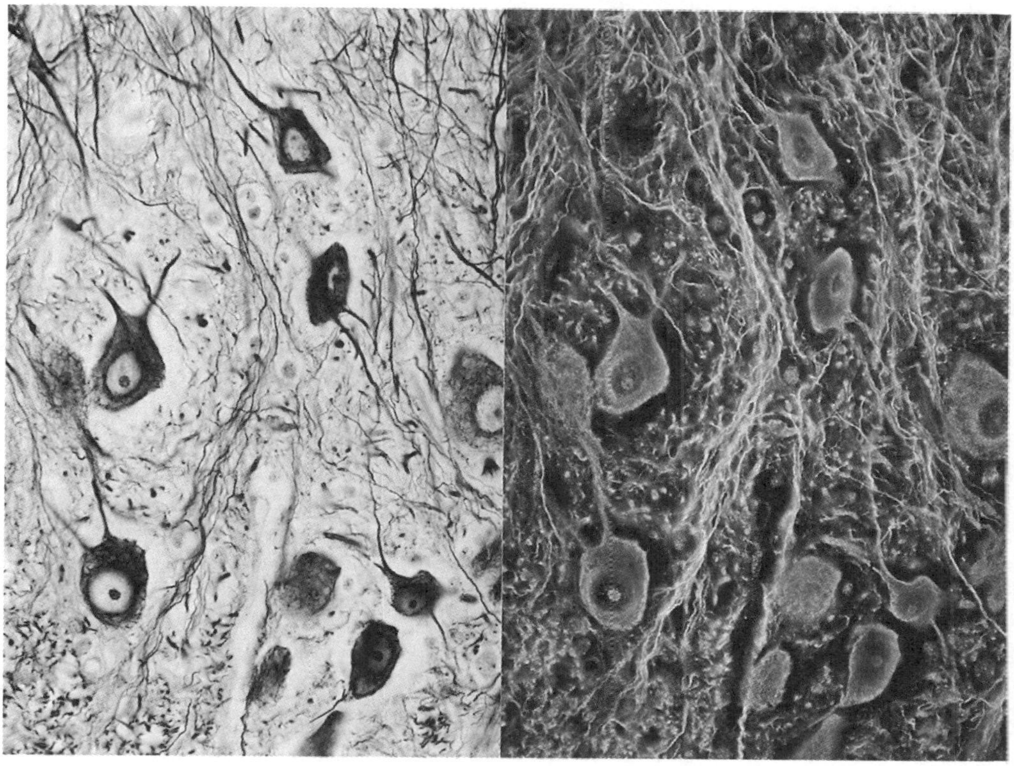

Fig 9.2. Comparison of brightfield (left) and darkground (right) microscopy at high magnification. Field size 260 μm × 170 μm. Transverse section of spinal cord, showing motor nerve cells. Zeiss *Universal* microscope, immersion darkground condenser, objective 40× planapo oil-immersion NA 1·0, Ilford *Pan F film*, *ID11* developer.

The theory of darkground microscopy

In darkground microscopy, the specimen is illuminated by a hollow cone of oblique rays of light that do not enter the objective directly, but may be reflected, refracted or diffracted into the objective by the specimen. Since no direct light enters the objective, an empty field appears black, and a specimen appears brightly illuminated against a dark background. This is the reason for the name 'darkground'. The method requires no more than a stop in the condenser blocking out the central rays of light that would enter the objective while allowing the peripheral rays to illuminate the object. The aperture diaphragm of the condenser must be fully open.

The required stop in the condenser can be built-in, supplied as an accessory, or fitted to the revolving turret of a phase-contrast or multifunction condenser. A simple stop (a patch stop) can be made and fitted into the filter holder, if there is one, underneath the condenser (see Chapter 4).

Figure 9.3. shows that the numerical aperture (NA) of the condenser must exceed the NA of the objective, so that the illumination cone passes outside the objective. In view of the importance of obtaining high NAs of the objective, this might seem a rather severe restriction on the usefulness of darkground, but the main usefulness of this technique is to obtain contrast rather than minimum resolved distance. In practice, a variety of condensers will be needed to enable darkground to be achieved with an assortment of objectives. It should be remembered that even the simplest two-lens 1·25 NA Abbe condenser is designed for immersion of the condenser top lens to the slide (this is true of any condenser with an NA exceeding 1·0), so that the maximum NA of such a condenser will be attained only with immersion. A particular advantage of the technique is that low-power objectives may enable good observation of a specimen which in brightfield requires higher magnification.

The specimen must be spotlessly clean; darkground is the technique of choice to *show* dust or other inclusions. Be very fussy with the selection of slides and coverslips and the filtering of mountants. Particulate preparations should be sparse, considerably diluted if necessary.

Darkground microscopy in practice

The patch (darkground) stop

A brightfield condenser can be converted to a low-power darkground condenser quite easily, using a patch stop (Fig 4.8). The simplicity of this modification, and the fact that patch stops are not sold by the more prestigious instrument manufacturers, should not deter the photomicrographer from attempting to make and use a patch stop. A method for construction of a patch stop is described in Chapter 4. The same principles are also applied to Rheinberg filter techniques (see below).

Low-power darkground condensers

Some manufacturers market special dry darkground condensers, which are much more convenient than the homemade patch stop for achieving darkground. To avoid the chromatic aberration inherent in refracting systems, better-quality darkground condensers consist of concentric reflecting, ie mirror, surfaces, using cardioid (Fig 9.3) or paraboloid construction. They are not cheap, being about six times the price of a normal condenser, and their use is limited to low-to-medium powers, with NA up to about 0·65, ie objectives in the 4× to 40× magnification range. They can also be used with a special oil-immersion objective fitted with an adjustable iris to limit the NA. As a technique, darkground has a reputation for being both messy and excessively fastidious; a dry darkground condenser will dispel these misgivings. Start with the microscope properly centred using a normal condenser, then insert the dry darkground condenser, increase the lamp intensity (possibly near to maximum), and focus the condenser to superimpose the field iris on the specimen. As different parts of the specimen are examined, minor changes may need to be made to the condenser focusing, to maintain image brightness and evenness of illumination.

Oil-immersion darkground condensers

Invariably, these are of mirror construction, in earlier times described as paraboloid or cardioid, indicating the geometric shape of an internal mirror surface. When held to the eye, an immersion darkground condenser appears to be completely dark, letting no light through. Because of the extreme obliquity of the rays emerging from the top of the condenser, total internal reflection occurs at the glass–air boundary. To avoid this glass–air interface, condensers of this type must have their top lens immersed to the slide. As the top lens may have a diameter of 12 mm or so, several drops of oil are required to cover this large area, and it takes some practice to immerse the condenser while avoiding air bubbles. Should air bubbles be included in the oil, we recommend that you remove the oil, wipe clean the glass surfaces, and start again.

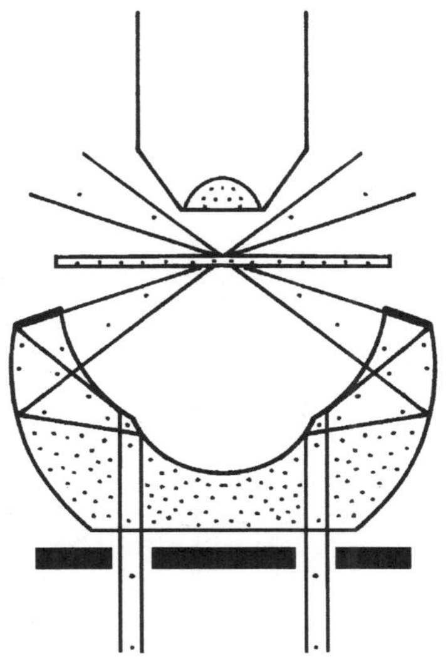

Fig 9.3. Diagram of low-power darkground (cardioid) condenser. Two mirror surfaces concentrate light onto the specimen. No direct light enters the objective.

Phase-contrast condensers

Darkground illumination can be obtained using a phase-contrast condenser (see Chapter 10) with a phase annulus of high aperture (eg for 100× objective). An advantage is that the patch stop in the condenser can be centred. This technique is very useful.

Oil-immersion objectives for darkground

These are immersion objectives with a built-in iris diaphragm. Typically, the cone of light emerging from the immersion darkground condenser has an NA of 1·4 (outer edge of the cone) to 1·2 (inner edge of the cone). Since darkground requires the NA of the condenser illumination (1·2 in the example just given) to be greater than the NA of the immersion objective (at least 1·25, possibly as high as 1·4), some mechanism is needed to reduce the effective NA of the objective. This mechanism is an iris diaphragm in the back focal plane of the objective. For brightfield immersion work, the objective is used with the iris fully open, but for darkground work, the objective iris is closed sufficiently to achieve darkground. If the iris is opened further, direct light will enter the objective thus destroying the darkground effect; if the iris is closed further than the position at which darkground is achieved, although contrast will be increased, it will be at the expense of resolution. An immersion objective with iris diaphragm performs everything that a normal immersion objective would be expected to do; it is an expensive duplication to possess both kinds of immersion objectives.

Epi-illumination darkground systems

Special objectives (Fig 9.4) are required if darkground is to be attempted with incident illumination. It is a variation on the patch stop principle in that an annular mirror is used, the mirror contained within a 'darkground block' that is built-in or inserted in the epi-illumination housing. A ring of light obliquely illuminates the specimen, which then reflects some of the light back into the central part of the objective.

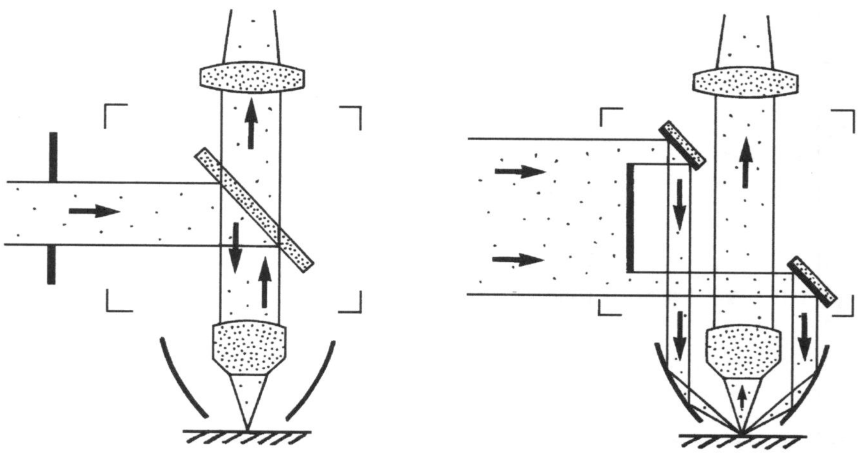

Fig 9.4. Diagram of a special objective for epi-illumination using either brightfield (left) or darkground (right) illumination.

With such a system, conventional brightfield epi-illumination is possible by replacing the annular mirror with a semi-reflector. The objective is designed to function also in brightfield, and so is described (by Zeiss) as an *HD*, *Hellfeld–Dunkelfeld* or *brightfield–darkfield* objective. The objective can also be used for a range of transmitted-light techniques, the whole system now lending itself to quite imaginative microscopy such as a combination of epi-illumination, darkground, with a filter of one colour, simultaneously with transmitted-light illumination, brightfield (or polarisation, etc), with a filter of another colour. Examples of results obtainable are shown in Figs 9.5 and 9.6, and Plate 13.

Biological material generally is poorly reflecting, so that very high intensities of illumination are a requirement. On the other hand, metallic objects, especially as used in the semi-conductor industry, or silver grains in radioautographs, or gold particles attached to immunoreagents, are often highly reflective and are suitable specimens for epi-illumination darkground.

Rheinberg illumination

Rheinberg illumination (Plate 4) is a variation of the darkground patch stop photographers and art directors. If the opaque central disc of a patch stop is replaced by a coloured filter (eg deep blue), the specimen will be observed in a blue brightfield; if the outer clear annulus of a patch stop is replaced by a filter of another colour (eg bright red), the specimen will be observed as a red-coloured darkground image. The red and blue acting together as a Rheinberg filter will transform a dull colourless specimen into a bright red object against a dark blue background, the kind of picture that colour supplements are made of.

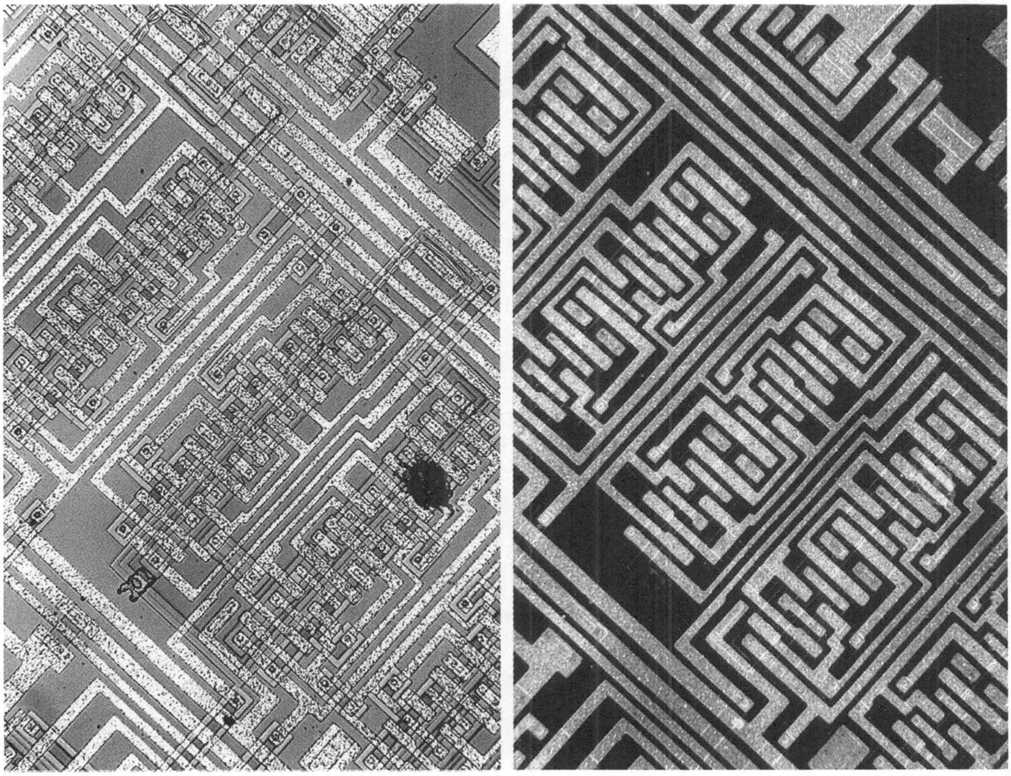

Fig 9.5. Epi-illumination, brightfield (left) and darkground (right) illumination of a microchip. Zeiss *Universal* microscope, patch stop in epi-illuminator, objective 16× *HD Epiplan*, Ilford *Pan F* film, *ID11* developer. Field size 0·75 mm × 1·2 mm.

It is not possible to buy Rheinberg filters; they have to be home-made on the principles that have been given for patch stop construction (see Chapter 4). Imaginative variation of these filters is possible, eg quadrants of alternating colours (see Plate 4) rather than a simple outer annulus, and a huge variety of colours can be used. Polycarbonate filters as sold to the television studio lighting industry are heat resistant and eminently suitable for construction materials, a free-sample swatch being exactly the right size and price for experimentation! A collection of brightly coloured gelatine filters is available from Cokin.

right size and price for experimentation! A collection of brightly coloured gelatine filters is available from Cokin.

Fig 9.6. Epi-illumination, brightfield (left) and darkground (right) illumination. Portion of printed letter 'i' on paper. Zeiss *Universal* microscope, darkground epi-illuminator, objective 6·3× *HD Epiplan*, Ilford *Pan F* film, *ID11* developer.

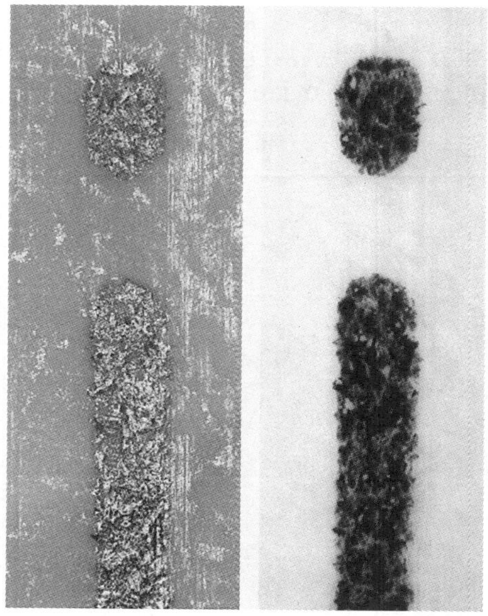

Darkground photomicrography

There are several difficulties associated with attempts to photograph darkground images:

- They are of low intensity (sometimes very low), making it difficult to measure the exposure accurately (see Chapter 16).
- They do not conform to the normal 18% averaged grey tone on which exposure meters are calibrated (see Chapter 16).
- There may be excessive contrasts which can not be accommodated by normal photographic processing methods (see Chapter 18).
- Prolonged exposure times involve film reciprocity failure (see Chapters 16 and 18).

In determining the required exposure, appropriate compensation is required for the proportion of light and dark in the field (see Chapter 16). A dark background implies a need to shorten the indicated exposure; reciprocity failure requires that the exposure should be increased. Just occasionally, ignorance of the quite complicated set of guidelines will lead to a perfectly exposed picture!

If the field is predominantly dark, the processing laboratory may have difficulty identifying the frame (picture) borders on the film, and may cut them inappropriately. Having an initial brightfield frame helps. The safest practice is to have the processed film delivered uncut, and to cut and mount the frames (chips) yourself.

10
Polarisation, phase contrast and DIC

This chapter deals with methods for increasing the contrast of images by making use of optical polarisation and interference. Phase-contrast and interference-contrast microscopy are used to reveal detail of colourless or low-contrast objects (such as living cells), by converting phase retardation (which cannot be perceived by the eye) to differences in brightness. Examples with comparisons are shown in Fig 10.1 and Plates 10–12.

Polarisation microscopy

This section is likely to have special appeal to many, for the sheer aesthetic pleasure derived from polarisation images. The pleasure should be maintained even though the theory and uses of polarisation microscopy are complex and are a part of the domain of optical crystallographers and mineralogists. The present work does not attempt to give any real understanding of polarisation microscopy. A few definitions and descriptions are given so that some working knowledge may be gained of the conversion of a brightfield microscope into a polarisation system. General introductions to polarisation microscopy are given by Oldfield (1994) and Robinson & Bradbury (1992).

The additional equipment required to adapt a microscope for polarisation microscopy is in principle only a pair of polarising filters. These can be obtained quite cheaply in sheet form and cut to size. One filter (the polariser) is usually placed either over the field diaphragm on the base of the microscope or in the filter holder under the condenser. The other filter (the analyser) in a binocular microscope is best fitted in the body tube under the prisms of the binocular head, and in a monocular microscope is usually most conveniently fitted in the eyepiece.

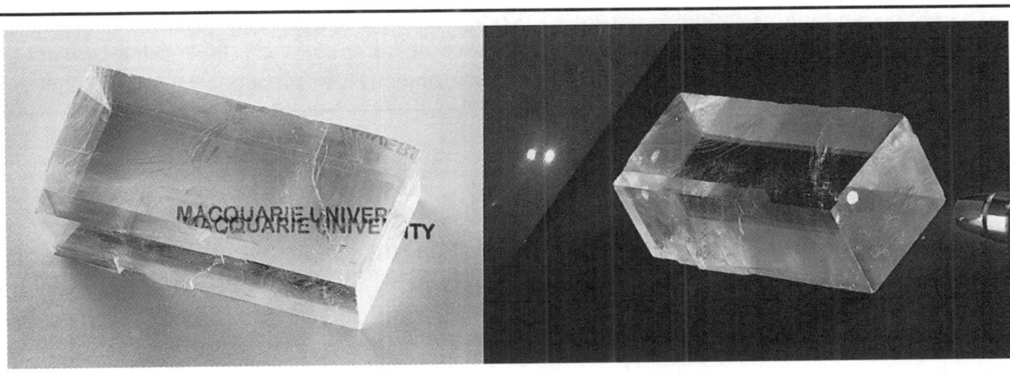

Fig 10.1. Double refraction in a calcite cleavage rhomb. Left, two images of the printing at different depths in the crystal. Right, the crystal produces two images of a single laser beam. In both cases, the two images are plane polarised at 90° to each other.

Double refraction

Many transparent crystals display the property of dividing incident light into two different paths, plane polarised at right angles to each other, and having different refractive indices associated with them. Calcite is the best known of these doubly refracting materials, recognised as producing two images from a single object (Fig 10.1). The rays are of two kinds: *ordinary* rays of constant velocity and *extraordinary* rays in which the velocity changes with the direction of transmission in the crystal. The difference between the maximum and minimum refractive indices, a number, is called the *birefringence*. The phenomenon is called double refraction; birefringence is a physical property that is a helpful characteristic for identifying each doubly refracting crystal.

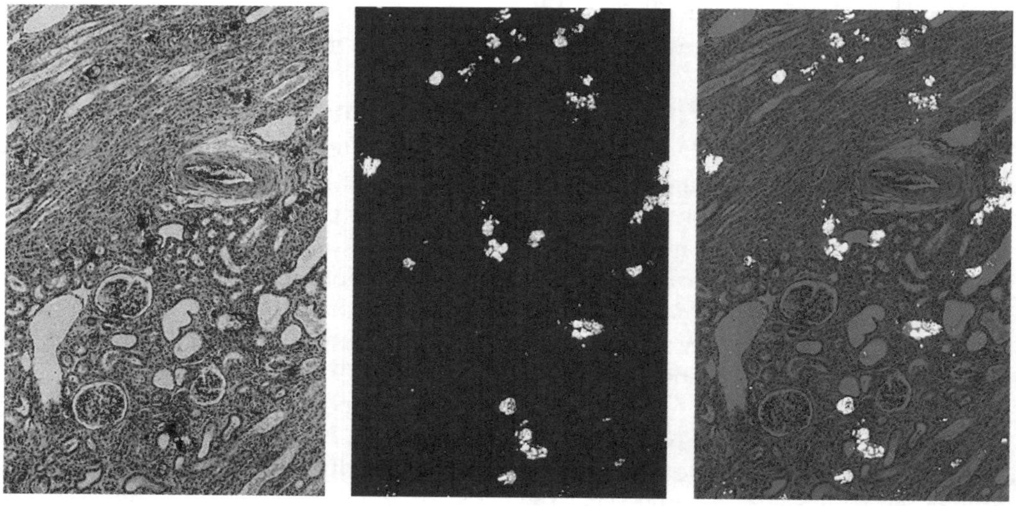

Fig 10.2. Crystals ('stones') in a stained section of human kidney tissue. Haematoxylin & Eosin stain, field size 0·9 mm × 1·4 mm. Left, a normal brightfield image. Centre, the same field is shown with crossed polars: crystals ('stones') are revealed, but the tissue stain is entirely masked. On the right, the polars have been partially uncrossed, revealing some detail of the stained tissue, but still emphasising the presence of crystals. One advantage of this technique is that rapid scanning is permitted. Very low magnifications, ie large fields of view, quickly show to the untrained observer the presence or absence of crystals. Zeiss *Universal* microscope, attachment polariser and insert analyser, objective 4× planapo, NA 0·14.

Polarisers

Any device that produces linear- or plane-polarised light is termed a *polariser* or *polar*. The word *Polaroid* is also used, for products of the Polaroid Land Corporation. By plane-polarised light is usually meant light in which the vibration directions of the electric vector of the electromagnetic radiation are confined to one plane, in a direction called the optical transmission axis of the polariser. Previously, polarisers were made from specially cut and re-cemented crystals of calcite. The polarisers of today are filters, made of foils in which millions of microcrystals (or polymeric iodine molecules) are embedded with a very high degree of orientation. The crystals are doubly refracting, but the ordinary rays are absorbed, and only the extraordinary rays are transmitted. The foils are enveloped in a protective cover of glass or similar material. Polarising filters are of two kinds: linear polarising and circular polarising; these are intended to provide linear and circular polarisation, respectively.

Crossed polarisers

Two good-quality polarisers with transmission directions at right angles to each other will together block all the light. This is the condition of *crossed polarisers* (*crossed polars*) that is used in the polarisation microscope (Fig 10.2). Lesser-quality polarisers will not have complete extinction of the rays; in some, for instance, much blue light passes through, and the background is never completely as black as it should be. Lenses or prisms that have strain in the glass will not permit a completely black field, and therefore strain-free objectives are made and specified for high-quality polarisation microscopy.

The polarising microscope

A microscope intended for serious polarisation studies has the following modifications (Fig 10.3), but elegant photographic work can be effected with lesser-quality accessories.

- All optical components of the condenser, the objectives, and the binocular tube should be selected as strain free. This adds considerably to the price of the optics.
- A *polariser* is located in a mount beneath the condenser. The polariser can be inserted or removed from the light path, and is capable of rotation, with click stops in N–S and E–W positions.
- The stage is capable of rotation through 360°, with a vernier measurement of the rotation. The stage should be able to engage 45° click stops from any position of rotation of the stage (Fig 2.4a, right).
- Between the objective nosepiece and the eyepiece another polariser, called the *analyser,* can be inserted or removed. In instruments meant for quantitative polarisation microscopy, the analyser is capable of rotation, with vernier measurement of that rotation. Immediately below the analyser, and often a part of its housing, is a slot for the insertion of compensation plates or a quartz wedge.
- A polarisation microscope has a *Bertrand lens* that can be inserted within the microscope tube, for convenient examination of interference figures which are formed in the objective back focal plane.

The minimum requirement to convert a biological microscope into a polarisation instrument (Fig 10.3) is the addition of a polariser beneath the condenser, and an analyser (preferably in a mount placed in a slot in the microscope tube) in a position somewhere between the specimen and the eye. Such an instrument, although inadequate for crystal optics, will give convincing polarisation images even with normal biological objectives. The polariser and analyser should be crossed to give maximum extinction when there is no specimen in the field. The prisms of a cheaper binocular tube may contribute to some deterioration of the extinction of crossed polars. A rotating stage is highly desirable. For 'pretty pictures' with biological specimens, a one-wavelength (1λ; also called *first-order red*) compensation plate (see below) is essential. The polarising microscope is first set up as any other microscope, paying attention to Köhler illumination. Then the polarisers are crossed to give maximum extinction (darkest background).

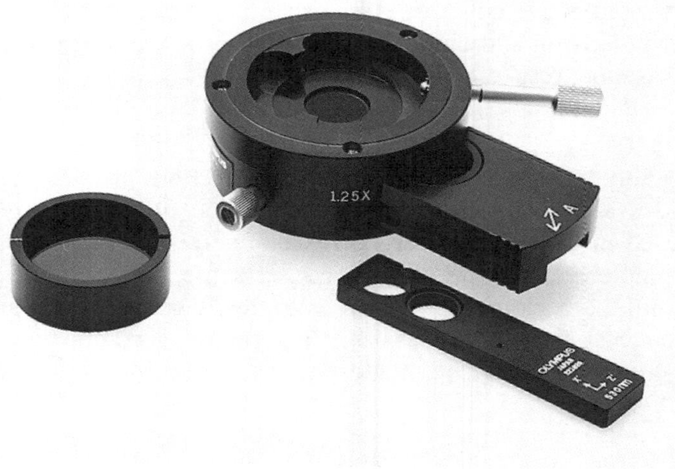

Fig 10.3. Accessories for polarising microscopy. Left, a polariser (polar), which is placed below the condenser. Top right, a fitting which is inserted between the objective and the eyepiece to house the (removable) analyser and the compensator. Bottom right, the compensator. The orientation of the housing is usually determined by a guide pin. The polariser is oriented at 90° to the analyser; the compensator is then at 45° to both polariser and analyser.

The one-wavelength (1λ) compensation plate (Fig 10.3) is a device for serious polarisation microscopy, assisting in the determination of the optical properties of anisotropic material, and thereby permitting discrimination between minerals. Usually cut from quartz or calcite, the plate thickness is such that the ordinary and extraordinary rays that pass through it have an optical path difference of 550 nm, ie one wavelength of green light. If the plate is inserted at 45° to crossed polars, green light is extinguished, leaving the blue and red. The field appears magenta (but is called red by optical mineralogists!). When weakly-birefringent biological material is examined, compensation effects transform colourless images into brilliant polarisation colours (yellow, orange, blue, and red against a magenta background) that produce genuine excitement in the observer. The colours change as the stage is rotated. The reason for these colours is given in the works cited above, but the theory is not simple.

Anisotropism

Material that is doubly refracting, such as most crystal sections or a length of hair, is recognised as anisotropic by showing up brightly in the crossed polars setting. As the stage is rotated, the hair will show four positions of darkness at settings separated by 90°, and intermediate positions with maximum brightness at 45° to the positions of extinction. Thicker material or crystals of higher birefringence will show bright colours that change with rotation. In thicker material still the colours will be muted.

Photographing the polarisation image

Most enthusiasts are so overcome with the incredibly beautiful images that can be produced in the polarisation microscope that they forget the normal and quite basic requirements of Köhler illumination. Often, it is the lowest-magnification objectives that are needed, which may require an ultralow-power condenser. If the field is filled with colours (as when the 1λ compensation plate is used), there should not be any particular problems with measuring exposure. Autofocusing may be affected. If there is a considerable area of blackness occupying the field, then negative compensation (less exposure) will need to be considered (see Chapter 16). It is a wise precaution to ensure that a heat filter (eg Schott KG1) is present, because crossed Polaroids transmit infrared light, which is measured by the camera exposure meter, leading to considerable underexposure of the polarisation image.

Phase-contrast microscopy

In brightfield microscopy, considerable emphasis is placed on making the image a faithful representation of the object, and assessment of the equipment and its operation might be made by judging how closely the image represents an enlarged duplication of the specimen. Living material is often of such low contrast that the image, because it is a faithful rendition of the object, is quite useless. If staining of the specimen is an unacceptable procedure, one way to increase contrast is to partially close the aperture diaphragm, which has the undesirable effect of limiting the resolving power of the system. Phase-contrast microscopy *modifies* the way in which the image is formed, by optical means, so that invisible structures are made visible (see Plates 10–11), while maintaining the full numerical aperture (NA) of the objective, ie maximum resolution (Fig 10.3). For this invention, the Nobel prize was awarded in 1953 to the Dutch physicist Frits Zernicke (1888–1966).

The theory of phase-contrast microscopy

When light passes through slightly differing thicknesses of a transparent material, there is a corresponding difference in phase between the two emergent rays. Because the eye is unable to detect phase differences, such *phase specimens* (if uncoloured) in the microscope are indistinguishable from the clear mountant in which they are placed. On the other hand, if there is a difference in the absorption of rays by the two thicknesses, the eye is very efficient in detecting that difference, which it perceives as contrast. The features of such a specimen, an *amplitude* specimen, can be well discriminated in the microscope.

Phase contrast, by optical means, changes small differences in phase to differences in amplitude, which show as differences in contrast. A theoretical explanation of phase-contrast microscopy is beyond the scope of the present text, but there are teaching models from which a reasonable understanding of the principles can be gained (Oldfield, 1994).

Phase-contrast microscopy employs a condenser that illuminates the specimen with a hollow cone of light, as in darkground microscopy. However, the cone of light is narrower and enters the objective. Within the objective is a glass plate with a ring-shaped (annular) structure, the phase plate, that both reduces the intensity of the light and introduces a phase shift of a quarter of a wavelength. Light diffracted by the specimen passes predominantly inside or outside the phase ring, and is therefore not affected by it. In the final image, the direct light (retarded $^1/_4$ wavelength) and the diffracted light are combined and interfere, constructively or destructively, thereby creating differences in amplitude. This technique causes minute variations of refractive index or thickness in a transparent specimen to become visible.

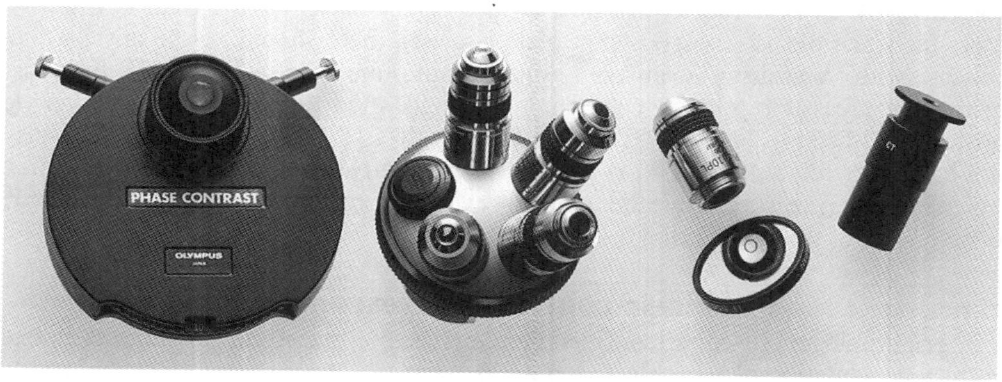

Fig 10.4. Accessories for phase-contrast microscopy. From left to right, a phase-contrast condenser, special objectives with a darkened phase ring (as seen reflected in the green filter), and a centring telescope.

The commercial product

Special accessories are required to achieve phase contrast, which normally take the form of a special phase-contrast condenser and special phase-contrast objectives (Fig 10.4).

The condenser needs to have a *phase annulus* (*annulus*, plural *annuli*, is Latin for *ring*) in its front focal plane, the plane where the aperture iris diaphragm is normally situated. A range of different annuli is required, the size of each annulus matching one or more phase objective NAs. Most commonly, a phase-contrast condenser has a rotating turret bearing an iris diaphragm in one position to permit normal brightfield observation, and three or four phase annuli occupying other positions (having no iris). The simplest systems have a number of separate annuli, as attachments, to be placed in a holder near the aperture iris. The iris itself must be fully opened for phase-contrast observation. Modern universal condensers have the possibility of inserting up to seven modules, as chosen by the user (Fig 10.6); these separate inserts may be for darkground, phase or differential interference contrast (DIC). Phase-contrast condensers are available in a range of optical corrections, from the basic Abbe construction to aplanatic-achromatic systems; and also with a long working distance to cope with thick containing vessels.

An objective for phase contrast has a *phase plate* in the back focal plane. Although a phase-contrast objective will have some notation inscribed on the barrel to indicate that the lens is meant for phase (eg Ph, PL, NH), it is most easily identified by holding the objective up to a bright light and recognising the dark annulus inside the objective – the phase plate (Figs 10.4, 10.5, 10.7). Less commonly, the phase plate may be outside the objective but in a plane conjugate with the objective back focal plane, in which case normal objectives can be used for phase. The range of phase-contrast objectives is considerable, including: achromatic, fluorite or apochromatic correction; with or without flat-field correction; with or without coverslip correction collar; dry, water-immersion and oil-immersion.

Positive and negative phase contrast. Some manufacturers have offered up to four kinds of phase-contrast objective, varying in sign (positive or negative, see Plate 11) and degree of contrast (high or relatively low). In *positive* phase contrast (the most commonly marketed variety), optically dense parts of the specimen appear dark against a lighter background; in *negative* phase contrast, relatively dense components appear bright against a dark background, rather like darkground. Optical density (optical path length) is dependent on specimen thickness and refractive index. In fact, the specimen appearance in phase contrast is much more complicated than stated here, which applies only to specimens with quite small differences in optical path. The annulus of the phase plate appears dark because of an absorptive layer included in it. The density of this absorptive layer affects the contrast of the final image; some manufacturers provide alternatives of higher and lower contrast for both the positive and the negative phase-contrast systems. Phase-contrast systems used for biology are typically high-contrast positive systems.

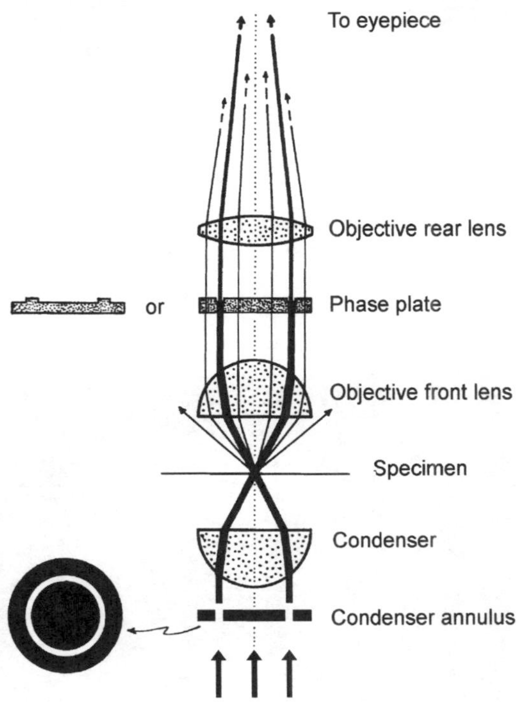

Fig 10.5. Diagram of a phase-contrast system. Two forms of phase plate for the objective are shown, and a plan view of the condenser annulus.

Setting up the phase-contrast microscope

Remove the normal objectives and condenser and attach the phase condenser and phase objectives. Set the condenser turret to the brightfield position (ie with iris) and achieve Köhler illumination. It may be helpful to use a well-stained specimen for this initial centring. When a phase image is required, choose the appropriate phase objective and match the phase annulus of the condenser turret to the objective that has been chosen. For photography, immerse the condenser if it is an immersion condenser (NA 1·0 or more). The phase condenser annulus requires accurate alignment with the objective phase plate. For this purpose a centring telescope, also called an auxiliary microscope, is provided – it replaces one of the eyepieces and is focused on the two annuli, namely the bright ring of the condenser and the dark ring of the objective phase plate. The bright ring of the condenser should appear superimposed on, and completely within, the dark ring of the objective. If the bright and dark rings are of unequal size the correct condenser annulus has not been chosen, or the condenser has been incorrectly used.

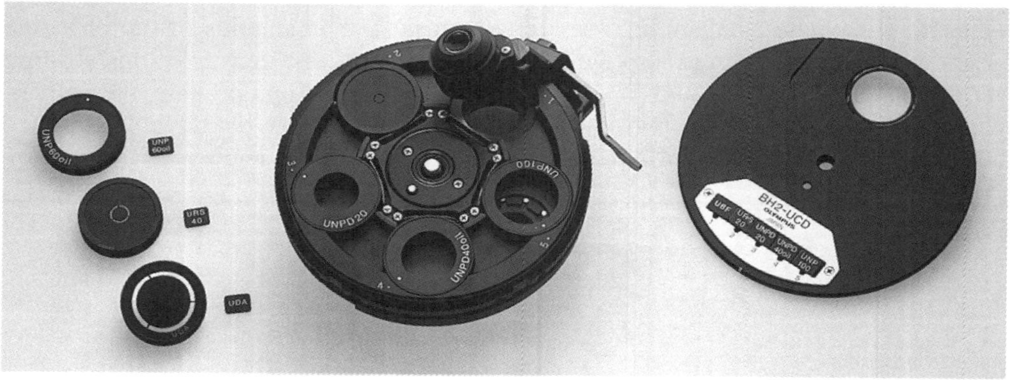

Fig 10.6. A universal condenser with cover plate removed. This Olympus model has the possibility of five inserts. Three inserts are shown separately, each for a specific compatible range of objectives: from top to bottom, DIC, phase contrast, darkground. A removable polariser is also built-in.

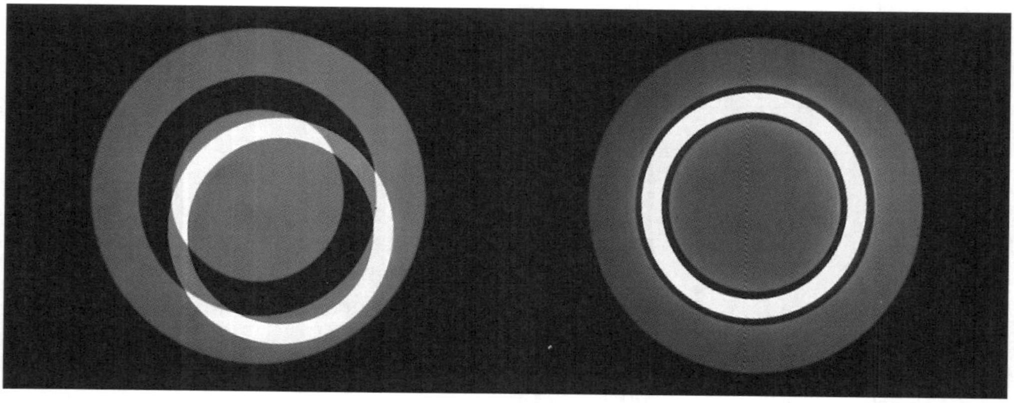

Fig 10.7. Phase rings as seen in the objective back focal plane. Phase rings off-centre (left), and properly centred (right). These views may be obtained with a Bertrand lens, or by removing an eyepiece and looking down the tube with or without a centring telescope.

The phase condenser will have adjusting screws to enable centring of the phase-condenser annulus to the objective (Fig 10.7). After centring of the annulus, the eyepiece is replaced and phase-contrast observation is possible. More sophisticated instrumentation has a Bertrand lens built-in to the microscope to facilitate observation of the objective's back focal plane.

A green filter is normally considered part of the phase-contrast set. This is consistent with theoretical considerations for maximum contrast with this technique. It is reasonable to use phase objectives for normal brightfield work, although the image will be somewhat soft. For photography, there is an advantage to having separate sets of phase and brightfield objectives, although this may be considered an extravagance for routine laboratory observation.

Attributes of the phase-contrast image

Changing the condenser annulus to the zero or brightfield position, and adjusting the aperture iris, enables a quick comparison between brightfield and phase images. Especially when photography is required, phase contrast transforms the image of unstained (or poorly stained) biological specimens. Attempts to giving meaning to intensity variations across the image may be difficult. The most obvious feature of the phase image is the *phase halo*, an anomalous intensity variation at the sites of abrupt optical density change. Large areas with unchanging optical path exhibit the *shading-off* effect (Fig 10.8). The halo and shading-off effects contribute to uncertain interpretation, and the interpretation of thick specimens requires caution. Phase contrast is seldom advantageous with well-stained material. Comparisons with DIC are given later in this chapter.

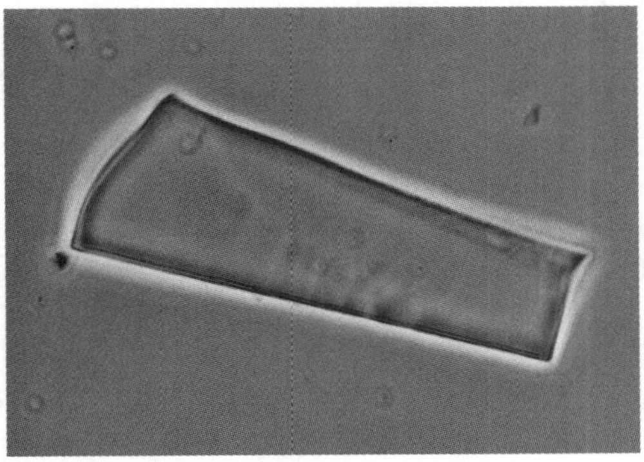

Fig 10.8. Artefacts of phase contrast showing in a glass coverslip fragment immersed in oil. Field size 100 µm × 140 µm. A *phase halo* shows at the specimen–oil boundary. From the dark rim of the glass there is a lightening of intensity to the grey centre, which matches the intensity of the immersion fluid, although the optical density of the glass is reasonably constant across the specimen. This is the *shading-off* effect.

Darkground with the phase condenser

By choosing a phase condenser annulus that is 'too large' (ie of greater diameter than is appropriate for the phase-contrast system) the annulus behaves as a darkground patch stop (see Chapter 9). With the 4× objective in position, bring the annulus for the 100× objective into the light path, set the condenser for high-power work (if it has that option) and increase the lamp intensity. Transparent material, even if out of focus, is now imaged brightly against a dark background, and can be more easily located and focused. The effects may be quite good enough for high-quality darkground photography, if a darkground condenser is not available. Some experimentation will be needed to establish the best choice of an annulus for a particular low-power objective. Immersing with oil an immersion phase-contrast condenser is an additional possibility to improve the quality of a darkground image.

Photographic considerations for phase contrast

Because of the absorptive layer in the phase plate of the objective, the phase-contrast image will be very much darker than equivalent brightfield images. As a consequence, faster film may be essential to obtain exposures short enough to avoid blurred images due to movement in living material. Even with a 100 W tungsten–halogen illuminator, a 25/15° ISO film will need an exposure of 30 seconds or so with high-power immersion phase systems.

With some manufacturers the 10× phase objective is the lowest magnification available. Often there is a requirement for larger fields, which can be achieved only with low-power eyepieces. Such eyepieces exaggerate the need for even illumination and for flat-field correction of the objectives.

Apart from the possibility of reciprocity failure in the film (Chapters 16, 18), it is some comfort that no other compensation needs to be considered, for the brightest part of the positive phase image is the phase halo; the background conforms almost exactly to the 18% grey (as in 18% reflectance) for which the exposure meter is calibrated. Negative phase contrast is less frequently used, but in such a circumstance negative compensation (less exposure) is appropriate, countered by positive compensation (more exposure) for reciprocity failure.

Fresh biological material, for which phase contrast is always a distinct possibility, is more than likely to be too thick for best imaging, ie the total thickness of coverslip, mountant and specimen exceeding 0·17 mm. One must endeavour to control the specimen thickness, and to remember that low-power oil-immersion objectives are more tolerant of errors in coverslip thickness. Long-working-distance condensers and long-working-distance phase objectives are also available in a low- to medium-magnification range for difficult specimens and containers, and have particular application in inverted microscopes.

In black-and-white (B&W) recording of phase contrast, the green filter, preferably a narrow band interference green filter, is an important and essential accessory to maintain full contrast. In desperate situations, such as with moving specimens, there will be a temptation to omit the green filter, for it requires a fivefold increase in photographic exposure. In colour photography, the green filter gives a green cast to the entire picture and is normally inappropriate.

Differential interference-contrast (DIC) microscopy

DIC microscopy is another technique that is used to introduce contrast, and sometimes colour, into specimens which lack contrast. Its usefulness parallels that of phase-contrast microscopy, and inevitably the two systems have to be evaluated against each other.

The theoretical aspects of phase contrast are a proper component of a senior optical physics syllabus, but for a number of years simplified models have been available that a non-mathematical biologist might be expected to understand. DIC is even more complicated, and lacks simple and convincing teaching analogies. The reader is directed to other works for more detailed theoretical information (eg Oldfield, 1994); this chapter aims to give some practical advice for operating a Nomarski-type DIC system.

The theory of Nomarski DIC

DIC (Figs 10.9, 10.10, Plates 6 and 12a) is a shearing technique in which two sets of rays pass through or onto the specimen. Shearing of the light source is effected by a polarisation method, doubly refracting crystals re-cemented to give ordinary and extraordinary rays separated by a distance less than the resolving power of the objective. The beam splitter is a modification by the French physicist Georges Nomarski, of prisms designed by William Wollaston, hence the name Nomarski DIC. The two rays, both passing through closely adjacent regions of the specimen, are recombined in another, similar, set of prisms. If the two rays have different path lengths, that region will show lighter or darker than those areas of the specimen and the mountant that do not have changing thickness or refractive index, hence the name *differential interference contrast*. By lateral displacement of the second, or combining, prism the differential between the two sets of rays can be changed to alter the contrasts or colours in the final image.

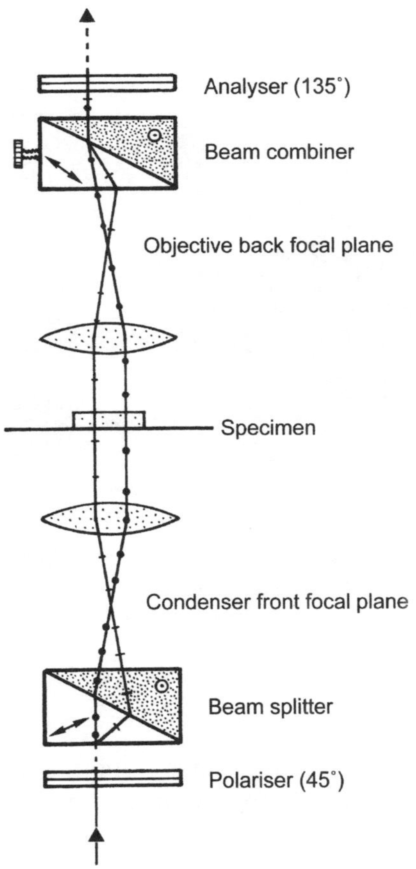

Fig 10.9. Diagrammatic representation of a differential interference-contrast (DIC) system for transmitted light.

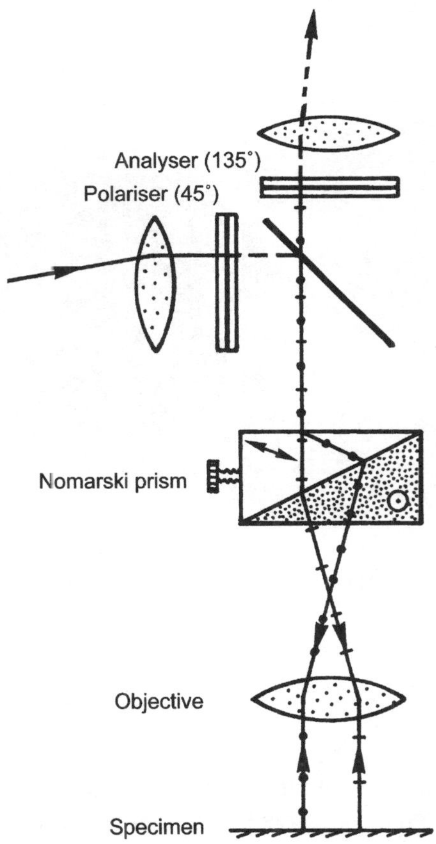

Fig 10.10. Diagrammatic representation of a DIC system for epi-illumination.

The Nomarski DIC microscope

The beam-separating prisms, one for each objective (more strictly one for each range of NAs) are held in a turret beneath the condenser lenses, in the same way that phase annuli are positioned. In some systems DIC prisms and/or phase annuli as chosen by the user are inserted in the one *universal condenser* (Fig 10.6). A polariser is introduced into the light path beneath the beam-splitting prisms, but removed for brightfield or phase-contrast observation. An aperture iris diaphragm is present and fully functional for both brightfield and DIC, but removed for phase. If the condenser permits (NA more than 1·0), immersion to the slide demonstrably improves the image quality.

Special attention needs to be given to the selection of good-quality slides and coverslips, because wedge-shaped glass will give irregularity to the image.

The objectives for DIC (Fig 10.11) need to have a fixed position for their back focal plane, with a special relationship to the upper beam combining prisms. Not all modern objectives will meet this requirement; the DIC catalogue or manual of a particular manufacturer needs to be consulted for the information as to which of an existing set of objectives may be suitable for DIC.

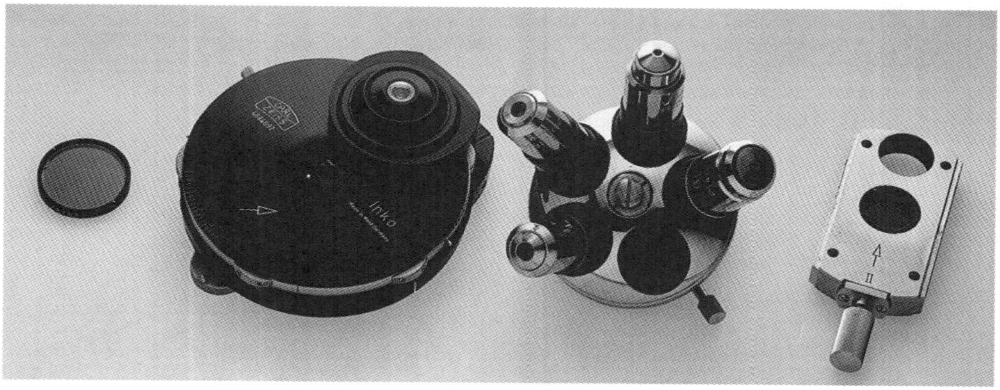

Fig 10.11. Accessories for DIC, for the Zeiss *Universal* microscope. From left to right, polariser, DIC condenser, planachromat objectives on nosepiece, beam combiner.

Often, one beam combiner (Fig 10.11) suffices for the full range of objectives. The prisms are mounted in a slider that fits above the nosepiece of the microscope. Immediately above the prisms is an analyser, normally part of the DIC beam combiner. There is a lever or screw that effects a lateral sideways shift to the beam-combining prism; this prism changes the path difference between the two beams coming from the specimen, thus changing the appearance of the background from dark, through greys, to light, and then the familiar colours of polarisation microscopy. The specimen can be made to look darker or lighter than the background, or of a different colour. For phase or brightfield microscopy the beam combiner is removed from the path of the light.

DIC with epi-illumination

The semiconductor industry has been an important user of DIC for quality control, checking for defects. The technique reveals *optical path gradients* that result from surface topographical changes or from phase changes at reflection boundaries.

For an appropriate set of objectives for epi-illumination there is a Nomarski prism module interposed between objective and nosepiece, the prisms acting initially as a beam splitter, then as a beam combiner for the rays reflected from the specimen. Lateral movement of the prism (Zeiss), or rotation of the analyser with or without a 1λ compensator (Olympus), causes a change in the optical path difference between the two sets of rays, enabling control of intensity and colour (Fig 10.10 and Plate 6).

A comparison of phase contrast and DIC

The DIC image is characterised by a pseudo-relief, an apparent representation of three-dimensional topography, but only rarely is the image truly representative of topographic profiles. The DIC image distinguishes localised sites in which there is a gradient of changing thickness or refractive index. DIC is an expensive attachment, and is very demanding of technical skills and manual dexterity, initially in the DIC setup, then in the continuous manipulation of specimen focus, of the aperture iris, of the stage rotation, and the lateral displacement of the beam combiner.

As an accessory, phase contrast is comparatively cheap, and once aligned, the microscope can be comfortably and effectively operated by quite inexperienced users. The image shows sites of abrupt refractive index or thickness change. The phase halo is characteristic, sometimes useful, sometimes a considerable disadvantage (eg, in determining boundaries for measurement).

DIC is very demanding on light intensity; an absolute minimum for photography is a 100 W tungsten–halogen lamp. One advantage of a photograph is that detail too dark to see in the microscope is more easily recognised in a print. The DIC image is direction dependent, phase contrast is not. For maximum detail in DIC, linear structures need to be oriented at right angles to the direction of shear (the shear direction is often NW–SE). It is highly desirable to have a rotating stage for photography to check on the most favourable specimen orientation, but most users of the microscope find rotating stages very uncomfortable in that the operation of the mechanical stage requires an awkward bending of the wrists.

In DIC the aperture iris diaphragm remains fully functional; closure increases contrast and maximises depth of field, but at the expense of good resolution. A particular benefit of DIC is the ability to achieve optical sectioning in thicker specimens, minimal depth of field giving cleaner images. Thick specimens do not lend themselves to good phase-contrast images, because the image in a particular plane of interest is seriously impaired by out-of-focus refractive index boundaries, boundaries in the specimen above or below the plane of focus.

The usefulness of phase contrast is confined to specimens with poor contrast. DIC can cope with both stained and unstained specimens. Because DIC is based on polarisation phenomena for beam splitting and beam combining, specimens that are themselves anisotropic (see section on Polarisation) may give unwanted effects. For the very smallest phase shifts (eg thinnest structures), phase contrast is likely to give more contrast than DIC.

The displacement of the beam combiner in DIC gives additional control and contrast variation, from dark backgrounds to light backgrounds, to multi-coloured effects. To be able to get a really high-quality darkground is a sign that the instrument is set as well as possible, but specimen relief is most apparent on either side of the darkground setting, and is usually preferred. However, the colours that are introduced by increased displacement of the beam combiner are a favourite for magazine colour supplements and journal covers.

Photography of DIC

As with phase contrast, the ability to get sufficiently low magnification may be limiting. With some manufacturers, the 10× objective is as low as is it possible to use (6·3× with older Zeiss systems). Low-power eyepieces have the disadvantage of showing up deficiencies in the flat-field correction of objectives, and are much more difficult to illuminate evenly.

If the medium-grey DIC settings are chosen, as mentioned in the text, exposure compensation is not necessary. Neither is it necessary for the colour settings. A major problem, however, is the comparatively low intensity and long exposures at high magnifications, 1 minute exposures being normal with 50/18° ISO film. Reciprocity failure needs to be considered (see Chapter 16).

In scientific photography, it is conventional to have the main light coming from the top left of the picture. There is some advantage in conforming to this convention in published DIC images, ie having the 'shadows' on the lower rather than the upper sides.

The unpredictable effects of infrared radiation on exposure measurement in systems using polarising filters are eliminated if a heat filter (eg Schott KG1) is always in place.

Other optical-contrast techniques

Special attention has been given in this chapter to phase-contrast, polarisation and DIC methods of microscopy as these are the most commonly used. Some less commonly used techniques are mentioned below. As far as photography of the images is concerned, these techniques have no special problems compared with those already discussed in this chapter.

Varicolor is a phase-contrast method that produces coloured images from uncoloured objects. Zeiss Jena marketed variable-contrast phase contrast in the 1960s, a technique re-introduced by Carl Zeiss in 1997 but modified by the possibility of oblique illumination and called *Varel*. Especially for inverted-microscope observation in which plastic culture vessels are routinely used, Varel is a much cheaper, simpler and more effective contrast mechanism than polarisation-based DIC.

Similarly, the Hoffman modulation-contrast method, which uses oblique illumination together with an amplitude filter in each objective's back focal plane, has the advantage of not requiring polarisation beam separation. Compared with phase contrast, Hoffman modulation contrast is quite expensive, simply because few sets are manufactured. As with DIC, phase gradients in the specimen are converted into visible, amplitude (intensity) variations imparting pseudo-relief to the image. There is no halo as in phase contrast. The system, with others, was reviewed by Pluta (1989).

11
Fluorescence microscopy

Fluorescence microscopy shows objects that are either fluorescent (such as many specimens of plants and minerals), or can be made so by staining with fluorescent reagents (as in immunofluorescence). Fluorescence is normally observed as luminosity on a dark background (Fig 11.1 and Plate 7). Therefore, fluorescence microscopy offers high sensitivity to detect substances even in extremely small amounts. Optical specificity is obtained by appropriate choice of filters. This chapter describes conventional fluorescence microscopy: laser-scanning confocal fluorescence microscopy is described (briefly) in Chapter 17.

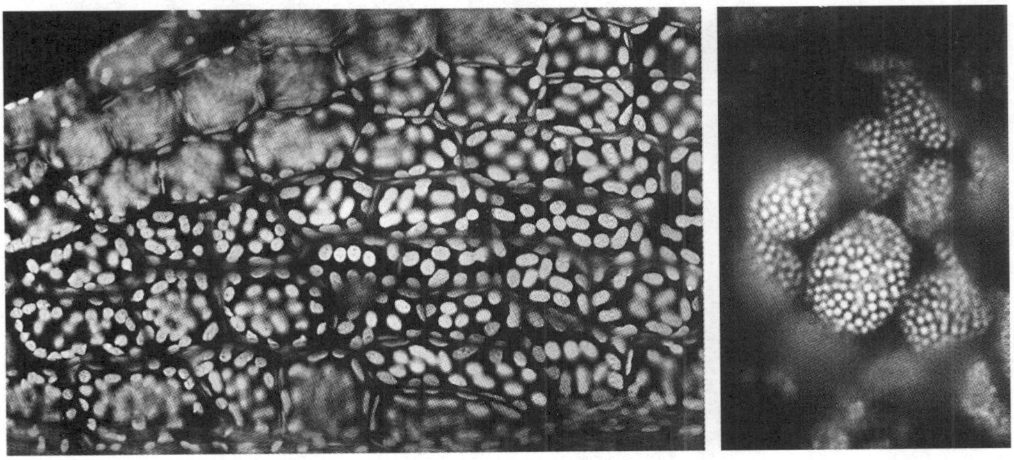

Fig 11.1. Fluorescence photomicrographs, low and high magnifications, showing red autofluorescence of chloroplasts (main picture) and grana in them (inset). Field sizes: left, 230 μm × 310 μm; right, 30 μm × 20 μm. Olympus *BH2-RFCA* microscope, blue excitation (as for FITC), epi-illumination, *PM-10ADS* photomicrographic system, Kodak *Technical Pan* film rated at 25 ISO developed in *Technidol* liquid developer. This film was used because of its extended red sensitivity. Main picture, *Funaria* (moss) leaf mounted in water. *S Planapo UV* 20× oil-immersion objective, NA 0·8. Inset, *Agapanthus orientalis* leaf section mounted in glycerine. *D Planapo UV* 100× oil-immersion objective.

In a fluorescence microscope (Figs 11.2. 11.3), the specimen is illuminated with light of a short wavelength, usually ultraviolet or blue. Part of this light is absorbed by molecules in the specimen, which become excited; this means that they are raised to a higher energy level. Part of this energy is re-emitted as fluorescence. The re-emitted light has a longer wavelength than that of the incident light, and its intensity is less. To enable the comparatively weak fluorescence to be seen, the light used for excitation is filtered out by a secondary (barrier) filter placed between the specimen and the eye (Fig 11.2). This filter should be fully opaque at the wavelength used for excitation, and fully transparent at longer wavelengths to transmit the fluorescence. The fluorescent object is therefore seen as a bright image against a dark background (Fig 11.1 and Plate 7).

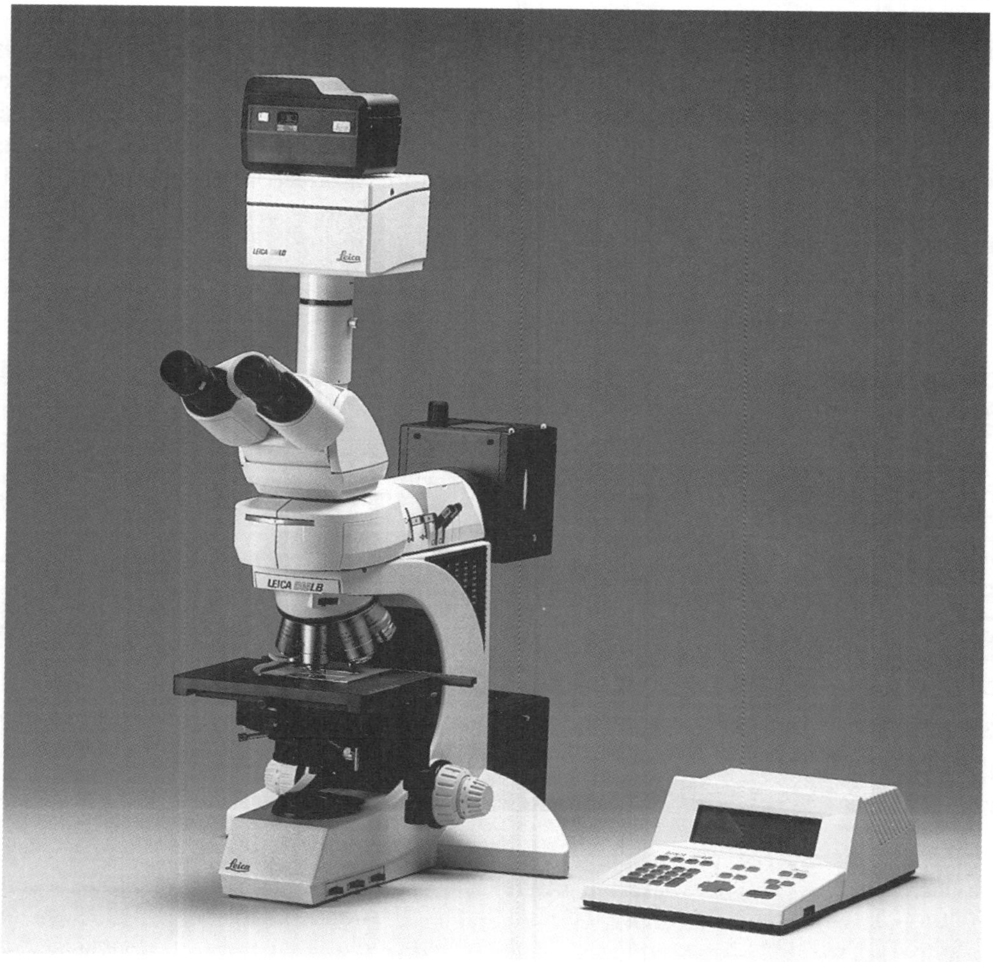

Fig 11.2. The Leica *DM* microscope with *4-lambda* epi-illumination fluorescence attachment and Leica *DMLD* automatic camera system for 35 mm and large format. The same camera module fits a range of Leica microscopes and macroscopes. Photograph courtesy Leica Microsystems Wetzlar GmbH, Wetzlar, Germany.

Epi-illumination

Opaque or very thick objects can be examined using epi-illumination (described in Chapter 7), a technique whereby the light for excitation is reflected downwards through or around the objective onto the specimen (Figs 11.2, 11.3). Although this technique is only essential for the examination of opaque objects, it has major advantages also for the more conventional transparent specimens. It is particularly suitable for use at high and medium magnifications, and can easily be combined with simultaneous or alternate transmitted-light techniques such as interference-contrast, phase-contrast and darkground illumination. Therefore, most modern fluorescence microscopes employ epi-illumination.

Co-author Fred has found that the intensity of excitation can be increased by placing a plane mirror underneath the substage condenser, to reflect light that has passed through the specimen back to the specimen again.

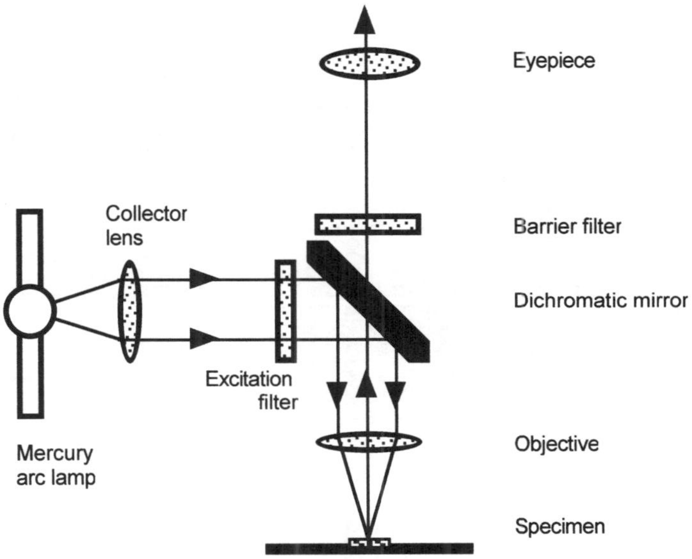

Fig 11.3. Diagram of fluorescence microscope with epi-illumination.

Special instrumental requirements for fluorescence microscopy

A modern fluorescence microscope (such as that shown in Fig 11.2) has, in addition to normal equipment, an epifluorescence unit with a powerful light source (typically a 100 W or 50 W mercury arc lamp), and an interchangeable filter block containing the excitation filter, dichromatic mirror and barrier filter.

For photomicrography of fluorescence, it is important that the body tube has provision for all (100%) of the light to pass up to the camera. Some makes of microscope have only a beamsplitter, so that some of the light is always diverted into the observation tubes, and the full amount of light from the objective is not available for photomicrography.

The optical arrangement of a fluorescence microscope is shown diagramatically in Fig 11.3. The lamp should be a powerful light source, rich in short wavelengths: high-pressure mercury arc lamps are the most common. A *primary* or *excitation filter* is placed somewhere between the lamp and the specimen. The filter, in combination with the lamp, should provide light over a comparatively narrow band of wavelengths corresponding to the absorption maximum of the fluorescent substance (fluorophore).

The *secondary*, *barrier* or *suppression filter* prevents the excitation light from reaching the observer's eye, and is placed between the specimen and the eye (preferably in the body tube). Its transmission should be as low as possible in the range of the light used for excitation, and as high as possible within the spectral range of the emission from the specimen.

The functions of the excitation and barrier filters may be more clearly demonstrated with the aid of Fig 11.4. The figure relates to a hypothetical fluorophore (fluorescent substance or object) that absorbs in the blue and fluoresces in the green. The emission spectrum is an approximate mirror image of the longest-wavelength peak of the absorption spectrum.

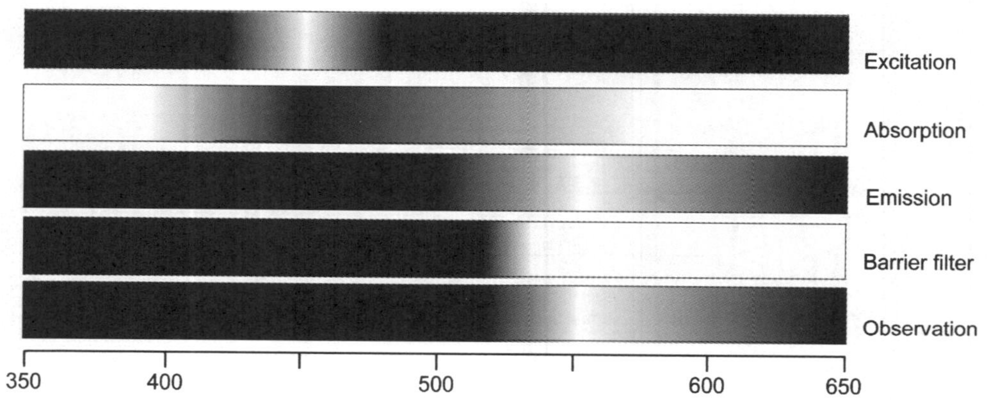

Fig 11.4. Diagram explaining the filter system used in fluorescence microscopy. The scale is of wavelength in nanometres (nm), from ultraviolet (left) to red (right). From top to bottom:

- The excitation filter transmits short wavelengths (here blue, centred on 450 nm).
- The absorption spectrum of the fluorescent substance, strongest in the blue.
- The emission spectrum (predominantly green) of the fluorescent substance.
- The transmission of long wavelengths by the barrier filter. The cutoff here is at about 520 nm.
- The wavelengths of emitted light observed through the barrier filter by the eye or camera.

Dichromatic mirror

Because the excitation and emission are at different wavelengths, modern epi-illumination mirrors are designed to reflect preferentially at the excitation wavelength, and to transmit preferentially at the fluorescence wavelength.

These mirrors are variously known as mirrors or as beamsplitters; those that reflect or transmit preferentially at different wavelengths are variously called 'dichromatic' or 'dichroic'. The latter term is unfortunate, as the word 'dichroic' normally refers to a quite different property, related to polarisation. Since the functions of the mirror or beamsplitter are primarily to reflect light down through the objective, and secondarily to refrain from posing an obstruction to light passing up from the objective, we prefer the term mirror, without having any real objection to the other term. Therefore, in the present work, the term 'dichromatic mirror' is used.

A dichromatic mirror gives a significant increase in efficiency, which can be explained as follows. First, consider a mirror that reflects 50% and transmits 50% at all wavelengths, with no absorption. Then the intensity of the excitation will be reduced by 50% at reflection, and that of the fluorescence will equally be reduced 50% on transmission. This results in a total reduction to 25%, compared with the ideal mirror reflecting 100% at the excitation wavelength and transmitting 100% at the emission wavelength. Therefore, a fourfold increase in efficiency would appear to be possible; in practice, a threefold increase can be obtained.

The dichromatic mirrors used in epi-illuminators are constructed in the form of interference coatings on glass, which must be of excellent optical quality because it is placed in the magnification system between objective and eyepiece. Each mirror is characterised by a wavelength, above which it preferentially transmits and below which it preferentially reflects. The transition wavelength must lie between those of the excitation and barrier filters. Manufacturers usually designate mirrors according to this wavelength, possibly preceded by letters to indicate the type or make of filter.

Special difficulties

Fluorescence microscopy has some particular problems, apart from the purely technical one of having the necessary equipment. The fluorescence image as seen in the microscope is weak compared with that obtained by almost all other kinds of microscopy. This makes particular demands on the efficiency of the system, so as not to waste light, and may lead to difficulties in photography as well as difficulties in interpretation due to difficulty in seeing properly at low light levels. To make matters worse, the specimen usually photobleaches (fades) under irradiation, and may fade too quickly to be photographed. Photobleaching can be reduced by using as little irradiation as possible, choosing optimal wavelengths for excitation, and appropriate choice of mounting medium (for details see Rost, 1991). The image seen in the microscope may consist of only a few small fluorescent areas in an otherwise black field. To enable the specimen as a whole to be visualised, and to show the position of fluorescent areas in relation to the rest of the specimen, fluorescence microscopy is sometimes supplemented with other forms of microscopy such as phase-contrast, DIC, or darkground illumination (see below, Combined techniques).

Setting up the fluorescence microscope

It is of major importance that the microscope be set up optimally for the specimen. The process (summarised in the Box on the next page, and described in detail by Rost, 1992) generally involves the following steps:

- Initial adjustment of the microscope using conventional transmitted-light microscopy, with a conventional slide as a test specimen.
- Setting up the microscope for fluorescence microscopy, with a fluorescent test slide.
- Selecting the correct filter combination for the fluorophore (or fluorophores) to be examined.
- Adjusting the microscope for optimal visualisation of the fluorescence.

Setting up a fluorescence microscope

It is best to set up the microscope on a vibration-free bench (see Chapters 3 and 15), in a room capable of being almost completely darkened.

1. Attach the epi-illuminator and light source, if they are not already in position.
2. Ensure that the shutter in the illuminator unit is closed, or that the mirror-house is set to block the light from the arc lamp.
3. Check that the nominal running hours of the mercury arc lamp have not been exceeded (if so, change the lamp). Switch on the mercury arc lamp (this usually needs to be done 5–10 minutes in advance of microscopy).
4. Set up the microscope for conventional transmitted-light microscopy. Use, if possible, a test slide that is also fluorescent, eg fluorescent pigment granules mounted in DePX, so that the same preparation can be used later for checking fluorescence, without re-focusing.
5. Ensure that the appropriate filter block is in place (or separate excitation and barrier filters and dichromatic mirror).
6. Ensure that the aperture and field diaphragms of the epi-illuminator are fully open.
7. Unless simultaneous transillumination is required, switch off or block the transmitted-light source.
8. Remove any DIC fittings or polar above the objective.
9. Open the shutter for the excitation light, and look through the eyepieces at the fluorescent test slide.
10. Adjust the epi-illuminator as necessary, including the field diaphragm and its centration, and the aperture diaphragm (which is normally left fully open).
11. Adjust the lamphouse controls (centration of lamp, mirror, collector lens) as necessary.
12. Unless simultaneous transillumination is required, place a light-trap under the stage, to prevent light being reflected back. If a light-trap is not fitted to the microscope, lower the condenser and place a piece of black cardboard or cloth under the stage; or, close the condenser aperture diaphragm and place a black object below the condenser. Alternatively, place a mirror below the condenser to reflect excitation back up again!
13. Close the shutter, and exchange the test slide for the specimen.
14. It is usually best to locate the relevant area of the specimen using visible light, possibly using phase or interference contrast, or darkground illumination.
15. Switch off the transmitted-light, phase-contrast (or whatever) lighting and open the shutter to examine the specimen by fluorescence.
16. If it is necessary to change the wavelength of excitation, the focusing of the collector lens may require a minor adjustment.

Every effort must be made to obtain the brightest possible image on the film for a given amount of excitation light. The objective's numerical aperture (NA) should be as high as possible; this may be limited by a requirement for depth of field. Objectives whose effective NA can be varied by an iris diaphragm may be helpful. An efficient barrier filter, transmitting most of the fluorescence, is important; if the cutoff of the filter is at too long a wavelength, not only will the colour be distorted, but also the intensity of the image will be reduced because only the long-wavelength tail of the fluorescence is transmitted by the filter.

It must be emphasised that time spent in preliminary adjustment of the microscope with conventional lighting (brightfield transmitted light) is always worthwhile, since it is easier to check for cleanliness, focus the condenser, and so forth using conventional brightfield illumination. Maintenance of the microscope and particularly of the mercury arc lamp is discussed in Appendix A1.

Selection of filters

In modern fluorescence microscopes, the excitation and barrier filters and dichromatic mirror are grouped together as a unit, in a metal block. Interchangeable blocks are provided for use at different wavelengths for different purposes. Special filter sets are available for examination and photography of double or triple labelling. The best filter sets are 'wedge-free', meaning that blocks can be interchanged without risk of the image being displaced; this means that sequential photomicrographs can be taken.

For photomicrography in colour, the correct filter combination is the same as for visual observation. However, because film is sensitive to ultraviolet (UV) and relatively more sensitive to violet than the eye, it is particularly important that the barrier filter should block short wavelengths adequately. If in doubt, an additional UV-blocking filter should be added to the barrier filter; if the main barrier filter is yellow, orange or red, the UV-blocking filter should be placed with the excitation filter (if possible) to block UV that may otherwise cause autofluorescence in the barrier filter.

Initially, an empirical approach is often best, trying different filter combinations to see which gives the best results. Logical selection of filter combinations requires a knowledge of the excitation and emission spectra of the fluorophore (see, for example, data given by Rost, 1995), together with a consideration of the aims or objectives of the microscopy. A record should always be kept of the *wavelength band of excitation* and the *barrier-filter cutoff wavelength*, and these data included in any publication.

Adjustments for optimal visualisation

The adjustments that are usually required are minor adjustments to the focus of the collector lens to give brighter or more even illumination, reduction of the field diaphragm opening, and sometimes a change of filters.

Evenness of illumination

Uniform illumination of the microscope field is notoriously difficult to obtain, especially with low-power objectives. It requires careful adjustment of the positions of the arc lamp, the reflector and the collector lens. If these adjustments fail, a diffusing 'filter' can be used, at the expense of some loss of brightness.

The aperture of the condenser, ie the aperture iris diaphragm of a substage condenser for transillumination, or the exit pupil of the objective for epi-illumination, must be reasonably fully and evenly filled with light. In the case of epi-illumination, the matter is complicated by variations in diameter of the exit pupil of different objectives. In principle, the collector lens needs to be readjusted each time the objective is changed.

Immersion oil

The immersion oils as now sold by the major optical houses may be expected to be adequate for fluorescence work. Cargille recommend *Type FF*, having virtually no autofluorescence, for fluorescence microscopy; or *Type DF* for highest resolution, meeting exact DIN specifications for refractive index and dispersion, but with slight ('very very low') greenish autofluorescence.

Combined techniques

The fluorescent image seen in the microscope may consist of only a few small fluorescent areas in an otherwise black field. To enable the specimen as a whole to be visualised, and to show the position of fluorescent areas in relation to the rest of the specimen, fluorescence microscopy is sometimes supplemented with other forms of microscopy such as transmitted light (possibly with the aperture diaphragm of the substage condenser partially closed to increase contrast), phase-contrast, DIC, or darkground illumination. These techniques can be applied either simultaneously or alternately with fluorescence microscopy. Alternatively, the autofluorescence of the specimen itself may be examined, using UV excitation, but the UV may cause fading of the specific fluorescence being studied. To avoid masking the fluorescence using a simultaneous technique, co-author Fred finds it essential to tint this additional illumination to a colour that contrasts with the fluorescence. Because of the barrier filter, the contrasting colour has to have a longer wavelength than the fluorescence. With blue, green or yellow fluorescence, co-author Fred has usually employed red for contrast. Red has the great advantage that, even if the light is quite bright, it does not spoil dark adaptation of the observer's eye. With red fluorescence, good colour contrast is more difficult to achieve. The intensity of the background illumination must be adjusted to balance the brightness of the fluorescence. The filter for the contrast colour need not be elaborate; suitable filters can be obtained from a photographic supply house (see Chapter 8). At a pinch, coloured *Cellophane* may serve. Where required, the special objectives for phase contrast or DIC must be used for fluorescence as well as for the special optical-contrast technique.

Photomicrography of fluorescence

The low light intensity of the fluorescence image leads to two major difficulties in photography: measurement of the exposure (requiring a sensitive photometer) and the length of the exposure time. The former is a merely technical problem, solved by appropriate equipment that is commercially available. The long exposure, however, usually results in fading of the fluorescence under the prolonged irradiation. Fading of the specific fluorescence is often faster than that of the background, so that the photograph suffers from loss of contrast. There is a serious complication, due to the properties of the photographic emulsion: as the length of the exposure increases, the sensitivity of the film decreases, so that a still longer exposure is required to compensate, and during this additional exposure there is more fading, giving a vicious circle of fading, longer exposure required, loss of film sensitivity, longer exposure required . . . A further difficulty is that the specimen typically shows small areas of fluorescence against a predominantly black background; this complicates the determination of the correct exposure.

The ideal specifications of a photomicrographic camera for fluorescence

The ideal photomicrographic camera for fluorescence should have the following characteristics (besides those listed in Chapter 2; see also Chapter 14). Some of these features may not be practicable for a particular application, on economic grounds.

- High light transmission: no beamsplitters, zooms, etc. The body tube should send 100% of the light to the camera.
- Low camera magnification. The film format should cover only a little less than the objective's field of view; indeed, for black-and-white (B&W), the format need not even be fully filled. The format should be as small as practicable (normally 24 mm ×36 mm on 35 mm film).
- Illuminated graticule for focusing and composing the picture, for visibility against a dark background, preferably visible in both normal eyepieces. The illumination should preferably be variable in intensity, possibly red in colour (to avoid spoiling the eye's adaptation), and with an on/off switch so that the graticule does not disturb normal observation. The illuminated graticule may be in one or both eyepieces (best), although some users prefer an illuminated graticule in a viewing telescope of the camera unit.
- Variable magnification of the focusing graticule – high magnification for focusing, low for composing the picture. Possibly an automatic focusing mechanism, operative even at low light levels, with manual override, would be helpful.
- Photometer of adequate sensitivity, optional integrated measurement or spot measurement from a defined moveable spot.
- Exposure control system with provision for setting ISO film speed over a wide range (especially high ISO values), compensation for proportions of bright and dark (see Chapter 16), and compensation settings for reciprocity failure characteristics (see Chapters 16 and 18). Bracketing should be easy.
- The control and exposure information of the exposure control unit should be clearly visible under low illumination levels. Any lamps or illuminated displays should not dazzle the eye, and preferably be in red colour to maintain dark adaptation.
- The film format should be as small as practicable, in order to minimise the magnification required to fill the picture with the desired object, and thereby to maximise the intensity of the image. Therefore, 35 mm cameras are almost universally used. Larger formats should generally be avoided (however, some Polaroid films are fast enough to be useable). Still smaller formats, such as the APS format (16·7 mm × 30·2 mm), would give shorter exposure times (given an appropriate projective).

Photomicrographic technique

The procedures required in taking photomicrographs are summarised in Table 11.1. Efforts must be concentrated on minimising the exposure of the specimen to irradiation both before and during photography.

Table 11.1. Basic fluorescence photomicrography

1. Switch on the arc lamp at least several minutes before commencement.
2. Block the light used for excitation.
3. Find the area of interest in the specimen without using fluorescence (use brightfield, phase contrast, DIC, darkground, etc).
4. Select the appropriate filter combination for the specimen.
5. Using fluorescence, confirm that the desired area is selected and focused.
6. Measure the exposure.
7. Block the light used for excitation, while checking what correction is to be made for reciprocity failure. Adjust the camera system accordingly.
8. Using fluorescence, take the photograph. Probably bracket the exposure; take the shortest exposure first, the longest last.

Focusing and composing the picture

The object to be photographed is first selected, taking care not to fade it unnecessarily. This is best accomplished by placing a neutral-density (grey) filter in the excitation light path, so that the specimen is observed with dim light. Preliminary focusing and location of the specimen without fluorescence excitation can be undertaken by methods outlined above (see above, Combined techniques).

The size of the field of view to be photographed should be selected by choosing the appropriate objective. Remove any magnification changer or zoom, or set it to minimal magnification. An illuminated graticule in the viewfinder eyepiece is helpful.

Exposure time

The principles of measuring exposure are summarised in Chapter 3, and dealt with in detail in Chapter 16, which discusses the problems specific to low light levels.

The correct exposure time is determined by a combination of many factors. They may be summarised as: the brightness of the fluorescence, the extent of fading during exposure, the magnification of the image onto the film, the amount of light loss in the optical system, and the sensitivity of the film under the prevailing circumstances.

The brightness of the fluorescence is maximised, and fading minimised, by methods that have been described by Rost (1992). Obviously these techniques are of particular importance for photomicrography. The magnification of the image at the film plane affects the intensity of the image; the latter is inversely proportional to the magnification. To minimise the magnification required to fill the picture with the desired object, the film format should be as small as practicable. 35 mm cameras are almost universally used for fluorescence photomicrography. Larger formats should be avoided (but see comments above on Polaroid films). Still smaller formats, eg APS, used with an appropriate projective, could give shorter exposure times.

Strictly, the above remarks concerning the effect of magnification on image brightness apply only to images of areas, and do not apply in the special case of point sources of light, ie an object consisting of unresolvable minute particles. In such cases, the images of the particles should, if sharply focused, be diffraction-limited and their dimensions independent of the magnification.

Loss of light in the optical system, always unfortunate in fluorescence microscopy, is to be avoided at all costs for fluorescence photomicrography. Causes of light loss peculiar to photomicrography are: a beamsplitter in the phototube of the microscope, which reflects part of the light into the eyepieces (use only a trinocular tube with provision to transmit 100% of the light to the camera), and a beamsplitter in the camera to reflect light to an exposure-measuring device.

High sensitivity of the film implies loading the camera with high-speed film (B&W or colour; if the latter, the film must be of the daylight type). It may be possible to raise the speed at which the film is rated, by a suitable developer (eg *Microphen* for B&W) or increased development time ('pushing') or pre-exposure (see Chapter 18).

Taking the pictures

To take a picture, if the camera has shutter speeds set manually: with the full excitation, operate the photometer to determine the brightness of the image. Block off the excitation while calculating the exposure to be given. Set the exposure to be given, open the excitation shutter, and shoot. Record the exposure in your notebook.

It is usually necessary to bracket the exposures, ie take additional exposures at shorter and longer exposure times, to ensure the best results. With colour film, take two additional pictures, one each about 0·5 to 0·7 and 1·4 to 2·0 times the calculated optimal exposure (ie 1 to $^1/_2$ stop; $^2/_3$ stop is convenient for instruments calibrated in $^1/_3$ stops). For B&W, give 3 to 4 times less and more; or take a series of pictures at 1 stop intervals. Because of the fading problem, we usually give these exposures in the following order: middle (expected to be correct), shorter, longer; or alternatively, start with the shortest and then take progressively longer ones. Thus, suppose that using Ilford *HP5* film at ISO 400/27°, the exposure meter indicates 12 seconds. From the reciprocity data supplied by the manufacturer, the corrected exposure is 30 seconds; so one can give 30 (or 32) seconds, 8 seconds, and 2 minutes. If fading is severe, after each exposure one should measure the exposure again, or choose a different field. The meter reading and the exposures given should be recorded, and later correlated with the results.

Pictures of control preparations must always be taken at the same exposure time as the 'test' pictures. This is particularly important in immunofluorescence, if 'positive' and 'negative' preparations are to be photographed. The correct procedure is to photograph the positive preparation first, noting the exposure given, and then to photograph the control specimen under exactly the same conditions and with the same exposure time. A fully automatic camera (determining the exposure for itself) can be used; but, for any control preparation, the automatic system must be overridden and the same exposure time given as for the test preparation. Otherwise, the automatic camera will give a negative control preparation a much longer exposure, in an attempt to make it appear as bright as the positive specimen!

Infrared and red fluorescence

Fluorescence emission in the infrared is widely known in chlorophylls, and has been observed from blue and green dyes such as Indocyanine Green. The fluorescence is invisible to the eye, but can be recorded on infrared-sensitive photographic film (see Chapter 12). For the fluorescence of chlorophyll (Fig 11.1), normal B&W film is inadequate even for the visible red component of the emission, and you should use a film with extended red sensitivity, such as Ilford *SFX* or Kodak *Technical Pan*.

Flash-fluorescence photomicrography

Photomicrographs of fluorescence can be made using an electronic flash as the light source. Electronic flash has spectral characteristics that are essentially those of a xenon arc, but giving only a brief flash rather than continuous output. Flash duration of conventional flash units is of the order of 0·1 ms to 1 ms (1/10 000 second to 1/1000 second). In the ordinary circumstances of a non-motile specimen, more than one flash can be given as multiple exposures on one frame of film to achieve the required exposure. Because of an effect similar to reciprocity failure, an intermittent exposure of this type may not equal in effect one longer flash of energy equal to the sum of the shorter flashes. Also, reciprocity failure occurs at very short exposures such as may be given by a flash unit. On the other hand, use of flash for fluorescence should assist in minimising fading.

Video-intensification fluorescence microscopy

Fluorescence microscopy is most easily accomplished by examining the image with some form of video (closed-circuit television, CCTV) system (see Chapter 17). This technique is now generally known as video intensification microscopy (VIM), so named by Willingham & Pastan (1978).

There are several advantages specifically for fluorescence microscopy. Firstly, the picture produced on a monitor screen is much brighter than the view in the microscope, obviating the necessity for a darkened room and dark-adapted eyes, and the greater sensitivity allows reduction of the intensity of irradiation, thereby reducing fading and damage to living tissues. Secondly, the screen can easily be viewed simultaneously by two or more observers. Thirdly, the camera output can be recorded on a video recorder or with a computer frame grabber, or, alternatively, the screen can be photographed; the exposure required is much shorter than direct photography of the fluorescence, and the exposure time is constant. Finally, use of a video camera expands the useable emission wavelengths to beyond the visible, to the UV and infrared, eg the infrared fluorescence of Indocyanine Green (Moneta *et al*, 1987).

For further information, see Chapter 17 and the books by Herman (1998) and Rost (1991).

Further reading

The current standard textbooks on fluorescence microscopy are those of Rost (1991, 1992, 1995). Anyone seriously involved in fluorescence microscopy should have at least vol 1 of Rost's *Fluorescence microscopy* (Rost, 1992, reprinted with additions 1996). There are also useful booklets by Herman (1998) and by several microscope manufacturers. Applications to a wide range of fields were reviewed by Rost (1995).

12
Infrared and ultraviolet microscopy

Photomicrography in infrared (IR) and ultraviolet (UV) light presents special problems, for two main reasons. IR and UV are invisible to the eye, and optical equipment is usually not corrected for these wavelengths. In addition, IR requires special film, and UV requires special UV-transmitting optics.

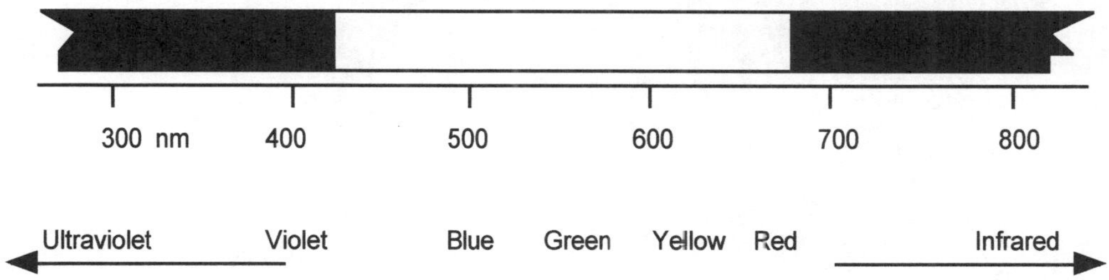

Fig 12.1. Diagram of a spectrum, showing relation of UV and IR to visible light. The diagram shows the approximate range of visible light, wavelengths in nanometres, and corresponding colours.

Infrared

Infrared (IR) light has wavelengths longer than those of visible light, ie greater than about 750 nm (0·75 μm), and extending up to about 40 000 nm (40 μm). Photomicrography with IR appears to have been first carried out by A. Köhler in 1921. Infrared photography can be carried out with an ordinary microscope, but has three major difficulties: the image is not visible to the eye, ordinary lenses are not corrected for the IR wavelengths, and special IR-sensitive film must be used.

Light sources and filters

Ordinary tungsten–halogen lamps, arc lamps and sunlight have plenty of IR. All hot or warm bodies emit IR. Heat-absorbing filters (ie IR-absorbing, such as Schott KG1) must *not* be used, and if present must be removed (remember to replace it for all other applications!).

For photography in pure IR, it is necessary to use a filter that blocks visible light and transmits IR. Such filters are supplied by (among others) Kodak (88A, 87C) and Hoya (R72, RM90). More commonly, a red filter is used, blocking most of the visible light (eg Kodak Wratten 25 or Wratten 29 red filters). A filter is always required to block UV and blue light. See Anon (1990).

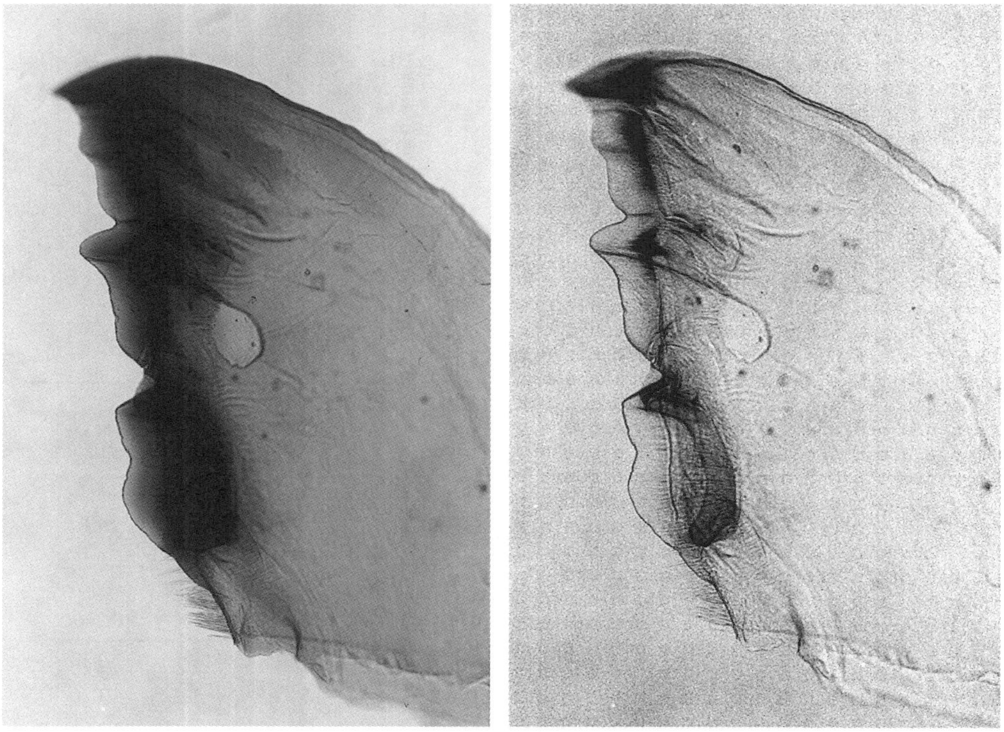

Fig 12.2. Photomicrographs in transmitted visible light (left) and infrared light (right). Cricket mandible, field size 2·3 mm × 1·6 mm. Olympus *BH2* microscope, 4× planapo NA 0·14 objective, *PM-10ADS* camera. Visible-light image: Ilford *Pan F* film, deep yellow G15 filter. IR image, Kodak *HIE* Infrared film rated at 4000 ISO, Hoya RM90 filter.

The camera

Equipment should be checked for its opacity to IR; black plastic and bellows are notoriously liable to be translucent to IR, even if appearing quite opaque in visible light. All equipment must be kept cool to prevent IR radiation, which might reduce contrast or spoil the film. Some single-lens-reflex (SLR) cameras with plastic components in their bodies cannot be used with IR film, because the plastic is not opaque to IR and the film can be fogged. Cameras with metallic bodies (eg Nikon SLRs) are safe in this respect.

The exposure meter may not give the correct exposure for IR, because of non-linear spectral sensitivity. Photomultiplier tubes tend to be less sensitive to IR, whereas semiconductor (solid-state) devices tend to be relatively more sensitive in the IR.

Lenses

All microscope and photographic lenses transmit at least the shorter IR wavelengths, but few are corrected for this region. All but the most highly corrected optical systems show a marked shift in focus from visible to IR light. Mention must be made of the special objectives made by Olympus, Nikon and Zeiss for IR. A small numerical aperture (NA) may be used to increase the depth of focus, if resolution is not a problem, to minimise focusing error.

The only immersion fluid currently available that is suitable for IR microscopy is paraffin oil. Ordinary immersion oil is not suitable.

Focusing

Because the IR image is invisible to the eye, composing and focusing the picture is carried out either with visible light (eg, using phase contrast), or (better) with the aid of an IR-sensitive video camera. Phase contrast or interference contrast may be useful if the specimen is transparent in the visible spectral region.

If focusing is carried out with visible light, it is necessary that the lens be sufficiently well corrected for chromatic aberration (axial colour) that the focus does not shift significantly between visible and IR light. An apochromatic objective is therefore advantageous. The visual focus of a normal achromatic lens is not correct for IR, the focal length usually increases. The correct focus must be determined by trial-and-error, by taking a number of photographs at various focusing settings (note the readings on the fine-focus adjusting knob).

Many modern microscopes have multiple camera ports, with the various images all conjugate with each other. This feature facilitates infrared focusing, for a conventional video camera is quite sensitive in the IR, and its image on a monitor will establish the correct focus also for the image in the camera.

Infrared film

Special films are available with extended sensitivity in the far red and infrared. Silver halide emulsions (see Chapter 18) are basically sensitive only to the high-energy (blue) end of the spectrum: the construction of red-sensitive (panchromatic) films require the addition of an organic dye that absorbs in the red and transfers the photon energy to the silver halide. IR film is of course also sensitive to visible and UV light. Both black-and-white (B&W) and false-colour versions are available.

IR film must be kept cool, and should be stored in a refrigerator. Because of ‘light piping’ (light piped along the film base through the film leader), IR film should be handled in the dark only, implying that the loading and unloading of a camera should be carried out in the dark (possibly in a changing bag).

Kodak *Ektachrome* infrared film is a reversal film for transparencies, giving false colours, of which cyan is the infrared record. The emulsion layers are sensitive to green, red and infrared rather than the usual blue, green and red. Its IR sensitivity extends to about 900 nm. It must be exposed through a deep yellow (minus-blue) filter, such as Wratten 12. Other filters can be used for special effects. Processing is by the E-6 process. It should be loaded into the camera in total darkness.

Kodak *High-Speed HIE Infrared* film (B&W) is sensitive to IR radiation to about 900 nm, with highest sensitivity from 750 to 840 nm. It is usually used with a red filter (25) or an IR filter (87, 87C, 88A or 89B).

Konica *Infrared 750 nm Professional* film is a B&W film. Its spectral sensitivity range is from 400 to 500 nm, then a gap from 500 to 640 nm, and then it is sensitive again in the IR with a peak at 750 nm. It can be loaded into the camera in daylight.

General-purpose B&W films with extended red sensitivity are uncommon, but include Ilford *SFX* and Kodak *Technical Pan* film.

Exposure

Exposure has to be determined by trial-and-error. In principle, an exposure meter can be used, but requires re-calibration. The meter scale is not calibrated for IR, for which photomultipliers are less sensitive and solid-state sensors are generally more sensitive. After initial experimentation, a conversion graph or table can be constructed (see Fig 16.2). For the Olympus *PM-10ADS* metering, the speed rating of Kodak B&W IR film, nominally 100 ISO, becomes 4000 ISO. In any case, IR film has limited latitude, so bracketing will be needed, $\pm^1/_3$ stop.

Applications

Objects that can be photographed are those that either reflect IR when illuminated, or emit IR because they are warm or because of IR fluorescence. Green plants appear white on B&W IR film because the green pigment, chlorophyll, reflects IR well (chlorophyll also fluoresces in the IR region). Medically, IR has been used to photograph blood vessels of the skin, which is to some extent transparent to IR, particularly if the skin is rubbed with glycerine or oil to make it more transparent (Longmore, 1955; Bollinger & Fagrell, 1990). Some materials, opaque to visible light, are transparent to IR. This enables the photography of internal structures of insects (see Fig 12.2). For other examples see Casida (1968) and Farrell (1969).

Fluorescence emission in the infrared is widely known in chlorophylls, and has also been observed from blue and green dyes such as Indocyanine Green. The fluorescence is invisible to the eye, but can be recorded on infrared-sensitive photographic film (Elkin & Park, 1975; Puchtler, Meloan & Paschal, 1980) or examined with an infrared-sensitive video camera (Moneta *et al*., 1987).

Further reading

Photomicrography with IR has previously been described by Pluta (1989) and (briefly) by Lawson (1972). For further information on IR photography in general, see Anon (1973), Gibson (1980) and Ray (1994a).

Ultraviolet

Ultraviolet (UV) light has wavelengths shorter than those of visible light, ie with a wavelength shorter than 400 nm. Photography with UV involves illuminating the specimen with UV light, and photographing though a special filter that blocks visible light and transmits only UV. The main complications are, firstly, that UV light is invisible and so the image cannot be focused by visual means, and, secondly, that ordinary optical systems do not readily transmit UV light.

Care should be taken to distinguish between photography in UV light (this chapter) and photography of fluorescence using UV excitation (Chapter 11). In techniques that use UV for the excitation of *fluorescence*, all visible light is prevented from reaching the specimen by filtration, but only the longer (visible) wavelengths of fluorescence take part in image formation and recording. *UV photography* implies UV radiation of the specimen, but other visible wavelengths may also reach the specimen; before or after the specimen, a UV-pass filter is required to remove all the visible wavelengths. The UV forms the recorded image.

Light source and filters

The main sources of UV light are xenon arc lamps and mercury arc lamps (see Chapter 8). Electronic flash is equivalent to a xenon arc; there may be difficulties due to the cover over the flash tube, which may not transmit UV. For work below 365 nm, xenon arc lamps are usually used, as they have relatively more UV below 365 nm than mercury arcs.

A filter must be placed somewhere in the system to eliminate visible light. Suitable filters include Kodak Wratten 18A and 18B, or a combination of Schott UGI + BG38, or a 365 nm interference filter. In principle, the filter should be placed in a position to eliminate any visible light emitted as fluorescence by the specimen or the optical system (and dust thereon). Do not use a filter that has previously been used as an excitation filter in a fluorescence microscope, because its optical quality will have been spoilt by the heat.

Lenses

Ordinary optics can generally be used at 365 nm. Older lenses may have a higher transmission than modern lenses with many elements and dense glass.

Special optical systems for UV are made by Leica, Nikon and Zeiss. Because ordinary optical glass does not transmit below about 350 nm, all optical elements in the illumination system must be made of quartz (fused silica), fluorite or other UV-transmitting materials. Mirror lenses with no glass elements are also suitable, particularly as mirrors have no chromatic aberration.

The specimen and its mount

In setting up the specimen, it may be necessary to remember that ordinary glass and plastics are opaque to UV radiation shorter than about 365 nm. If it is necessary to cover or contain the specimen, quartz or fused silica must be used instead of glass. UV-transmitting microscope slides and coverslips are available, but are very expensive. To reduce the expense, the slides are made much smaller than standard, just large enough for the specimen, and are themselves mounted in a metal holder. Naturally, slides and even coverslips are usually too expensive to use only once, and are cleaned for re-use.

The mounting medium and immersion fluid (if used) also need to be transparent to UV. Useful substances include water, glycerol, and liquid paraffin, which are transparent to UV and non-fluorescent. Glycerol and water can be mixed (eg 90% glycerol, 10% water by volume).

Focusing

Because the UV image is invisible to the eye, composing and focusing the picture is carried out either with visible light (eg, using phase contrast), or (better) with the aid of a UV-sensitive video camera (see the corresponding section on IR, above). Phase contrast or interference contrast may be useful if the specimen is transparent in the visible spectral region. If focusing is carried out with visible light, it is necessary that the optical system be sufficiently well corrected for chromatic aberration (axial colour; see Chapter 6) for focus not to shift significantly between visible and UV light. If necessary, the correct focus must be determined by trial-and-error, by taking a number of photographs at various focusing settings, noting the readings of the fine-focusing scale.

Film

A high-contrast B&W film is the most appropriate, eg Kodak *Technical Pan* film. Many films, especially daylight-balanced slide films, have a barrier overcoating to absorb UV. This may make them unsuitable for some UV photographing techniques. If a colour transparency film is to be used, one balanced for tungsten light is usually preferable, because these films are designed for full sensitivity at the blue end of the spectrum and do not have the UV-absorbing overcoat. Exposure has to be determined by trial-and-error (see Chapter 16).

Further reading

Photomicrography with UV has previously been described (briefly) by Lawson (1972). For further information on photography in UV generally, see Morton (1984) and Arnold *et al*. (1971).

13
Stereomicroscopy

Our perception of objects as three-dimensional depends primarily on binocular vision; each eye produces an image of the subject as seen from a different position. Complex image processing in the brain results in perception of three dimensions. This is known as binocular vision. A similar effect, called *stereoscopic vision*, can be achieved by taking two photographs (a *stereo pair*, Fig 13.1) from positions a little apart, and then presenting each image to the corresponding eye; the left-hand picture is seen by the left eye, while the right-hand picture is viewed simultaneously by the right eye. A stereoscopic view from photographs of an object is not quite the same as a binocular view of the same object, because in the latter, when looking at objects of different distances, the eyes vary in convergence and accommodation, whereas in stereoscopic viewing these parameters remain constant.

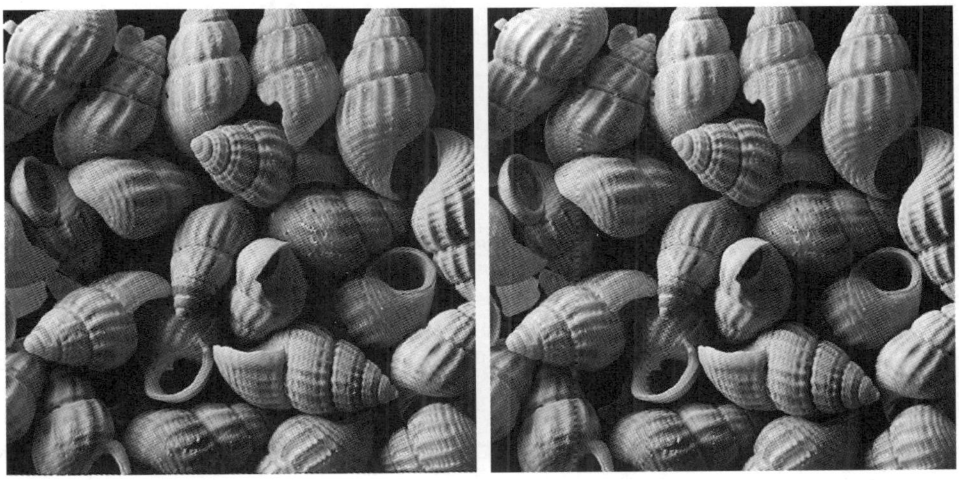

Fig 13.1. A stereo pair (low power) of tiny seashells, *Alvania novarensis*, from Botany Bay, taken with the microscope shown in Fig 13.3, and the tilting board shown in Fig 13.5. Ilford *Pan F* film, developed in *ID11*. Field size 7 mm × 7 mm.

Stereomicroscopes

For the observation of surface relief, and for many tasks such as dissection that demand manipulative skills, optical instrumentation is required that gives binocular vision, magnification, and a long working distance between lens and specimen. For manipulative work, the image should be 'correct' in the sense that the specimen's left–right and top–bottom relationships need to be maintained. Stereomicroscopes have been designed for this purpose. Corresponding photomicrographs can be obtained that, when examined in a stereoscopic viewer, give the impression of relief.

Stereomicroscopes provide separate optical paths for each eye, and are designed to provide a true binocular image; ordinary microscopes do not provide such an image. Porro prisms in the stereomicroscope tube act on the image so that it is viewed erect and laterally unreversed. Stereomicroscopes are of two main designs (Fig 13.2), namely the *Greenough* and the *common main objective* (CMO) patterns.

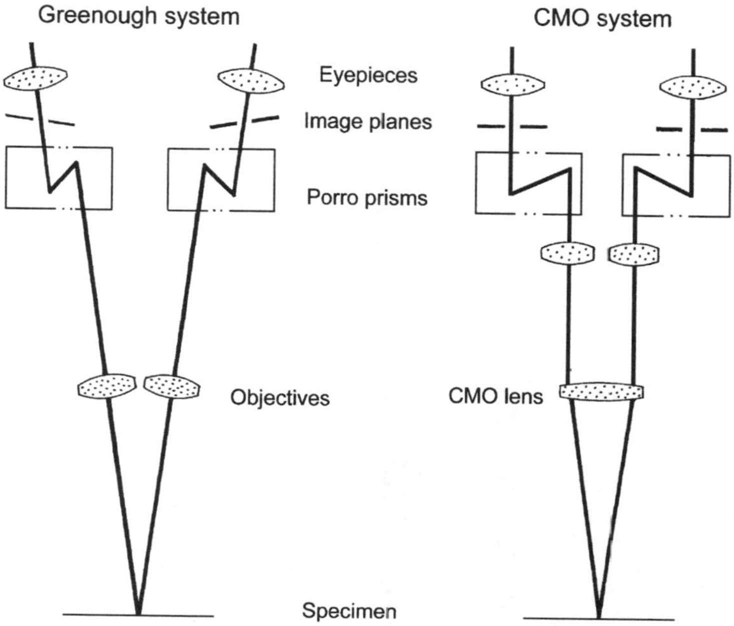

Fig 13.2. A diagrammatic representation of the two major kinds of stereomicroscope. The Greenough type (left) has two optical systems inclined at an angle of about 15° to each other. In the CMO type (right), parallel beam paths above a common main objective have some design advantages for accessory attachments.

Greenough systems

Figure 13.2 shows two different approaches to the provision of a stereoscopic view. On the left is the Greenough type, which consists of two quite separate microscope systems, side by side, but inclined to each other by about 15°. This design followed a proposal by Horatio Greenough, a zoologist, who conceived the idea of obtaining enlarged stereoscopic views of small objects by combining two compound microscopes side by side, one for each eye, modified to give an erect image. This concept was adopted by Zeiss for manufacture in 1895. The advantages of this system include that high numerical apertures (NAs) can be achieved, and that a very high degree of chromatic correction can be realised. A characteristic feature of the Greenough system is convergence of the eyepieces, a feature that to some users is disturbing. Because the axes of the two optical paths are not normal to the object plane (ie not at 90° to it), the planes of focus of each half of the instrument are inclined at an angle of about 7°–8° to the plane of the stage, and therefore it is impossible to focus the whole of a large flat object. This is not usually a problem during visual observation, but for monocular photography it may be necessary to tilt the specimen.

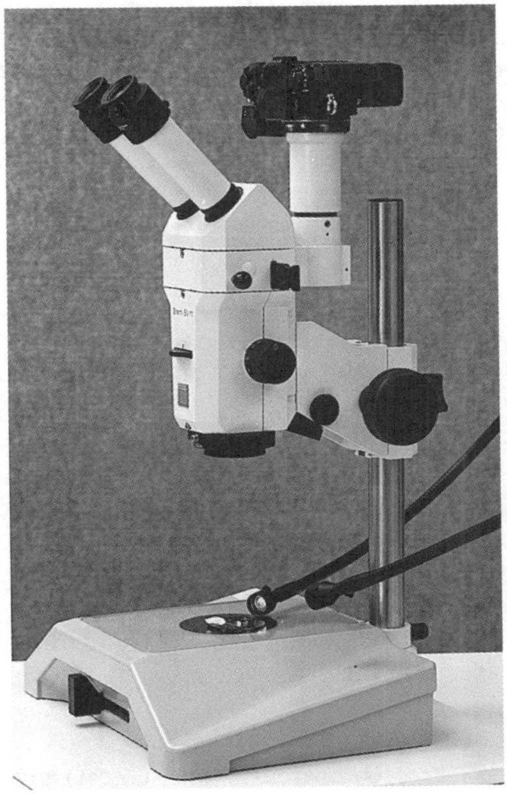

Fig 13.3. A Zeiss CMO stereomicroscope with zoom magnification changer and camera attachment. Note the single objective lens, twin eyepiece tubes, and separate tube for the camera. The specimen is illuminated by a twin-arm fibre optics light source, which is comparatively heat-free. The base illuminator enables brightfield, darkground or oblique transillumination. The fibre optics and the base have independent variable-intensity power supplies. Such lighting equipment may cost half as much again as the stereomicroscope! See also Fig 15.3.

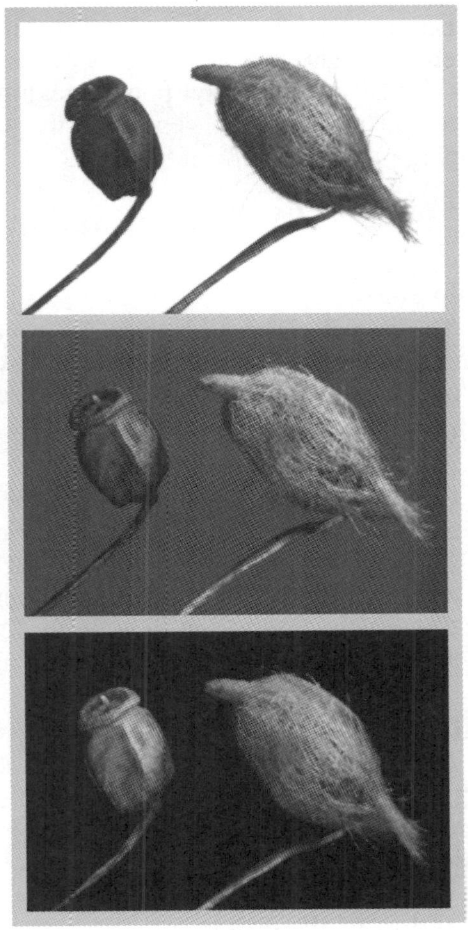

Fig 13.4. Examples of backgrounds for black-and-white photography. The dark moss capsule on the left and the much lighter, fibre-covered capsule on the right present a difficult choice if a plain background is to be used. Field size 8 mm × 13 mm. These photographs were taken with the equipment shown in Fig 13.3.

Common main objective (CMO) systems

In common main objective (CMO) systems, introduced by Zeiss in 1946, the two optical paths share a common front lens, the common main objective (CMO) (Figs 13.2, 13.3, 15.3). The diagram (Fig 13.2) shows, in a CMO stereomicroscope, parallel rays that facilitate the incorporation of accessories such as magnification changers, zoom optics, and drawing and polarisation attachments, thereby increasing the versatility of the design. Interchangeability of viewing and/or photographic heads is more readily possible. Unlike the Greenough design, the CMO optical axis is normal to the specimen, so that one can focus over the whole field. However, optical correction of CMO systems is more difficult, because the axes of the two optical systems pass through the margins of the front lens (the CMO) rather than its centre. This leads to relatively poor imaging, and limits the NA of the system. For photomicrography, the centre of the CMO lens can be used, thereby improving imaging.

Illumination of the specimen

Light source

The first decision to be made is usually whether the photograph is to be taken using continuous lighting or flash. Except in those rare cases where sunlight or daylight can be used, the basic choices are:

- Continuous lighting for focusing and composing only, flash for photography, and daylight-type film.
- Continuous tungsten lighting for focusing and composing and for photography, and black-and-white (B&W) or artificial-light colour film.
- Continuous tungsten lighting for focusing and composing and for photography, and daylight colour film with a colour-correction filter.
- Continuous fluorescent lighting for focusing and composing and for photography, and daylight colour film with a colour-correction filter.

Diffuse and small-source illumination

Diffuse illumination, from a large source (large compared to the subject) gives soft, even illumination, with soft-edged shadows. *Small-source illumination*, from a source that is small compared to the subject, gives hard illumination, with sharp-edged shadows.

Direction of illumination

There are four main choices for the direction of illumination: any one, two or more can be used simultaneously.

- Transmitted-light illumination from below.
- Darkground illumination, obliquely from below.
- Oblique illumination from above. Special case: edge-lighting.
- Frontal (axial) lighting.

Transmitted-light illumination for stereomicroscopes is usually rather primitive. Köhler illumination is not considered a realistic possibility with stereomicroscopes, owing to the large field areas to be covered (cf Chapter7, Adapting the illumination to the objective) and the double optical system of stereomicroscopes. The illumination system would need to be very large. In practice, for transmitted light, there is usually a mirror under the stage, to reflect light from a diffusing screen illuminated by a lamp. In some cases, the transmitted-light illuminator is a separate unit on which the stereomicroscope proper is fitted when required.

Darkground illumination is possible; some instruments have built-in provision for this.

For solid three-dimensional objects, such as molluscan shells or many fossil specimens, the illumination is 'an art in itself and perhaps demands the skills of the professional photographer rather than those of the classical microscopist' (Watts, 1982). Fibre-optic illuminators are generally favoured, partly for their intensity, partly for their low heat output. An alternative is a set of two or three small spotlamps on adjustable arms, possibly attached to the microscope itself (Fig 15.3), but the heat generated in the specimen is considerable. The older method of using a lens to concentrate light onto the specimen is shown in Fig 4.9. Frontal (axial) lighting does not show texture; the more oblique the illumination, the more conspicuous texture becomes. Epi-illumination (see Chapter 7), possible only with the CMO design, is particularly effective for microchips.

Fluorescence microscopy is possible. The Leica *MZFLIII* stereomicroscope is specifically designed for fluorescence microscopy.

Backgrounds

If the subject does not entirely fill the field, the background should be chosen appropriately (see Fig 13.4).

A black background usually gives the most dramatic effect and avoids unnecessary glare, but a succession of pictures with a black background may become boring. A black background may consist either of a matte black material (black cotton velvet is the classical material), or (usually better) the object can be supported on a clear glass sheet with black velvet or other light-trap underneath. The glass must be exquisitely clean (try soaking it in dilute acetic acid), and reflections in the glass are difficult to eliminate.

A white background can be obtained with a white background suitably illuminated, or by using the instrument's transmitted-light illumination system. A shadowless white background can be obtained by illumination from beneath, ie using the instrument's transmitted-light illumination system, or a sheet of white opal plastic or glass with appropriate lighting behind it. For the background to appear white in the photograph, it must be illuminated sufficiently strongly to register as such on the film. Its colour temperature should approximate to that of the main lighting, but moderate errors will not appear if the exposure is sufficient.

A bright background, white or coloured, shining into the lens creates glare. This is best controlled by limiting the size of the background, masking it to the least size needed for the job, using a field iris diaphragm (if there is one) or any improvised method such as a piece of black card with a hole in it to accommodate the specimen.

A coloured background can be obtained with an appropriately coloured background (eg of paper or card) illuminated with white light, or with a white background illuminated with coloured light, or by using the transmitted-light illumination system with a coloured filter. The actual colour chosen is very significant in that it should complement the subject matter. This is an important aesthetic judgement.

Photomicrography with stereomicroscopes

Low-power non-stereoscopic photomicrography

Usually the photograph required is of a single, non-stereoscopic view. In some instruments, the CMO lens may be laterally displaced, enabling use of the better performing axial region of the objective. However, compared with Greenough stereomicroscopes, the CMO intermediate lenses are still restrictive of the instrument's NA.

Stereomicroscopes of the CMO variety commonly have a trinocular head (Fig 13.3), just as in an ordinary microscope; the optical path for the camera passes through the centre of the objective. A standard photomicrographic camera attaches to the phototube, and the photograph is taken in the same way as for any other microscope.

Stereophotomicrography

For photography of stereo pairs (co-author Fred cannot understand why this is not done more often; Ron says that with proper lighting, stereo presentation is unnecessary!), using a normal (non-stereo) camera, the camera system must be positioned first over one side and then over the other. Some CMO microscopes have provision for this. If a stereo camera is used (see Morgan & Lester, 1954) with the Greenough type it is necessary to fit prisms in front of the lenses to accommodate the inclined optical axes of the stereomicroscope. Sometimes the microscope is re-focused between shots, to increase the apparent depth of field.

There are three ways in which a stereo pair can be taken using a microscope:

- Using a stereomicroscope, and with the subject fixed, the camera is moved from one side of the microscope to the other and photographs are taken in succession from each side (or the two pictures of the stereo pair are taken simultaneously with a stereo camera). In a Greenough microscope, there will be differences in focus because of the tilted axes.
- With the camera fixed, the subject is tilted about a horizontal axis (ie an axis in the plane of the stage) through an angle of about 7°–8° each way (Fig 13.5). This produces the same effect as taking two photographs with a Greenough microscope. This technique is used in electron microscopy.
- With the camera fixed, the subject is moved a short distance. The problem here is that part of the specimen may be moved out of the field.

Macroscopes

Macroscopes (photomacroscopes), a more recent and expensive innovation, are low-power microscopes of higher NA than normal stereomicroscopes. They are not stereo instruments. To control (increase) depth of field, an aperture iris diaphragm is incorporated into the body of the instrument.

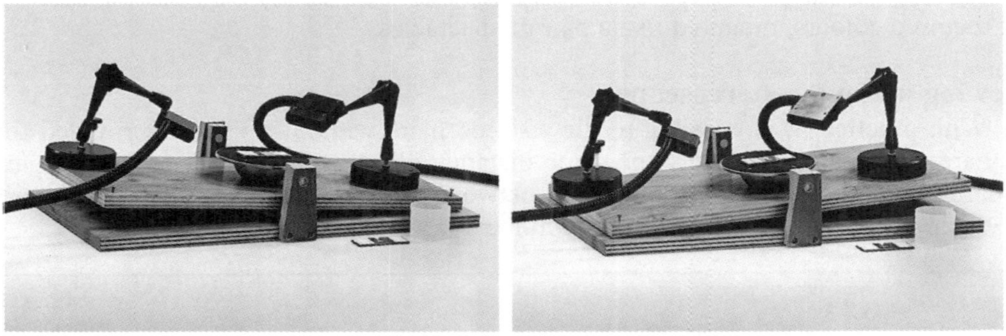

Fig 13.5. A home-made tilting board for stereo photography, designed for medium-sized specimens. The camera (stereomicroscope) position is fixed; two photographs are taken with the board tilted first one way and then the other, approximately 7° – 8° away from horizontal on each side, a total tilt of about 15°. The surface of the specimen should be level with the pivot. Note the lamps, carried on the board so that the direction of lighting does not alter with the tilt.

Confocal microscopy

High-power stereo pairs are most easily achieved with a laser scanning confocal microscope (see Chapter 17).

Mounting and viewing a stereo pair

If the pictures are not wider than 75 mm, they can be mounted or printed side by side (as in Fig 13.1), with their centres separated, if possible, by 65 mm (taken as the normal interpupillary distance). Traditional stereo views are prints about 75–80 mm square, mounted side by side on a piece of cardboard approximately 90 mm × 180 mm.

There are several mounting systems for colour transparencies. For 35 mm stereo transparency pairs, standard stereo mounts measure $1^5/_8$ inches high by 4 inches wide (41·3 mm × 101·6 mm), with two apertures having their centres about 63 mm apart. Several varieties are or have been made, differing in the dimensions of the apertures for different formats, or with different separations for distant, medium distance, or close-up photographs. The standard size frame is 24 mm × 24 mm, but some cameras take a larger size. The mounts which co-author Fred has used have apertures measuring 28 mm × 23 mm and their centres are 63 mm apart.

Stereoscopes

A stereoscope (Fig 13.6) is a device for viewing a stereo pair of pictures using binocular vision so that a three-dimesnional effect is obtained. It typically consists of two lenses that enable the eyes to focus on the two pictures, held at a short distance in front of the eyes, while the eyes themselves are relaxed and focused to infinity. If the prints are too big to be placed side by side with their centres at a distance similar to the interocular distance, mirrors are incorporated to enable the prints to be placed further apart. Red–green stereo viewers usually consist merely of a pair of filters of the required colours, mounted like a pair of spectacles.

Viewing without a stereoscope

With practice, it is possible to view stereo pairs without a viewer, provided that they are placed approximately the same distance apart as the viewer's eyes. A piece of cardboard, about 250 mm long, held between the viewer's nose and the pictures, may help the viewer to acquire the technique.

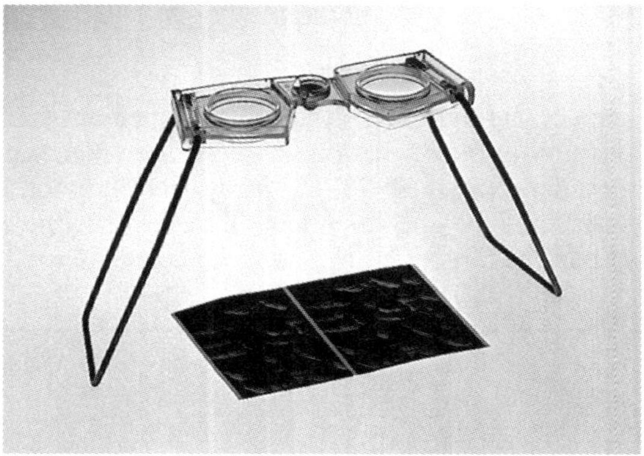

Fig 13.6. A simple stereoscope for viewing stereo prints. The instrument folds up for storage.

Red–green pairs (anaglyphs)

An anaglyph is a superimposed pair of pictures printed in red and green respectively, and viewed through a pair of spectacles with one red and one green glass on appropriate sides (red to port and green to starboard!), so that each eye sees only one image. The method is applicable only to monochrome prints, which must be printed in appropriate colours. Stereo vision using anaglyphs is not affected by red–green colour blindness. Anaglyphs can conveniently be made automatically from digital images (eg from a confocal microscope) and displayed on a colour monitor (see Chapter 17).

Further information

Photomicrography in stereo was described by Acharia (1975), Lester & Richards (1954), Delly & Brown (1980) and Blaker (1989). Stereo photography was described by, among others, Ferwerda (1987), Judge (1950), and Morgan & Lester (1954). The optics of stereoscopic systems was lucidly described by Ray (1994a), who gives further references. A comprehensive treatise on stereoscopy, including stereophotography, was written by Valyus (1966).

Part IV

Advanced photomicrography

This part describes photomicrographic techniques in detail. Chapters of this part assume the subject matter of Chapters 1–3 and of Part II. It is not necessary to have read Part III before Part IV.

- Aims: to describe techniques of photomicrography more advanced than the basic techniques described in Chapter 3.
- Prerequisite knowledge: This part assumes knowledge of Chapters 1–3. Chapter 15 assumes also knowledge of Chapters 6–8 and 14. Chapter 16 includes references to techniques described in Chapters 9–12.
- Exercises: see Appendix A3.
- Further information: see sections entitled Further reading, at ends of chapters.

14
Camera systems

To take photographs with any microscope, we need to add some kind of camera. The camera usually captures the image on film, but modern equipment may make use of a digital camera or a video camera, both of which are discussed in Chapter 17. The camera for photomicrography is usually specially constructed, made to suit the particular microscope, and mounted on the vertical tube of a trinocular head (Fig. 14.1). In microscopes specially designed for photomicrography, the photographic system may be incorporated into the microscope body (Fig 14.3), or form a substantial module attached to the top of the stand (Figs 11.2, 14.1, 17.5). An ordinary camera can be adapted, as described in Chapter 4, but is less convenient. There is a very large choice of photomicrographic cameras, most of which can give high-quality results. The choice will be made according to the volume of photomicrographic work, the versatility required of the instrument, the availability of existing cameras, and the cost and convenience of the attachments.

The ideal specifications of a photomicrographic camera

An ideal photomicrographic camera should have the following characteristics. Some of these features may not be necessary or practicable for a particular application, on economic or other grounds.

- For composition of the picture, a rotatable camera system (unless the microscope stage is rotatable). A well-centred rotation of at least 180° is required.
- High efficiency of light transmission. This implies the possibility of removing beamsplitters, zooms, etc.
- A viewfinder (focusing telescope) with an illuminated graticule for focusing and composing the picture, for visibility against a dark background; even better, the focusing graticule should be in one of the normal eyepieces. The graticule illumination should be variable in intensity, possibly red in colour (to avoid spoiling the eye's adaptation), and with an on/off switch so that the graticule does not disturb normal observation. The field-of-view markings must be precisely coordinated with the film frames.
- A graticule showing only the field actually photographed, as in a single-lens-reflex (SLR) 35 mm camera, would be preferred by one of us (co-author Ron).
- Variable magnification of the focusing graticule – high magnification for focusing, low for composing the picture, would be preferred by co-author Fred. Possibly an automatic focusing mechanism, operative even at low light levels, with manual override, would be helpful.
- Low camera magnification. If flat-field objectives are being used, the film format should cover only a little less than the objective's field of view.
- A photometer with an option for exposure measurement integrated over the whole field, or part of the field, or spot measurement from a defined moveable spot, or zone metering. High sensitivity is required for some applications involving dim light (eg fluorescence, darkground, coal reflectance). There should be provision for setting

film speed (manually and by DX coding) over a very wide range, from 6/9° to 4000/37° ISO values.

- A colour temperature meter to check the colour of the illumination.
- The control settings and exposure information of the exposure control unit should be clearly visible under low illumination levels. Any lamps or illuminated displays should not dazzle the eye, and preferably be in red colour to maintain dark adaptation. Count down during the exposure is very useful.
- A compensation facility for variation of the exposure (at least ±2 stops, or $^1/_4$× to 4×) according to the percentage composition of bright/dark areas in the field.
- Automatic compensation settings for film reciprocity failure characteristics.
- Provision for easy bracketing (preferably automatic). The step between exposures should be adjustable by $^1/_3$ stop or $^1/_2$ stop increments up to at least 1 stop, and the centre exposure value should also be adjustable (for colour transparency film one usually brackets the exposure mainly downwards, whereas for black-and-white (B&W) negative film one brackets the exposure mainly upwards). The number of exposures taken automatically should be adjustable between 1 (no brackets), 2, 3 and 5. Similar automatic bracketing is already available in the best SLR cameras.
- An exposure control system, including vibration-free shutter mechanism, with automatic and manual exposure controls for exposures from 0·01 second to at least 60 seconds (10 minutes for DIC and fluorescence).
- Provision for automatically taking a series of pictures at preset time intervals, for time-lapse photography.
- Choice of formats, including 35 mm (24×36 mm), medium format (6×6 cm or 6×7 cm on 120 roll film), large format (4×5 inches), and Polaroid formats.
- Interchangeable backs to hold the film.
- A data-back for recording identification and other data.
- A device for automatic insertion of a scale bar.

Adaptation of the microscope

Real and virtual images

Under normal (visual) conditions of usage, the microscope image is formed at infinity, and is a virtual image. This means that the image cannot be captured on a screen or piece of film. In the process of visual observation, parallel rays that emerge from the eyepiece are focused by the lens of the eye onto the retina. Without the lens of the eye a focused image will not form. This statement appears to contradict experience with projected images from the microscope, where it is evident that auxiliary lenses are not essential to form a *real,* projected, image. For projection, a focused image is formed by changing the distance between objective and specimen, ie by changing the focus of the microscope.

The objection to re-focusing the objective is that lens aberrations will be introduced, principally spherical aberration, and also curvature of field. As discussed in Chapter 6, microscope optics are skilfully designed to minimise aberrations; this can be accomplished for only one object distance.

In spite of this objection to the re-focusing of the microscope image, it is a method which has been, and is, commonly employed for photomicrography. Especially with low-power magnifications, the re-focusing required may be quite considerable. However, the recognisable quality of the photographs that can be produced bears out the acceptability of the technique (as discussed in Chapter 4). It is a matter of judgement, seeking out a compromise between financial cost and the highest picture quality.

There are four alternative methods of forming a real image, an image that can be photographed, through the normal microscope.

1. The normal lens of a camera is substituted for the lens of the eye, so that the microscope image, at infinity, is brought to focus in the film plane. Simply holding a camera with its lens over the eyepiece enables us to focus the microscope image onto the camera screen. The technique is discussed fully in Chapter 4.
2. For large-format bellows-camera photography (now quite uncommon), various modifications of eyepiece design with negative lenses and focusing top lenses were produced. These systems are no longer available, but a normal high-quality flat-field eyepiece is acceptable.
3. In simple instrumentation today, the normal eyepiece of the camera tube is replaced by a projective (see below) with a short projection distance.
4. In more sophisticated instrumentation, an auxiliary relay lens is added above the eyepiece to bring the emergent parallel rays to a focus in a specified and fixed film plane.

Eyepieces for photography – the projective

Specially designed eyepieces for photography are called *projectives*. They are designed for the short projection distance, often 125 mm, between the eyepiece exit pupil and the film plane of the camera. This projection distance differs from the normal visual conditions (infinite projection distance) for which ordinary eyepieces are optically corrected. Without a well-designed projective, curvature of field and distortion will be introduced into the image, no matter how perfect the correction of the objective.

The trinocular head

This was described in Chapter 2 (see Trinocular heads).

Ports for photographic and video cameras

A microscope designed for photomicrography should be equipped with both a binocular or monocular tube for observation and a separate monocular tube or camera port to accommodate the camera. A sliding mirror or beam-splitting device allows the light from the objective to pass alternatively to the observation tube or to the phototube or to both.

There are circumstances, especially fluorescence microscopy (Chapter 11), when the light-transmitting efficiency of microscope and camera is of vital importance. There is a particular advantage in being able to remove all beamsplitters, prisms and intermediate lenses to enable imaging rays to proceed unimpeded from objective/projective to film. On the other hand, in many circumstances the observer will want to observe the microscope image while the exposure is actually being effected. Some makes of microscope have only a beamsplitter, so that some of the light is always diverted into the observation tubes, and the full amount of available light cannot be utilised for photomicrography. This is unsatisfactory, having the effect of unnecessarily prolonging the exposure required. Also, if this kind of tube must be used, the eyepieces should be covered when not in use to prevent stray light from the room reaching the photometer and film.

In the photographic module, although it will add considerably to the cost of the optical system, the three-way mirror systems (reflecting 100% to the focusing telescope, or 100% to the exposure meter, or 100% to the film) associated with some specialised photomicrographic systems permit the most efficient distribution of the microscope image.

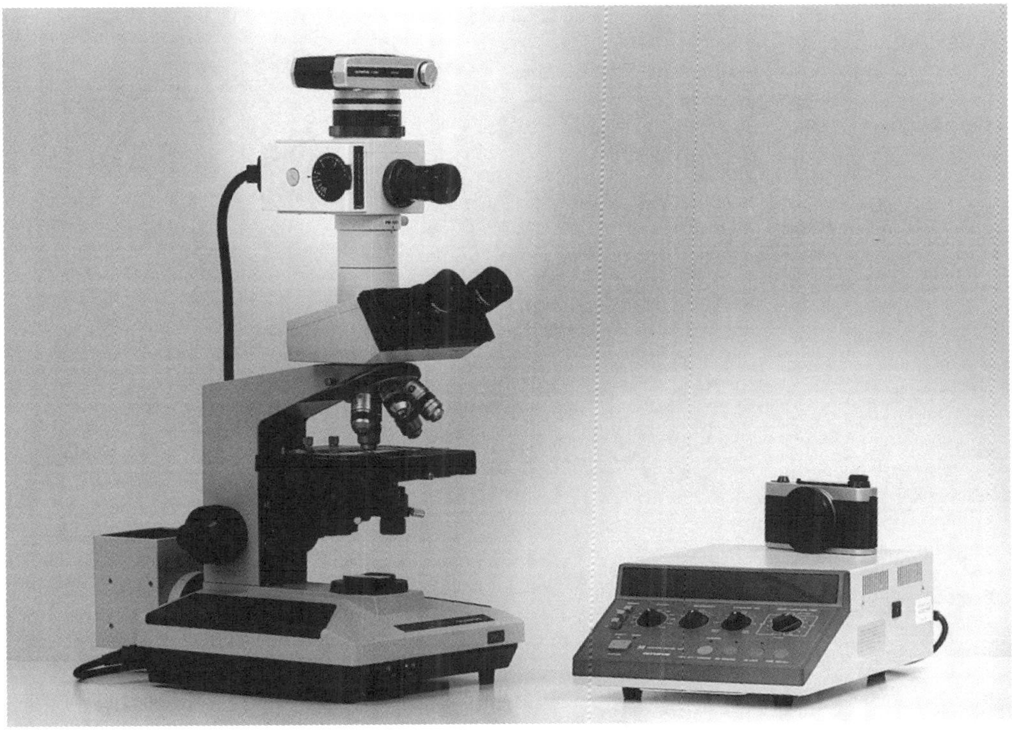

Fig 14.1. Olympus *PM-10ADS* photomicrographic attachment camera, on an Olympus *BH2* microscope. On the right, a spare camera body sits on the control box. In addition to the camera module's telescopic viewfinder, the microscope has a finder eyepiece with a graticule for photography. Either system can be used for composing and focusing the photograph. The trinocular head, carrying the camera, can be rotated through 360° if required.

Cameras for photomicrography

Photographic equipment for photomicrography falls into three classes:

- Normal cameras with an appropriate adapter to the microscope (Figs 4.1 *et seq*).
- Specialised photomicrographic cameras attached to the microscope (Figs 14.1, 14.2).
- Dedicated built-in photomicrographic systems (Fig 14.3).

Ordinary photographic cameras, particularly 35 mm SLRs, were discussed in Chapter 4.

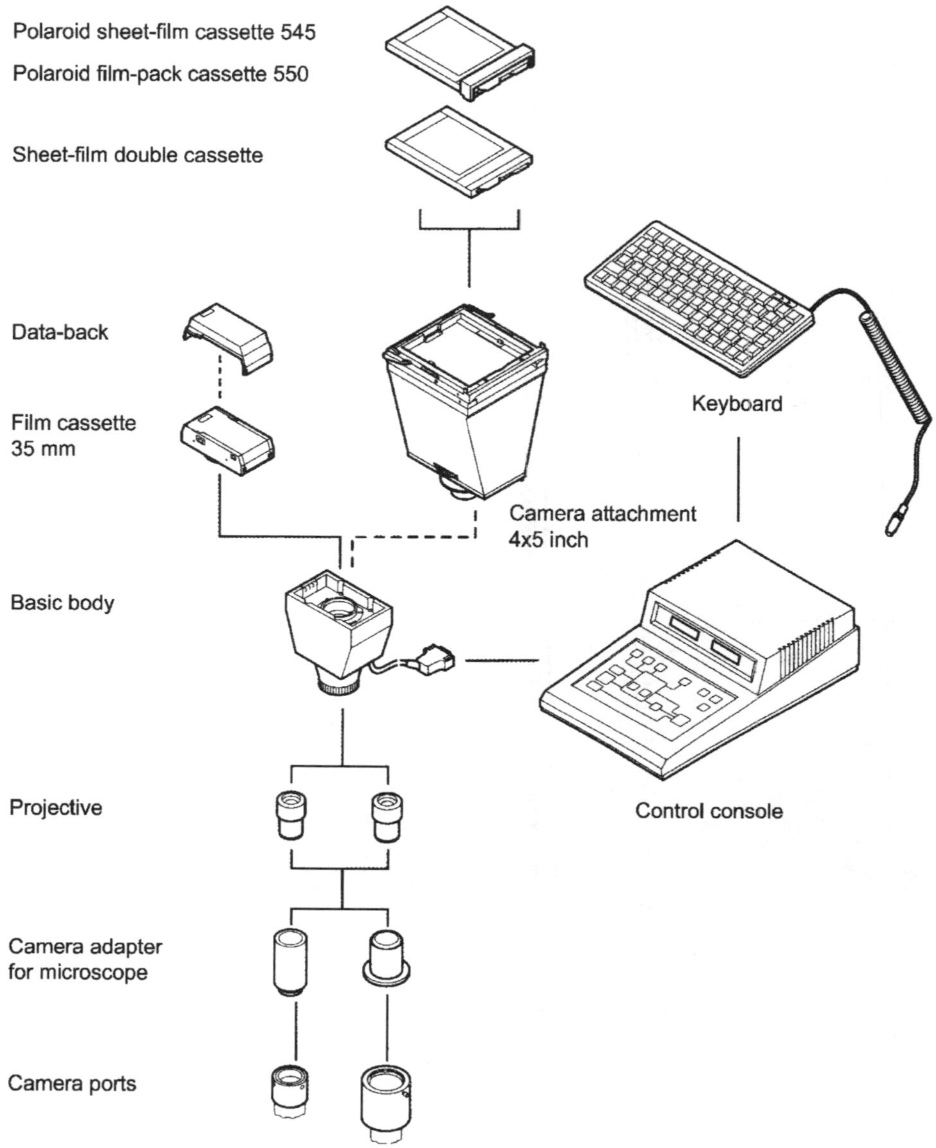

Fig 14.2. Schematic diagram of a modular photomicrographic system, showing how 35 mm, Polaroid and 4×5 inch films can be used. The diagram is based on the Zeiss *MC80DX* microscope camera system. Redrawn after a manufacturer's catalogue illustration, and reproduced courtesy of Carl Zeiss Pty Ltd, Sydney.

Attachment photomicrographic camera modules

An attachment photomicrographic camera is basically similar to an ordinary camera, the microscope optics serving as the lens. With considerable advantages for the microscopist, these systems are characterised by the possibility of special focusing devices, which were introduced and illustrated in Chapter 3; they serve to eliminate many of the difficulties associated with ground-glass screen focusing. The variations and comparisons between the available formats (film sizes) that were discussed above still apply. However, these attachments are limited to the task of photography through the microscope, possibly only with the microscopes of the same brand as the camera, and they may be expensive, the best being nearly ten times the cost of a conventional high-quality 35 mm camera. There is a wide range of quality and price in the units embraced in this class.

The simpler units (Fig 3.1) replace the normal eyepiece with one of a number of available projectives. Typically a 2·5× or 3·3× magnification is used, but higher magnifications are available (be careful of the limits of useful magnification in the finished print!). A telescope permits accurate aerial image focusing even at the highest magnifications, but camera vibrations may limit the usefulness of this possibility. Possibilities exist for the inclusion or not of a leaf shutter and/or an exposure meter. These units terminate in a T-mount fitting, permitting a wide range of 35 mm camera bodies to be attached, rather convenient for the user already in possession of such a camera. T-mount adapters are known to exist for Canon, Contax, Fujica, Minolta, Nikon, Olympus, Pentax and Ricoh camera body mounts.

It may be possible to use such a photomicrographic attachment on a variety of microscopes originating from different manufacturers; these attachments are usually cheaper than those from the major microscope makers.

Telescopic aerial image focusing

In these systems (Figs 3.1, 3.2, 3.3, 14.1) a prism diverts some or all of the light from above the eyepiece to a special focusing telescope. The telescope has in it a graticule that is conjugate with the plane of the film. With a built-in auxiliary magnifier, the eye first focuses on the graticule that has one or more pairs of very fine parallel lines to enable sensitive focusing. The microscope focus is then adjusted so that the specimen image is sharp and superimposed on a sharp image of the graticule. The graticule will also give an indication of the field of view that will be recorded; there may be several such fields indicated on the graticule, each set appropriate for a particular camera format or attachment, 35 mm, Polaroid, 4×5 inches, or other. The telescope eyepiece may be a source of stray light on the film plane if it is left uncovered and directed at a light source such as a window or desk lamp during photography.

More specialised photomicrographic cameras

There is a substantial price leap to the systems, as marketed by the major microscope manufacturers, that are now to be considered (Fig 14.1). These photomicrographic systems have telescopic aerial image focusing in the attachment unit (as discussed above), or in a *finder eyepiece* inserted in the binocular head. An option between the two finder/focusing systems may be offered. The size of the shutter control unit is comparatively unimportant, and bulky devices are happily tolerated in exchange for the other benefits conferred. The shutters are electromagnetic, and exceedingly well damped against vibration compared with a normal photographic camera.

In some photomicrographic cameras, the camera contains lenses that completely replace the eyepiece. Others employ a system in which an eyepiece resides at the top of the phototube, and the camera sits above that with additional lenses to form a real image. A range of projectives ('photo eyepieces') may be available with different magnifications.

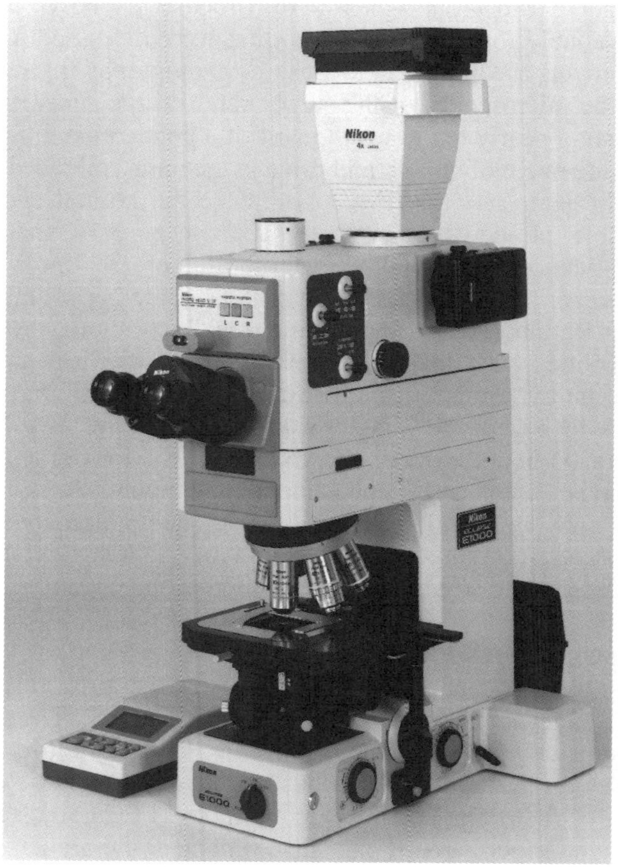

Fig 14.3. Nikon *Eclipse E1000 Biological Research Microscope*, with photomicrographic system including ports for 35 mm, 4×5 inch and video cameras. Photograph courtesy Laboratory Supply (Qld) Pty Ltd, Tingalpa, Queensland.

Finder eyepieces

Composing the field, and aerial image focusing for the camera is at its most effective when incorporated into the viewing eyepieces of the microscope. A special finder eyepiece must be employed; one of the eyepieces, most frequently the right-hand one, includes a graticule with a finely paired line or cross. First the focusing eyelens of the eyepiece is used to make the graticule lines sharp to the eye. Then the microscope image is viewed and focused in the normal way. Once again, the graticule will have fields delineated for the range of photographic eyepieces (projectives), one of which must be selected for insertion in the phototube.

There is likely to be a different graticule (or finder eyepiece) for each of the various camera formats compatible with the system. The orientation of the eyepiece and of the graticule within the eyepiece becomes significant, as does the orientation of the camera if this is not fixed by the manufacturer. To correctly align the eyepiece, it may have a grub-screw on the eyepiece barrel that fits into a slot in the eyepiece tube. If the screw does not fit into the slot correctly, the eyepiece is at a wrong height as well as a wrong orientation, and focusing will be incorrect, as the graticule is no longer conjugate with the film plane.

This kind of photomicrographic attachment is likely to function only for a particular brand of microscope, even only for a particular model. It is likely to be designed for a modified camera back (to hold the film) useful only for this attachment. This may be considered an advantage (the back is less likely to disappear) or a disadvantage (an additional expense). It is often desirable to have more than one back, so that different films can be exposed at will, eg B&W, colour negative, or colour transparency, or for keeping the peace between multiple users.

Because the eyepieces of a binocular system are separated to match the interpupillary distance of a particular user, special care may be needed to ensure correct use of the binocular head. Ideally, automatic tubelength compensation of the binocular system should occur with interpupillary distance change, a feature that minimises problems with the photographic image focus. In cheaper or older trinocular heads, tubelength compensation is achieved manually, not automatically. In such a case, both left and right eyepiece tubes have independent focusing mechanisms. The interpupillary distance of the user must be known, the tubes separated accordingly, and the focusing of each eyepiece tube set to match the interpupillary distance. This procedure, which is required to ensure a constant tubelength for the microscope, is simple enough to put into practice, in spite of what tends to be a wordy description. If the procedure is not carefully followed, image focus on the film plane will be incorrect. If the trinocular tube does not permit tubelength compensation, finder eyepiece usage is unlikely to be successful and is not recommended.

The alternative focusing possibilities

Three viewing and focusing alternatives may be offered in some photomicrographic systems – a (finder) eyepiece in the binocular head, a telescope in the attachment device, and a viewfinder in an SLR camera, a provision that seems to be a wasteful and expensive replication of optics.

It will be personal preference as to which finds favour. For convenience with routine photographic recording, the finder eyepiece in the binocular head would seem to be unrivalled. But experience with students suggests that the aerial image telescope of the attachment system is more free from focusing error, especially for inexpert users, or in those circumstances (eg polarisation, DIC) where rotation of the camera head relative to the stage is desirable for better composition of the microscope picture. If the telescope is not to be used, save money and do not buy it!

Photomicrographic camera modules

Photomicrographic camera systems (Fig 14.2) are commonly built up on a modular basis, to enable photographs in several formats to be taken using a variety of microscopes designed for different applications. Commonly, video equipment can also be added (see Chapter 17) in place of photographic modules.

Dedicated built-in photomicrographic cameras

Specialised photomicrographic cameras as an integral part of the microscope have been available commercially for many years, the pioneer being (we believe) the Zeiss *Photomikroskop*. A current (1999) commercial instrument of this type is illustrated in Fig 14.3. State-of-the-art systems made by the major manufacturers were such that the camera optical system(s), 35 mm or 4×5 inch, were actually incorporated into the body of the microscope itself. Not surprisingly, state-of-the-art systems invariably implied top-of-the-range prices!

It is possible that the peak of interest and development of built-in camera systems has passed. The authors have always believed that, although these systems were absolutely wonderful for the routine run of all kinds of research and laboratory microscopy, they were limited in their versatility for innovative or experimental techniques. Just putting a home-made filter (or a patch stop, or a photometer) in the light path became more and more difficult, if not impossible. The progress of major and rapid changes from silver photography to digital and computer-based recording systems, suggests that today's in-built novelty will be tomorrow's out-dated model; six months is a long, long time in the development of digital cameras. On the premise that no *one* recording device is optimum for all potential users, and will remain so, there is some advantage in fitting *external,* attachable, image-capture accessories.

This decision whether to buy a dedicated instrument or an attachable unit is likely to depend upon considerations of economics, including the availability of a suitable microscope to accept an accessory camera. In principle, a dedicated instrument should offer slightly higher quality in terms of mechanical rigidity and optical alignment. On the other hand, if the camera unit requires to be sent away for service, a dedicated microscope necessarily goes too, adding to the transport problem and depriving the laboratory of a microscope.

Choosing commercial photomicrographic cameras

The purpose of this section is to offer some guidance to the prospective purchaser as to how to set about choosing suitable equipment for a particular purpose. Published information on commercial microscopes is to be found mainly in manufacturers' catalogues, brochures and house journals. A review article by Cowen (1969), discussing instrumentation of the time (now obsolete) may still be of interest.

The choices to be made may be summarised as:

- The brand (marque) of equipment.
- Dedicated photomicroscope or separate microscope with attachable camera.
- The formats to be supported (35 mm, 4×5 inch including Polaroid, digital still and digital video, in B&W or colour).
- The amount of 'bells and whistles' included.

Brand of equipment

At the time of writing, the commercial microscope scene is dominated by four firms: Leica, Nikon, Olympus and Zeiss. Both of us have used equipment from each of these. The top-of-range equipment of all of these is capable of producing superb results. Considerations likely to influence the final decision will include:

- The in-house availability of existing microscopes of a particular brand, from which specialised accessories can be borrowed on occasion.
- The quality and cost of the after-sales service and support offered by the local representatives.
- The possible existence of the best instrument for the given purpose in a particular manufacturer's range.
- The local cost of the various instruments.
- The familiarity of the user with a particular brand.
- The likelihood that newly purchased equipment will remain compatible with future instrumental developments and innovations.

Checklist

Format(s)
35 mm, 4×5 inch, Polaroid, video (C-mount) port
Use of standard camera body or back

Focusing and composing
Graticules for different projectives
Illuminable graticule for fluorescence, darkground, etc
Autofocusing
Picture area only on graticule
Rotating stage, camera or image

Exposure measurement and control
Spot, integrated, centre-weighted, zone metering
Spot limited to centre of field only, or moveable
Sensitivity (eg for fluorescence, darkground, reflection)
Colour temperature metering
Automatic exposure
Manual exposure times in increments of 1 stop, $^1/_2$ stop, $^1/_3$ stop
Programmable automatic bracketing
Compensation settings
Correction for proportion of black/white
Automatic reciprocity failure corrections
DX sensing on 35 mm cassettes
Wide range of ISO film speed settings (eg 6/9°–3200/36°)
Manual setting for ISO (or ASA or DIN) film speed rating
Computer control
User-friendly keyboard

Photographic system
Interchangeable backs or magazines
Automatic or manual loading
Motor or manual wind
Motor or manual rewind
Data-back. Imprinting between frames and/or on frame
Scale bar insertion

15
Advanced photomicrography

The object of this chapter is to describe the finer technical points of obtaining first-class photomicrographs in black-and-white (B&W) or colour. This chapter supplements Chapter 3, which described the basic procedures involved. The steps outlined in Chapter 3 are listed in more detail in the box on the next page, and many of the points are amplified below. The measurement of exposure is dealt with separately in the next chapter (Chapter 16). For examples of good photomicrographs, see Plates 1–8 (colour) and 9–16 (B&W).

The basis for successful photography through the microscope is sound technique in both microscopy and photography. An important requirement is the perfection of microscope imaging, achieved by attention to matters such as the principles of Köhler illumination, the choice of objective, and considerations of numerical aperture (NA) and useful magnification.

Setting up the microscope

It is wise to place the photomicrographic equipment in a darkened room, or at least in a position where overhead lights do not directly illuminate eyepieces, telescopes or other viewfinder systems. It is possible for stray light to enter the microscope by these routes, and to find its way to the film, causing flare, fog or reduction in contrast.

Stability

The microscope bench itself must be vibration-free. This is a problem usually related to the floor on which the bench is located, a product of too-close positioning to ventilation or air-conditioning plants, or of heavy street traffic. A large bowl, developing dish or bucket filled with water and left to stand on the bench is an excellent means of gauging building vibrations – if the water surface has ripples, seek another site for your microscope bench! Ripples are best detected by reflecting a broad beam of light off the water surface onto a white screen. There exist vibration-dampening devices that are marketed or can be improvised. These consist essentially of a heavy base, on which the microscope sits, with flexible supports that allow the base to float relatively undisturbed while the surroundings shake. If possible, it is preferable to make careful and deliberate choice of a stable floor and a solid workbench. An office desk of substantial construction, provided that the legs are braced, is quite adequate as a workbench. It may be worth noting that equipment made in continental Europe is designed for a lower workbench than is typical of British laboratories, ie for a bench of desk height meant to be sat at on an ordinary chair. The microscope is often stood on a plastic mat, as a final precaution against vibration.

Procedure for photomicrography

Setting up the microscope

Check that the microscope is correctly set up, and that the optics and stage are clean. Check that a heat filter is in place.

Loading the camera

Select a suitable film (see Chapter 3, or Chapter 18 for details).
Load the film in the camera, following the manufacturer's instructions.
Set the film speed rating (ASA, ISO, EI) on the camera's exposure meter or control box.
Record the date and film type in your notebook. Possibly label the camera too.

Examining the specimen

Set up any special illumination or contrast system.
Turn the nosepiece to a low-power objective (4× or 10×), ie one with a reasonably long working distance.
Place the specimen slide on the stage, and centre the specimen under the objective.
Examine the specimen with the low-power objective.
Locate the area to be photographed.
Decide on the magnification to be used, and select the appropriate objective.
Adjust the Köhler illumination to optimal conditions (see Chapter 7).

Selecting the field of view to be photographed

Look in the viewfinder, and move the specimen until the desired composition is obtained.
Check that the magnification is appropriate. If necessary, change the objective and/or intermediate magnifier and/or projective.
Record, in your notebook, the specimen, subject, and magnification. Set the data-back (if available) for desired imprinting (if any).

Focusing the camera

Focus the graticule in the viewfinder for your eye (see Chapter 3). Adjust the microscope's fine focus until the aerial image of the subject coincides with the graticule.

Adjusting the illumination

Check the Köhler illumination for the objective in use (see Chapter 7).
If the field of view is small, adjust the field diaphragm until its image is just clear of the area to be photographed.
Select a filter (for B&W or colour as appropriate)
Turn up the lamp current to the preset value (may not be necessary for B&W).

Determining the exposure

The recommended exposure is read, using either full-frame or spot metering.
Compensation may be necessary in some circumstances (see Chapter 16).
In manual systems, the chosen exposure is set.

Making the exposure

Check that the light path is set to the camera, and gently press the button.
If in doubt of the exposure, bracket the exposures (see Chapters 3, 16).
Record, in your notebook, the exposure(s) given.
Is a scale required? See Chapter 3 for use of stage micrometer.

Cleanliness

The microscope should be maintained in a clean, dust-free and functional condition. Surfaces that, when dusty or dirty, are particularly likely to create imaging problems are the objective front lens, and all glass–air surfaces (even the internal ones) of the photographic eyepiece. Ask an expert to show you how to clean lens surfaces; any trained salesperson will be delighted to encourage such care by one of their customers. Further information on maintenance is given in Appendix A1.

Basic adjustment of the microscope

We will assume here that the microscope has been set up ready for use (for prodcedures see Chapters 2 and 7). It may be required to set up some special mode of microscopy, eg phase contrast or fluorescence, as described in Chapters 9–12. It is a wise precaution to ensure that a heat filter (eg Schott KG1) is present (particularly for polarisation and DIC microscopy, because the infrared light otherwise transmitted may be metered, so that the exposure meter measures more light than it should, producing underexposure).

Loading the camera with appropriate film

The selection of film (B&W and colour; negative and transparency) is described in Chapters 1 and 18. Of course, with a digital camera (Chapter 17) this step is not required! The film is loaded into the camera, following the manufacturer's instructions. The film speed rating (ISO or EI) is set on the camera's exposure meter or control box; this rating is not necessarily that marked on the packet (see Chapter 16, Exposure measurement). The date and film type should be recorded in your notebook or computer. If the camera has a data-back, the location of the imprint (on or between frames) and data to be imprinted (if any) should be chosen.

Examining the specimen, and selecting the field of view to be photographed

The specimen

A perfect specimen is the best starting point for a perfect photograph. This ideally implies a thin, flat section or smear, good contrast, lack of specimen movement, and control of coverslip/mountant thickness. Unfortunately, these important considerations are not always under practical control.

Selecting the field of view to be photographed

Action: one turns the nosepiece to a low-power objective (4× or 10×), ie an objective with a reasonably long working distance, places the specimen slide on the stage, and centres the specimen under the objective. The specimen is examined first with the low-power objective, to locate the area to be photographed. Sometimes this initial examination is carried out using a mode of microscopy different from that to be used for photomicrography (eg using transmitted light or phase contrast before fluorescence or darkground microscopy).

One must decide on the magnification to be used, and select the appropriate objective. Experience may be needed to determine the best magnification to use. Beginners are inclined to overdo the magnification, choosing an enlargement that is greater than that which best illustrates a given feature. Aesthetic considerations in selecting the field are discussed in Chapter 5. Look in the viewfinder, and move the specimen until the desired composition is obtained. Note that this process may include, not only movement along the *X* and *Y* axes, but also turning either the specimen or the camera. One should now record, in the logbook, the specimen, subject and magnification.

Focusing the microscope

Focusing was described in Chapter 3.

Depth of field

Depth of field and depth of focus were defined in Chapter 3, and discussed in detail in Chapter 6. If the specimen is at all thick, and particularly at high magnification, there may be insufficient depth of field. There are three ways to deal with this problem, all of which involve trading-off some loss of detail for increased depth of field. The easiest is to use a lower magnification. A better solution, if possible, is to change the objective to one of similar magnification but lower NA. If the objective has an aperture diaphragm (regrettably rare), the required effect can be achieved by partially closing that diaphragm until sufficient depth of field is obtained, or loss of resolution becomes unacceptable. Alternatively, in some modalities of microscopy, partially closing the condenser aperture diaphragm will produce a similar effect (see below). A confocal microscope (Chapter 17) is usually better able to cope with thick specimens than an ordinary microscope, and scanning electron microscopy may be more appropriate for opaque specimens. Finally, a drawing can be made of a specimen too thick to photograph (see Chapter 19).

Adjusting the illumination

The effects of closing the illumination aperture diaphragm may be summarised as follows. In all cases, the brightness of the image is reduced. The effects on resolution and contrast depend upon the modality of microscopy, as follows.

Closing the illuminator (condenser or epi-illuminator) diaphragm *decreases* the effective NA of the system, thereby increasing depth of field and contrast, in the following modalities:

- Transmitted-light brightfield ('normal' microscopy, for absorptive specimens).
- Transmitted-light polarisation.
- Transmitted-light interference contrast.
- Epi-illumination brightfield (reflective specimens).
- Epi-illumination brightfield polarisation.

Closing the illuminator (condenser or epi-illuminator) diaphragm does *not* affect the effective NA of the system; therefore depth of field and contrast are *unchanged*, in the following modalities:

- Transmitted-light fluorescence.
- Transmitted-light darkground (darkfield).
- Epi-illumination fluorescence.
- Epi-illumination darkground (darkfield).

Reducing the illuminator (condenser or epi-illuminator) NA is *not possible* in the following modalities:

- Phase contrast.
- Most darkground (darkfield) systems.

The illumination system

The illumination system is required, primarily, to provide uniform illumination across the field, and to have an appropriate NA to give the required resolution and contrast. The principles of Köhler illumination, dealt with in Chapter 7, need to be applied; this is usually a matter of consulting and interpreting the microscope's instruction manual. It is not usually necessary to set the illumination exactly until the appropriate magnification has been determined, since changing the objective may necessitate adjustment to the condenser aperture. The condenser setting will vary according to the microscope design, for there is a very considerable variety of systems, with auxiliary condenser lenses, removable top lenses to the condenser, etc. For serious microscopy, unless you are satisfied that Köhler illumination is achieved, it is not wise to proceed. Tests for satisfactory Köhler illumination are given in Chapter 7.

Surprisingly, it is the very low power (less than 4×) objectives that may prove the most difficult of all to use for photomicrography. Very few systems will permit true Köhler illumination, and in all such cases a special *ultralow-power* condenser, not cheap, is essential (see Chapter 7). Without the right equipment, ultralow powers may prove difficult, and very demanding of the illumination system to provide even illumination. It may be tempting to avoid ultralow microscope systems for photography, and to use macroscopic photographic systems instead, but if the specimen is flat and thin, the resolution that the microscope is capable of achieving is much to be preferred.

Condenser immersion

If the condenser has an NA greater than 0·9, it is specifically designed to be immersed to the slide. Immersion is essential if the full NA of the condenser is required, eg, for optimum resolution, or for an immersion darkground condenser (Chapter 9), and for DIC systems (Chapter 10). Many users, understandably, will prefer to avoid the immersion process, but it is the only way to achieve illumination apertures with an NA greater than about 0·9. One advantage of condenser immersion is that two air–glass interfaces, condenser and slide, often dirty and troublesome, are eliminated. The major disadvantage of condenser immersion is that the slide, stage and condenser, and perhaps also the condenser mount, will need cleaning afterwards.

Oiling the condenser is a messy process, always. Using a low- or medium-power objective, first find the approximate area of interest in the microscope slide, then lower the condenser and place three to four drops of immersion oil on the top lens of the condenser, very carefully avoiding any air bubbles. If air bubbles are seen, wipe off the oil and start again. Slowly raise the condenser until the oil makes contact with the undersurface of the slide, and proceed to set up Köhler illumination.

Adjust the field diaphragm until its image is just clear of the area to be photographed (Fig 3.2). Check that the illumination is uniform across the field.

Control of contrast

Contrast is controllable by the following means:

- Choice of modality of microscopy.
- Adjustment of the objective and condenser NAs (see above, Depth of field).
- Use (for B&W photography only) of coloured filters, as described below.
- Use of appropriate film (with high, medium or low contrast; see Chapter 18).
- Processing the film to the desired contrast (gamma, see Chapter 18).
- Printing on an appropriate grade of paper (see Chapter 18).
- Computer adjustment of a digital image (see Chapter 17).

Colour filters for black-and-white photography

In B&W photography, a coloured filter may be used to adjust the contrast of a coloured or stained specimen, or to emphasise or subdue one particular colour. The choice of filters for microscopy is quite complicated, and for B&W photography through the microscope, a box of filters and an understanding of their selection is essential knowledge. Types of filter are discussed in Chapter 8.

Since resolving power (minimum resolved distance, MRD) is at its best with short wavelengths (see Chapter 6), there is good reason to use a *blue* filter. However, since achromatic and planachromatic objectives are corrected for spherical aberration for the green part of the spectrum only, and since a narrow wavelength band of illumination will also remove chromatic aberration, there is good reason to use a *green* filter. The image from an achromat used with a green filter should approach the image quality of an apochromat, and at a very much reduced price. An attitude that has some merit is that the green filter should be left permanently in the light path (for B&W photography), and only if a reason is advanced should the green filter be removed.

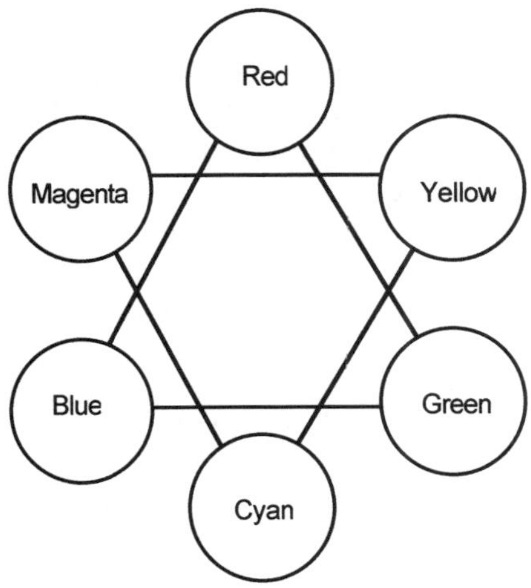

Fig 15.1. The selection of filters for B&W photomicrography. The 'Star of David' diagram. Complementary colours are opposite one another in the diagram.

There are *contrast* considerations also, related to the colour(s) of the specimen itself. From the foregoing, if the specimen is colourless, a green filter definitely should be used to minimise chromatic and spherical aberration. But not, of course, if the specimen itself is green. A filter that is the same colour as the specimen will reduce image contrast. To increase image contrast, frequently needed in biological photomicrography, a filter colour complementary to the stain is used (Figs 15.1, 15.2). The aim is to render the stained portion darker, to help to distinguish the stained portion from the unstained area. For example, contrast of a blue stain will be enhanced with a yellow filter. Since staining procedures for biological material routinely involve more than one colour, filter selection may not always be straightforward. For a red/blue combination of stains, a green filter should be chosen.

Occasionally, there may be overstaining of the specimen, and a need to reduce contrast. Under such circumstances, a filter of the *same* colour as the stain would be selected. This is called *detail* filtering, but the phrase is not an appropriate one.

The coloured filter needs to be placed in the light path of the microscope, usually between the specimen and light source. The microscope will have a special filter rest or holder, typically under the condenser or on the microscope foot, sometimes in front of the lamp. A filter holder on the foot is in an exposed, horizontal position, immediately adjacent to the field iris diaphragm, and since the field stop is superimposed on the plane of the specimen, the inevitable dust on the filter will be unacceptably more or less sharply imaged on the specimen. It may be useful practice to use a clear glass filter as a deliberate trap for the dust that falls on this field iris plane, but careful and frequent cleaning of the filter is then appropriate.

Measuring the required exposure

The problem of measuring the exposure may be very simple, or very difficult. This matter is therefore dealt with separately in Chapter 16. In many cases it is advisable to take two or more exposures at different exposure times (bracketing), and to select the best result.

Making the exposure

Check that the light path runs to the camera (this usually requires moving a slider), and press the button. If in doubt of the exposure, bracket the exposures, usually at 1 stop (2×) intervals (eg 2× and $^1/_2$×). If the specimen is not going to be available to re-shoot if necessary, take an additional exposure just in case of accidental damage to the negative or transparency. In these circumstances, and if the specimen is very important, co-author Fred never feels happy unless he has at least two shots on each of two separate rolls taken with different cameras. Record, in your notebook (or computer), the exposure(s) given.

Shutter release. Camera shake is a very real threat to sharp pictures in photomicrography. If the camera is not electrically controlled from a separate control box, a remote release (shutter release; see Chapter 4) should be used to avoid transmitting movement of finger or hand to the camera. There may be an advantage in aiming for exposures of several seconds rather than a fraction of a second, because a longer exposure is less likely to be affected by camera shake. However, longer exposures have complications in their effect on the speed and colour balance of photographic film (see Reciprocity failure, Chapters 16 and 18).

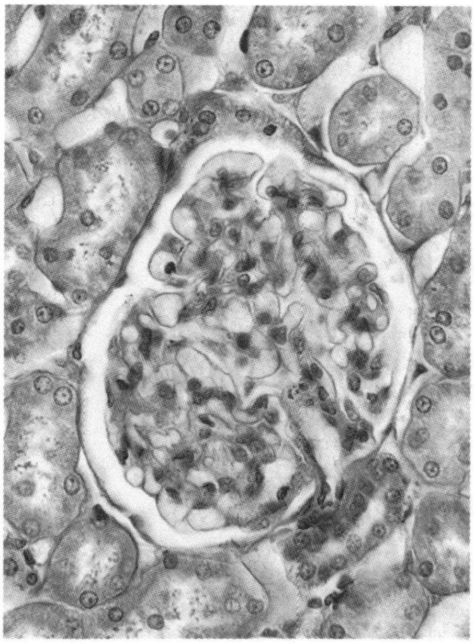

Fig 15.2. The effects of different coloured filters in black-and-white photography. Section of mouse kidney, stained with modified Masson's trichrome stain (red, orange and blue). Field size 260 µm × 160 µm. The same field is shown in colour in Plate 8. In this example, one filter is not 'better' than any other. The filter colour is chosen to subdue or emphasise a particular feature of the specimen. Zeiss *Universal* microscope, Olympus *PM-10ADS* photomicrographic system, Ilford *Pan F* film.

Left: without filter (ie 'daylight'), contrast enhanced photographically during printing (see Chapter 18).

Bottom left: blue filter (Wratten 45), photograph printed on normal-contrast paper.

Bottom right: orange filter (Wratten 22), photograph printed on normal-contrast paper.

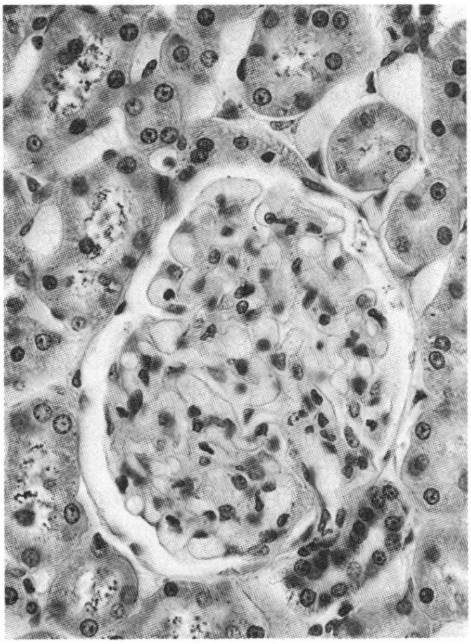

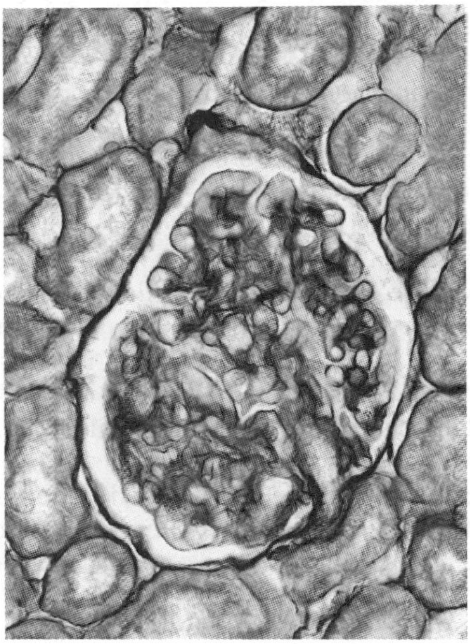

Troubleshooting

If the pictures do not come out well (see Figs A2.1 and A2.2 for horrible examples!), or cannot be taken at all because of technical difficulties, the fault may lie in the microscope, the camera, the film, or the processing of the film. Appendix A2 (Troubleshooting) offers some hints for identifying the cause or causes of the problem.

Colour

This section discusses those aspects of photomicrography that are peculiar to the use of colour, and assumes that the reader is already familiar with the basic procedures of setting up the microscope and taking photomicrographs. Examples of colour photomicrographs are shown in Plates 1–8.

Photomicrography in colour differs from photomicrography in B&W in four main respects, which are discussed in detail below:

- The illumination system (source and filters) must provide light whose colour temperature matches that of the film.
- A higher degree of correction of chromatic aberration is required.
- The exposure time is more critical than for B&W photography.
- The camera must be loaded with colour film.

Colour film

Colour film is described (briefly) in Chapter 1, and in more detail in Chapter 18.

Choice of film

The decision as to which type of film to use is not always easy. The basic decisions are: transparencies or prints? If transparencies, daylight type or artificial-light type? *Kodachrome* or E6-processing?

Transparencies are relatively inexpensive, easy to store, and suitable for use in lectures, and for publication. Prints or digital images can be made from them if necessary. Prints are usually needed only for inclusion in a thesis, or for display. Of transparency films, *Kodachrome* is generally regarded as having the greatest permanence, and the highest contrast. On the other hand, *Ektachrome* is more resistant to fading under strong illumination (ie while being projected) than *Kodachrome*. Films for which quick processing (eg E-6) is available may be more convenient or appropriate in many circumstances.

Our current favourite films include the following. Of daylight-type transparency film, *Kodachrome 25* (25/15° ISO) offers outstanding reproduction of colour and detail, and archival permanence; *Kodachrome 64* (64/19° ISO) has adequate resolution and its higher speed is often helpful. Fuji *Velvia* (50/18° ISO) can generally be processed more quickly, and its colour rendition is excellent for photomicrography – it seems to be the best film currently available for histological sections stained with Haematoxylin & Eosin. Among colour negative films, Kodak *Royal Gold 25* (25/15° ISO) is outstanding for fine grain.

Daylight or artificial-light film?

Daylight film is obligatory in some circumstances: for recording fluorescence, and for use with electronic flash or a xenon arc lamp. If daylight film is used for other purposes, it may be convenient to stock and use only one type of film. If both transparencies and colour negatives are required, use of daylight transparency film saves changing the colour temperature of the source between film types, since colour negative film requires daylight-type illumination.

Artificial-light film is in principle more appropriate for a light of low colour temperature, since film is naturally more sensitive to blue light; it seems a little illogical to use a blue filter to enable the use of film that has been artificially desensitised to blue light! However, there are several reasons why it is more convenient to use daylight-type conditions. One is that the eye can see the specimen better with daylight-type lighting than with amber lighting, and it is convenient to be able simply to push a button and obtain a picture. Artificial-light film is favourable for dim-light conditions, because it is more sensitive than the corresponding daylight film, but one can always use a more sensitive film if necessary.

Colour prints

Most workers shoot colour transparency (reversal, positive) film, this being usually the most convenient, the cheapest, and giving slides for projection or reproduction. Also, it is easiest to see how well the colours match the original preparation. Prints can easily be scanned for digital processing and printing (see Chapter 17).

If prints are required, there are three possibilities. Firstly, excellent, but expensive, prints can be made from transparencies. Secondly, prints can be made from an internegative made by rephotographing the transparency with colour negative film; we have found this method quite satisfactory for most purposes, using a fine-grain negative film and having the developing and printing done at the local mini-lab. Third, the photomicrographs can be taken directly on colour negative film. This gives best results, but it may be helpful or indeed essential to have transparencies as well so that the operator making the prints can be shown the correct colours.

Colour rendition

The following criteria may be laid down for good colour rendition in a photomicrograph taken by transmitted light:

- The (empty) background must be white, or at worst a pale neutral grey.
- The colours should be well defined and reasonably accurate.
- There should be sufficient overall contrast.
- A transparency should be exposed appropriately for its intended use.

Colour temperature

The concept of colour temperature (see Chapters 3 and 8) can be appreciated by watching the light from the tungsten-filament lamp of the microscope as the current is switched on and progressively increased by the rheostat. The filament, initially non-luminous, glows a deep red, then bright red, orange and finally becomes ‘white’ hot. Colour temperature meters operate by determining the ratio of red to blue content of the light, from which the colour temperature can be calculated. Such meters are built-in to some photomicrographic cameras.

Obtaining the correct colour

Before embarking on a programme of photomicrography, it is essential to calibrate the light source. This involves photographing an empty field under various conditions, to determine which conditions produce the correct balance of colour temperature, resulting in a neutral grey photograph (see Plate 1a). There are in principle two possibilities: either, with a given blue filter (or possibly no filter, given artificial-light film), one takes a series of pictures with varying values of lamp current; or, if the lamp current is fixed (eg by the lamp being run at maximum), the series of pictures is taken with a series of blue filters or filter combinations. If the camera has a colour temperature meter, it is necessary only to confirm that the meter reads correctly at the colour temperature required for the film type in use.

Obtaining a white background

The first and most important point to remember is that the background will come out white if, and only if, the film is sufficiently exposed. Even if the light is not correctly colour-balanced, so long as the exposure of background areas exceeds the latitude of the film, they will appear white. If the exposure is too short, the background will appear one of several colours: grey, if the light is correctly balanced; blue, if the colour temperature is too high; amber, if the colour temperature is too low; or some other colour, at long exposures, due to the addition of a colour cast induced by reciprocity failure.

For an attachment camera, using transparency film, the film speed rating that is given for pictorial work should be *decreased* to give $^2/_3$ stop more than the standard measured exposure. This is a consequence of the normal brightfield microscope image being rather brighter than the conventional 18% grey. For colour negative film, give 1 stop more (as for B&W).

Consistency of colour

If, for whatever reason, it is required to take a large series of photographs with a high degree of consistency in their colour, the following considerations need to be taken into account.

Reproducibility of illumination. This is the biggest problem. Using a tungsten-filament lamp, the lamp current needs to be set to the same value each time. We have heard that setting the current rather than the voltage gives greater reproducibility, but we do not know whether this is true or not. Tungsten-filament lamps become weaker and redder as they grow older. If the lamp is replaced, it will be necessary to re-calibrate for the correct colour temperature. A xenon arc or electronic flash gives greater reproducibility of colour temperature.

Reproducibility of film. It is essential to stick to the same type of film, as there are considerable differences in colour rendition between types. In principle, for greatest consistency, one should obtain a large quantity of film of a single batch, calibrate the film, and use only that batch for the project until it is exhausted, keeping unused film refrigerated. Such a procedure is unlikely to be necessary for photomicrography.

Reproducibility of processing. Assuming that one employs a commercial processing house, one can only choose a reliable one and hope for the best. Sometimes it may be possible to have special films put through early in a batch, but this is not relevant to continuous-processing machines.

Colour casts. If the exposures are not consistent in length, there may be colour variation due to reciprocity failure.

Exposure. The exposure of a transparency film needs to be appropriate for the intended use of the transparency. For projection, a fairly light transparency is usually best. For reproduction, a slightly dark transparency is better. Co-author Fred commonly takes two exposures, differing by about $^2/_3$ stop; the lighter one for projection, the darker one for reproduction. Bracketing may in any case be necessary to ensure that the correct exposure is given to at least one frame of film (see Chapters 3 and 16).

Taking the picture

Special effects

Sometimes the photographer will wish to reproduce an object in colours that differ from its natural ones, for aesthetic or other reasons.

Rheinberg illumination is a form of darkground illumination (see Chapter 9 and Plate 4). A special filter is placed in the aperture plane of the condenser. The Rheinberg filter has differently coloured segments, so that the specimen is illuminated with different colours in different directions.

Simultaneous epi- and trans-illumination (ie through the objective and through the condenser simultaneously; Plate 8b) in different colours is possible, eg to provide a coloured background for an opaque object.

Simultaneous fluorescence and transmitted-light (Plate 7a) is a special case of the above. Fluorescence is excited using epi-illumination in the usual manner (see Chapter 11). Simultaneously, the specimen is illuminated through a substage condenser, using either conventional transmitted light (Chapter 7), phase contrast (negative or positive) or DIC (Chapter 10), or darkground (Chapter 9). The illumination from below is coloured by a filter with a colour contrasting with that of the fluorescence and of a longer wavelength so as to be transmitted by the barrier filter. Use of a contrasting shorter wavelength requires double exposure, the second exposure (for dia-illumination) being taken with the excitation off and the barrier filter removed.

Troubleshooting

Colour pictures are subject to all the troubles that may plague B&W pictures, and have some faults of their own. If the pictures do not come out well, or cannot be taken at all because of technical difficulties, the fault may lie in the microscope, the camera, the film, or the processing of the film. Appendix A2 offers some hints for identifying and correcting the cause or causes of the problem or problems.

Use of flash (strobe)

Electronic flash (strobe) lighting has two advantages: it has a constant and reproducible colour temperature, and it generally gives a very short exposure that can be used to freeze the motion of living or mobile objects. As regards the latter, it must be admitted than sometimes more than one flash is required to obtain sufficient illumination. Normal lighting is additionally required for focusing and composition of the picture. For details of electronic flash, see Chapter 8.

Details of large objects

'It is not always possible to cut pieces off a specimen' (Lawson, 1972, p. 178).

If the specimen is too large to fit on the microscope stage, the microscope, like Mahomet, has to go to the mountain. There are several ways of achieving this. Firstly, though, it may be worthwhile considering whether photomacrographic apparatus might be more suitable (see the next section, Photomacrography versus low-power photomicrography). If not, then what about a stereomicroscope? These are commonly designed so that they can be supported over a specimen (Fig 15.3), instead of being attached to a stage and base. Photomicrography with stereomicroscopes is described in Chapter 13. Microscopes designed to be carried and used directly on large (eg metallurgical) objects are sometimes called *travelling microscopes,* although this term is more correctly applied to microscopes which travel on a slide and are used for measuring.

Large-specimen microscopes. Some microscopes are or were designed to accept large specimens, typically for industrial use. Most inverted microscopes will accept an object of unlimited size on the stage, provided that the weight is not excessive. Co-author Fred supposes that some such microscopes could be turned upside down (an upside-down inverted microscope!) to be sat on a specimen.

Footless microscopes. The Zeiss *Axiomat* microscope (now, alas, no longer made) was made in modular units sitting on top of each other, and it was possible for the body of the microscope to sit on a large object (such as the deck of a battleship) and examine it. Older-style microscopes, from the days when the body tube was moved up and down for focusing, can easily be adapted for this kind of work, the body tube and its focusing mechanism being attached to any convenient type of support (see Lawson, 1972, pp. 178–181).

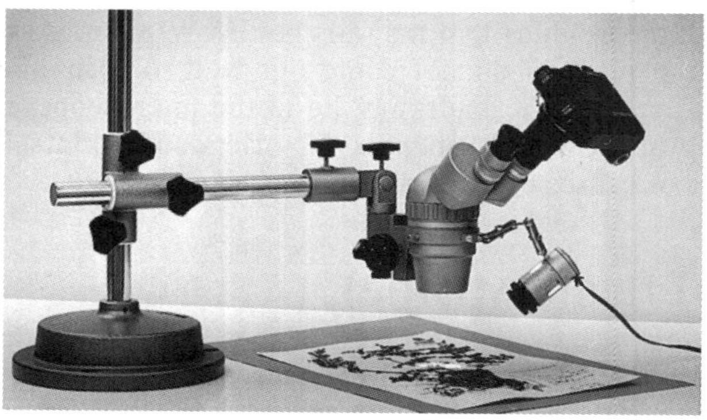

Fig 15.3. Photomicrography of a large object, using a stereomicroscope with a simple attachment camera. The extended arm on a heavy stand permits unobstructed examination of a herbarium sheet. Note the illuminator attached to the microscope body. Olympus *SZ3* stereomicroscope, with Olympus *OM4* camera.

Photomacrography versus low-power photomicrography

When photographing at a low magnification, one has (in principle) the choice of several techniques. With a conventional microscope, the lowest magnification objective that can conveniently be used is usually 4×, and this, used in conjunction with a 2·5× projective, gives a magnification (on 35 mm film) of 10×. Objectives are available with lower magnifications, down to 0·5× (Nikon), but their use requires a special condenser. In any case, the lower limit (so far as we know) is 2·5× overall. For low magnifications, one may prefer to use a device such as the Leica (Wild) *Photomakroscop*, which is specifically designed for low-magnification use (see Plate 3), or a stereomicroscope (Fig 15.3; see Chapter 13). An alternative is a photomacrographic system such as the Nikon *Multiphot*. For opaque objects, a simple photomacrographic system, such as an SLR camera (see Chapter 4) and a macro lens may be the most effective. Such a system, at least in the 35 mm format, can be expected to offer automation for focusing, exposure, and film winding, and an optional data-back. Objects to be photographed in transmitted light can be placed on a light box, but if no condenser is used, useful magnifications are limited to less than about 2×.

Coping with low light levels

This section deals with the special problems of those forms of microscopy that yield a dim image. These are, in particular, DIC, darkground, fluorescence, and reflection microscopy. The dimness of the image may also be caused or aggravated by a dark specimen, a weak light source, high magnification, and the use of strong filters (particularly crossed polarisers). The techniques that are useful in coping with dim images include:

- Optimising the efficiency of the optical system, to avoid wasting light.
- Use of fast film, possibly push-processed.
- Increased exposure time, with compensation for reciprocity failure.

Efficency of the optical system

Every effort should be made to maintain the efficiency of the optical system, to conserve light. This efficiency is required in both the illumination and magnifying systems. Useful methods include:

- Use of a trinocular tube that sends 100% of the light to the camera, rather than having a beamsplitter that sends only part of the light to the film..
- Elimination of unnecessary glass surfaces, eg zoom systems, magnification changers, filters.
- Use of objectives with high NA. This is assisted by using a low-magnification projective (or low camera magnification), enabling use of a higher-power objective for the same overall magnification.
- Use of coated optics.
- (Fluorescence microscopy only) Use of efficent filter systems (see Chapter 11).

Fast film

Exposure times can be much reduced by the use of a fast film. Using the 35 mm format, *Kodachrome 200* is particularly useful, but very fast colour films tend to be excessively grainy. If a film with the required speed rating is not available, the fastest available film can be push-processed (see Chapter 18) to compensate for underexposure.

Measuring low light levels

The measurement of the required exposure for dim images requires special attention: see Dim images, in Chapter 16.

Video intensification

Dim images can be examined by video-intensification microscopy (see Chapters 11 and 17); at present this technique is not readily adaptable to multicoloured images.

Applied photomicrography

The intention of this section is to provide some suggestions for dealing with particular problems of which we have had practical experience.

Stained biological specimens

Stained specimens are usually the easiest to photograph, as the contrast is generally quite high, and the specimen is generally a section or smear, so that it can be illuminated by transmitted light, and the problem of depth of field is minimised.

In B&W photomicrography of a coloured specimen, use may be made of filters to darken or lighten specific colours (see above). Generally, if the specimen has two or more colours, the stain that is the most important should be made darker by use of a complementary filter. Sometimes a change of mode of microscopy (eg, to fluorescence or darkground) may be helpful.

Eosin

Eosin is an acid dye, widely used as a stain for histological sections of human and animal material, usually in conjunction with Haematoxylin. Strictly, the term 'Eosin' refers to a group of related dyes. All are acidic and red, but there are several shades, of which at least two are commonly used: Eosin Y (yellowish) and Eosin B (bluish). An alternative red dye with similar histological characteristics is Biebrich Scarlet.

The red colour of Eosin is notoriously difficult to reproduce on colour film. It commonly reproduces as a pale pink, or may appear a quite different colour. Use of a didymium-glass filter (eg Schott BG20) is recommended. Eosin is reproduced by some colour films better than others; in co-author Fred's experience, Fujichrome *Velvia* is currently the best in this respect.

Ultrathin sections

In an electron-microscopy laboratory, a section of approximately 2 µm thickness is called a *thick* section; the same section by light microscope standards is considered an *ultrathin* section. The problem is that very little absorption of light takes place in the specimen even after histochemical staining, so that the image contrast for observation and photography is extremely poor.

The requirement often is for very high resolution of uncovered sections, ie sections attached to a microscope slide, stained and dried, but without a coverslip. A normal approach is to add a drop of oil and use an immersion objective. Sometimes, if further histochemical staining is expected, it is not appropriate to add oil directly to the section; in this case a high-aperture dry objective is warranted, but one which is designed for use without (or '0' thickness) coverslip. If such an objective is not available, one alternative is to put a drop of water on the section, and then a coverslip before applying immersion oil and using a conventional immersion objective. The water should be boiled first to minimise the chance of air bubbles forming during microscopical observation. We have had frustrating and unpredictable experiences with the oil or water alternatives suggested above. Differential expansion of tissues may occur, sometimes with oil, sometimes with water, with consequent buckling of the sections. A coverslip may help to suppress the buckling.

A stain that is commonly used is Toluidine Blue, which gives blue and pink colours. Although colour differentiation may be significant, it is quite difficult to achieve publication-quality results with colour film. Planapochromatic objectives come into their own, combined with an immersed achromatic aplanatic condenser. Apart from good microscopy and high-saturation colour film, there may not be much more that can be done.

B&W recording ought to be much more successful. Some experimentation with colour filters is advisable. Using Toluidine Blue, a combination of Wratten 15 (deep yellow) and Wratten 58 (green) filters will lift the contrast considerably; a powerful light source is necessary. In desperate cases, Wratten 22 (orange) may replace the yellow filter. Some increase in film contrast can be obtained with Kodak *Technical Pan* film and Kodak *HC110* developer in a medium-contrast range of dilution. Be generous with bracketing, at $^1/_2$ stop intervals around ISO 50/18° until experience has been gained. The resulting negatives can be expected to print on No 2 paper.

Unstained, colourless specimens

The primary difficulty with colourless specimens is that of achieving contrast. This normally requires a retardation technique such as phase contrast, DIC, or polarisation (see Chapter 10), or possibly a change of wavelength to ultraviolet (UV) or infrared (see Chapter 12). Using brightfield transmitted light, partial closure of the condenser aperture may assist (see Chapter 6). Darkground illumination may demonstrate intracellular structure (Plate 10).

Living material

With living material, the microscopist must adhere to the old medical principle, *primum non nocere* (*above all, do no harm*). This may involve keeping the light level low, particularly if fluorescence is involved (see Chapter 11), and avoidance of UV wavelengths.

Fast-moving specimens are best photographed using flash. Alternatively, a short exposure time is used; this may require the use of a fast film, or a really bright light (eg from a xenon arc) to be shone onto the specimen (briefly, so as not to damage it).

Most photomicrographic cameras have a fastest speed of about 1/200 second, rather slow by general photographic standards. SLR cameras (Chapter 4) have faster speeds, currently to 1/8000 second, but because the shutter blinds take longer than this to traverse the film (of the order of 40–200 milliseconds, or 1/50 to 1/300 second) the appearance or relative positions of moving objects are distorted. Moving subjects can also be dealt with using video techniques (see Chapter 17).

Further reading

Books which may be of interest for further reading on the finer points of photomicrography include those of Delly (1988), Lawson (1972), and Loveland (1970), and the Olympus booklet (Anon, 1984a).

16
Exposure measurement

The problem of measuring the exposure may be very simple, or very difficult, as was stated in the previous chapter (Chapter 15). The present chapter is therefore devoted to this subject. The correct exposure time is determined by a combination of many factors. The major factors are: the brightness of the illumination system, the density or reflectivity of the specimen, the magnification of the image onto the film, the effective numerical aperture (NA) of the objective, the amount of light losses in the optical system, and the sensitivity of the film under the prevailing circumstances. The exposure is usually determined by using an exposure meter to measure the brightness of the image, from which the duration of the required exposure is calculated having regard to the sensitivity of the film and the type of specimen. Even then, it is often advisable to take two or more exposures at different exposure times, and to select the best result.

Exposure meters

Photomicrographic cameras are usually provided with an exposure meter to measure the brightness of the field. For this purpose, light from the image is diverted to a photometer either by a sliding mirror that can be inserted into the light path, or by a permanent beamsplitter that reflects part of the light to a photometer. The latter arrangement is more convenient and allows measurement during the exposure itself (to allow for fading during exposure, which may happen in fluorescence microscopy), but has the disadvantage that the beamsplitter reduces the brightness of the image on the film, thereby necessitating a longer exposure. In ordinary cameras, another method is measurement of light reflected from the film (during long exposures), or from the blind of a focal-plane shutter (before short exposures). This, although a Minolta patent, was first introduced in the Olympus *OM1* camera. The reading on the exposure meter, taken in conjunction with the speed of the film and possibly other factors (described below), gives an estimate of the exposure to be given. This exposure is given either manually or automatically, depending upon the sophistication of the system.

Estimation of correct exposure

There are three ways in which the length of exposure can be determined: trial and error, brightness measurement before exposure, and continuous measurement during exposure.

Trial-and-error, as the sole method of exposure determination, may be acceptable for routine photography under highly standardised conditions, but otherwise is not satisfactory in our experience. The method involves first taking a series of trial exposures at various exposure times (each exposure say twice the previous); the exposure giving the best result is noted and made the basis of further photomicrography (see Fig 16.2). Exposures using this method should always be bracketed – that is, additional pictures should be taken, eg at double and half the estimated exposure. If the magnification is changed, corrections to the estimated exposure can be calculated or determined empirically. Long-term diminution in the light output from the lamp must be expected.

Measurement before the exposure is similar to the method usually adopted for conventional photography. The brightness of the image is measured, the exposure estimated and given. Again, the exposure should be bracketed, although usually a smaller range of exposures is required (eg a factor of 1·5 each way, above and below the estimated exposure). This method is much more accurate than the previous, but is still subject to error due to reciprocity failure during long exposures (see Chapter 18).

Measurement during the exposure is carried out by at least two automatic systems. This method compensates for fading of the specimen during exposure, as may occur in fluorescence microscopy.

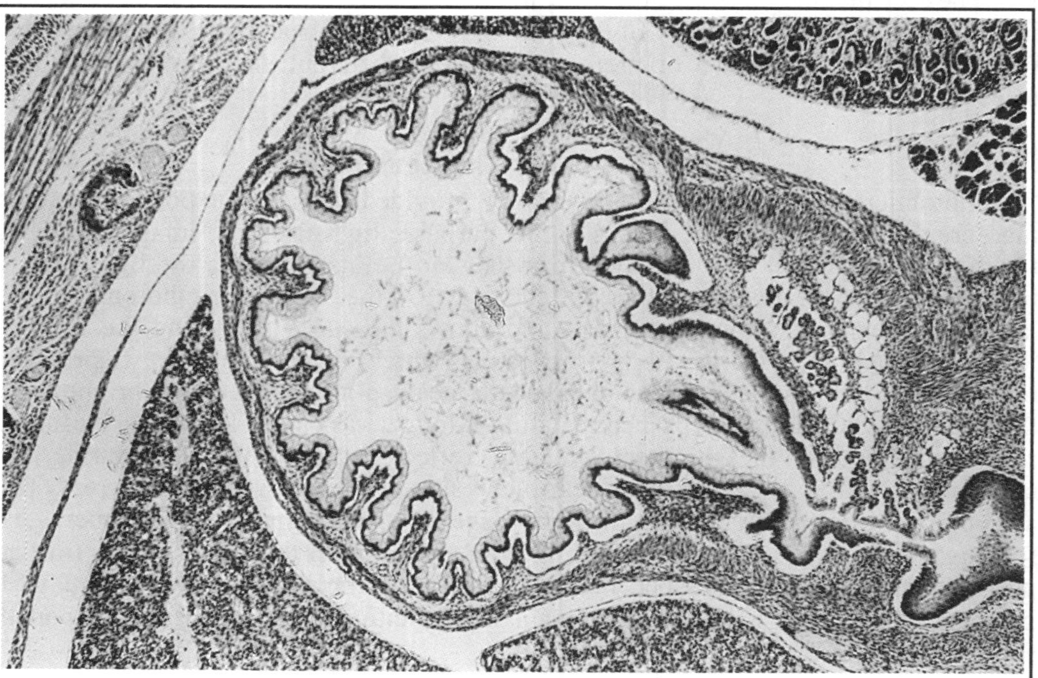

Fig 16.1. Histological section (mouse embryo, stomach) illustrating the problem of spot measurement. This kind of specimen needs spot measurement, but not in the exact centre of the field. Field size 2·8 mm × 1·7 mm. Cf Fig 3.4.

Spot and integrated measurements

Spot measurements, as their name implies, are made from a small area, usually in the centre of the field (Fig 3.4). Spot measurements are particularly helpful if the specimen contains substantial blank areas (Figs 3.4, 16.1). If the measuring spot is fixed in the middle of the field (Fig 3.4), necessitating moving the specimen to get a suitable area into the spot and then again to compose the picture (see Fig 16.1), this method is suitable only for those cameras that measure the exposure before opening the shutter. In a fully automatic camera measuring during the exposure, it is essential to be able to move the spot to a relevant area.

Integrated measurements are made by integrating (totalling) the light from the entire picture area.

Centre-weighted measurement is a form of integrated measurement in which greater emphasis is given to the brightness of the centre portion of the field. The calculation for correction of proportion of field is more difficult in this case.

Fully automatic cameras

Fully automatic systems in which the exposure is controlled automatically by a photometer may be convenient in some respects, and may be excellent for general-purpose photomicrography, but four problems may arise: (1) some light is lost by the beamsplitter reflecting light onto the photometer; (2) identical exposures cannot conveniently be given for test and control preparations; (3) with spot measuring systems, the area of the field from which the measurement should be taken may not be in the middle of the field where the measuring spot usually is; and (4) appropriate corrections may not be made automatically for reciprocity failure. It follows that such equipment may not be suitable for fluorescence, or at least must be operated with special care. Some modern photomicrographic systems provide a locking system for exposure times, to overcome problem (2) above.

Corrections by trial-and-error

Despite having an accurate photometer, some manual compensation is almost always required, based on experience. We recommend keeping a detailed record of all pictures taken. The record should include, besides the specimen and details of microscopy, the ISO film speed set, the photometer reading, the compensation settings (if any), and the length of the exposure given. Afterwards, when the pictures have been developed, note the ones that were correctly exposed. Co-author Fred has found it invaluable to plot a graph (Fig 16.2) showing, for all successful pictures, photometer reading plotted against exposure (or, with an automatic camera, ISO setting against actual exposure time). A separate graph is required for each film type, and usually for each modality of microscopy (eg transmitted light, etc). From this graph, one can estimate from a given photometer reading what the optimal exposure is likely to be. One can also estimate the likely amount of error, on which the bracketing exposures can be based. For an automatic camera, a similar plot of ISO speed against exposure time allows estimation of the ISO value(s) to be set. It is normal to expect up to a $^1/_2$ stop variation in exposure calibration due to changes in film batches and processing runs of colour films.

In a complicated field such as fluorescence, because of the considerable variation in images presented to the camera, co-author Ron is much more reliant on past experience than on photometer readings of (in his opinion) dubious value. But whatever the approach, detailed record-keeping is invaluable and should avoid the costly repetition of mistakes.

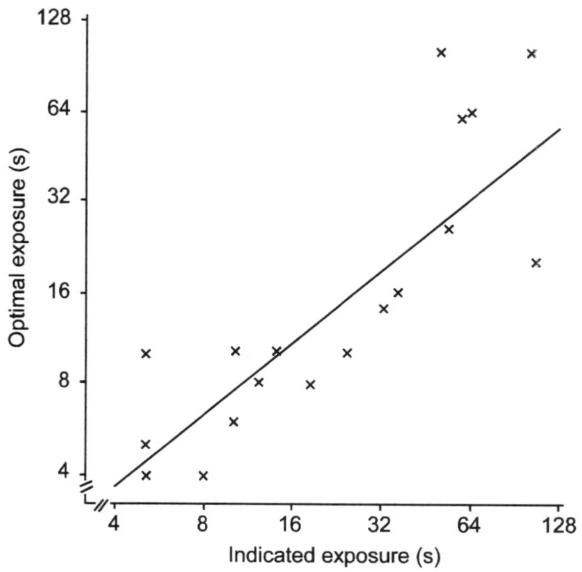

Fig 16.2. An example of a graph used for calibration of a photomicrographic exposure meter. Scales (in seconds) are logarithmic. Each cross on the graph represents one correctly exposed photograph; the circled cross represents two crosses on the same point. Data of photographs taken on Kodak *Ektachrome 200* film, of plant autofluorescence. The camera was an Olympus *PM-10ADS* system with the automatic reciprocity-failure correction set at '5' in accordance with the manufacturer's recommendations. The diagonal line is the calculated regression line (line of best fit). The long exposure times shown arise because the graph relates to fluorescence microscopy. Redrawn after Rost (1992).

Factors that affect the required exposure

The exposure required for a given specimen under given conditions depends, mainly, on the following factors:

- The brightness of the light used for illumination.
- The optical transmission (transparency) of the specimen (or reflectivity, etc, as the case may be).
- The amount of light gathered by the objective (related to its NA).
- The overall magnification from the specimen to the film.
- The sensitivity of the film.
- The desired tone (darkness or lightness) of the photograph.

The brightness of the specimen is determined by the illumination system, notably by the lamp current and the NA of the condenser.

The brightness of the image at the film plane is proportional to the square of the NA of the objective, and inversely proportional to the overall magnification. Using transmitted light, the effective NA of the objective is reduced if the NA of the condenser is less than that of the objective.

Strictly, the above remarks concerning the effect of magnification on image brightness apply only to images of *areas*, and do not apply in the special case of *point* sources of light, ie an object consisting of unresolvable minute particles. In this case, the images of the particles should, if sharply focused, be diffraction-limited and their dimensions independent of the magnification.

Distribution of light and dark in the specimen

It is necessary to distinguish three types of image., Firstly, there is the variety in which the image is of approximately the same density all over the field. Secondly, there is the image that consists of dark patches on a light background. Thirdly, there is the type with bright patches on a dark background, as is the case in darkground and (usually) fluorescence microscopy. The latter two types both give erroneous readings on an exposure meter, and need to be handled differently.

Figure 16.3 illustrates the distribution of light intensities in three types of image, On the left, a fairly uniform density is spread over the whole field. The two centre images have a few dark patches on a light background; the two images on the right have bright patches on a dark background. They might well represent images from the microscope, phase contrast (left), brightfield chromosomes or dark crystals (centre), and fluorescence or darkground (right). Since the page is uniformly illuminated, they should all be recorded with exactly the same exposure, but integrated exposure meter readings of each of the five fields will give five different exposure readings. As a particular example, the lower right image will have an intensity reading 13/2 times greater than the upper right image, but since each white area has the same intrinsic intensity, the two fields should be given exactly the same exposure.

It appears that there is a fundamental source of error in exposure values that are determined by photographic metering systems. Which exposure, if any, will be right?

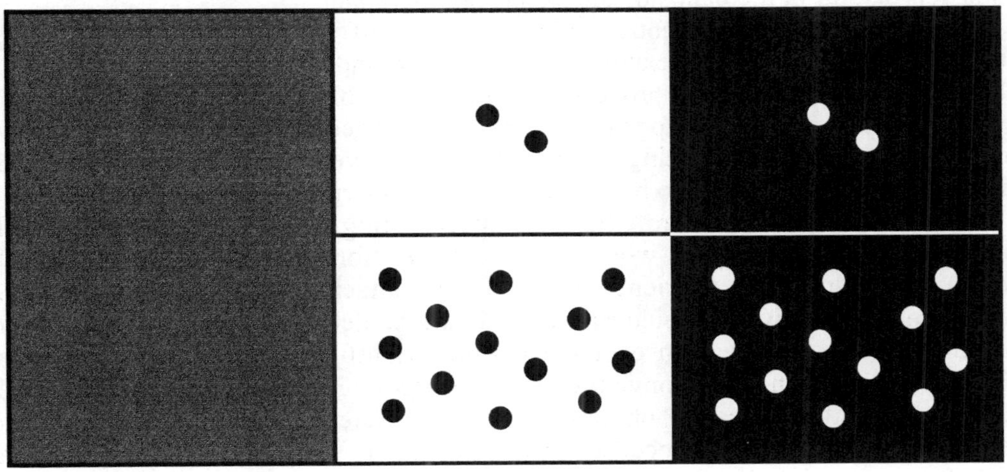

Fig 16.3. Hypothetical microscope fields, to illustrate the effects of black/white distribution on exposure determination. The field on the left approximates 18% grey (ie 18% reflectance); the white paper has a reflectance of about 90%. The four fields on the right all require the same exposure, but would give different readings on the photometer.

Camera exposure meters are calibrated to reproduce a scene as an averaged 18% grey (Fig 16.3, left). Any area that is to be photographed is considered to reflect, on average, 18% of the incident radiation, so that the intensity distribution averaged over the final photograph gives a uniform 18% grey tone. The assumption at first appraisal would seem to be quite unjustified, and yet experience shows that most pictorial photography conforms very well to the general rule. Confining our attention to pictorial photography, some exceptions to 18% averaged reflectance include snow or beach scenes (high reflectance) and scenes with heavy shadow areas (low reflectance). The photographer should recognise these exceptions, and modify the exposure accordingly. The snow scenes need more exposure, so that the snow appears white, and not 18% grey; the night scenes need less exposure, so that the night sky appears black, and not 18% grey. The careful photographer learns to avoid scenes with dominant bright areas of sky, or modifies the exposure for the scene as measured by the meter.

The normal brightfield microscope field is *not* an 18% grey, the averaged brightness being considerably greater than the equivalent of an 18% reflectivity. About the *only* microscope field that *is* middle grey is a phase-contrast image. Otherwise there is great variation, from brightfield images of chromosomes to darkground or fluorescence images of bacteria.

Some camera metering systems average out the various intensities over the whole field, all areas of the field contributing equally to the exposure determination. This is known as *integrated measurement*. In some cameras the centre of the field is emphasised, the measured exposure being *centre-weighted*. This may have some advantage for microscope work in which the specimen occupies only part of the field, although for aesthetic considerations the centre of the field is not always where such a specimen should be placed. The most expensive of cameras have a *spot metering* option, in which measurement is determined from very small areas of the field, and this is very useful in the hands of the expert photographer.

As suggested above, centre-weighting of itself is inadequate to establish unequivocally the correct exposure. In darkground, fluorescence, and some polarisation fields, the greater proportion of the field is black, highlighting small areas of specific interest. To the exposure meter, the averaged field intensity is very low, and the exposure correspondingly long. To avoid overexposure, the exposure as indicated by the meter needs to be *compensated*, as described below.

For an attachment camera, the film speed rating that is stated by the film manufacturer for pictorial work is excessive for conventional bright-field photomicrography. Our experience is that for an attachment camera the ISO film speed rating that is given for pictorial work should be decreased to give $^2/_3$ stop more exposure. This is a consequence of the normal brightfield microscope image being rather brighter than the conventional 18% grey. This correction is usually incorporated into dedicated photomicrographic systems. Further compensation, positive or negative, may be needed for a field that is much darker or lighter than usual. In any case, it is always necessary to take some test shots of the kind of material that one is using, and to compensate thereafter as necessary.

Dark on bright

A typical specimen viewed by transmitted light appears dark against a bright background. In the final picture, the background should appear either white or pale grey. In photography of this type, the required exposure is determined primarily by the brightness of the background. In the absence of a specimen, ie photographing the background only, the exposure meter will recommend an exposure that will make the picture 18% grey overall (as explained above). This is too dark, and so an increased exposure is required. For colour transparency films, an increase of $^2/_3$ stop is appropriate. This setting is normally satisfactory for well-stained histological sections, using an integrating exposure meter. For weakly stained specimens, no increase is required.

Bright on dark

Some modes of microscopy produce a bright image of the subject against a dark background – eg darkground (Figs 9.1, 9.2, 9.5, and Plates 2, 3, 10) and fluorescence (Fig 11.1 and Plate 7). Determining the exposure under these circumstances is more difficult. If the image consists of bright areas on a dark background, the exposure meter will be misled by the preponderant dark areas, and will suggest an exposure that is too long. If a bright object (eg fluorescence) occupies only a proportion of the field, the calculated exposure must be corrected accordingly (inversely in proportion to the proportional area of the specimen). Figures 16.3 and 16.4 illustrate the situation. The correction consists of a reduction in the exposure below that indicated *prima facie* by the exposure meter – if for example the fluorescence occupies 25% of an otherwise black field, the exposure should be reduced to 25% of that indicated. A similar correction can be applied to spot measurements if the object does not fill the spot. The proportion is difficult to estimate by eye, partly due to optical illusion – the bright objects on a dark background tend to appear larger than they really are. Figure 16.4 provides some standards for comparison; further standard diagrams are given by Rost (1992). These diagrams were produced by a computer, programmed to draw rectangles consisting of square blocks of white on black with specified proportions of white to black. The arrangement of the white blocks is random.

Table 16.1. Compensating factor for proportion of bright area

This table gives the compensating factor (*F*) by which the exposure must be multiplied, given the proportion (*P*) of the field that is a bright object of interest and the ratio (*R*) of the intensity of the background to that of the object. The figures are given to more decimal figures than are required for photomicrography, so that the significance of the numbers is clearer to the reader. The table is reprinted (with minor modifications) from Rost (1992).

Contrast ratio (*R*)		**1/2** **0·500**	**1/4** **0·250**	**1/8** **0·125**	**1/16** **0·063**	**1/32** **0·031**	**1/64** **0.016**
Proportion (*P*)		Compensating factor (*F*)					
1	**1·000**	1·000	1·000	1·000	1·000	1·000	1·000
1/2	**0·500**	0·750	0·625	0·563	0·531	0·516	0·508
1/4	**0·250**	0·625	0·438	0·344	0·297	0·273	0·272
1/8	**0·125**	0·563	0·344	0·234	0·180	0·152	0·139
1/16	**0·063**	0·531	0·297	0·180	0·121	0·092	0·078
1/32	**0·031**	0·516	0·273	0·152	0·092	0·062	0·046
1/64	**0·016**	0·508	0·262	0·139	0·077	0·046	0·031
1/128	**0·008**	0·504	0·256	0·132	0·070	0·039	0·023

Fig 16.4. Standard diagrams of white-on-black images, representing light objects of equal brightness, seen against a black background. These diagrams can be used for comparison with the specimen. The proportions occupied by the light areas are indicated. From a wider range published by Rost (1992, Fig 6.3), which includes diagrams for lower proportions of white.

A further factor to be taken into account is the brightness of the background. If the proportion of the field that shows a bright specimen is P, where $P \leq 1$, and if the ratio of the brightness of the background to that of the specimen is R, then the required compensating factor F is given by:

$$F = P + R(1 - P)$$

Values of F for various values of P and R are given in Table 16.1. For cameras (such as the Leica *Orthomat E*) that have a compensating setting for the proportion of bright field, the appropriate setting is given by $(F \times 100)\%$ light on dark.

Dark images

It is necessary to distinguish two types of image, both of which will give low readings on an exposure meter, and need to be handled differently. Firstly, there is the image that consists of bright patches on a dark background, as is the case in darkground and (typically) fluorescence microscopy. Secondly, the variety in which the image is dim all over. Fluorescence microscopy may produce a weak image in both categories.

If the image is dim all over, the following problems may arise: (1) the exposure meter may not be sensitive enough to give a reading, (2) the exposure may be inconveniently long, and (3) the exposure required will be additionally lengthened by reciprocity failure in the film.

If the exposure meter is not sensitive enough, there is little that one can do except either to obtain a more sensitive instrument or to manage without the meter. In the latter case, trial-and-error is the only possible course of action, taking careful notes so as to be able to repeat successful exposures. Sometimes it may be possible to use a standard bright specimen to calibrate the brightness of the illumination: eg, for fluorescence, a block of fluorescent glass or plastic; for reflection, a highly reflective object.

Reciprocity failure

For the definition of reciprocity failure, see Chapter 18. There are several ways to tackle this problem, namely:

- Measure the intensity of the image, and consult your calibration graph (Fig 16.2), from which the correct exposure can be estimated. The graph will automatically correct for reciprocity failure.
- Measure the intensity of the image, and calculate the exposure in the ordinary way. Then use reciprocity data of the film type in use to calculate the exposure to be actually given. (Such data should be obtainable from the film's manufacturer.)
- Some automatic systems have electronic compensation for reciprocity failure. The correct functioning of these systems for the film/developer combination in use must be checked by test photographs.
- Automatic systems without automatic compensation for reciprocity failure must be pre-set for a suitable compensation factor. It will be necessary to have some idea first of the approximate length of exposure to be expected. The relevant sensitivity rating (ISO, ASA, DIN, EI) for that film type at that approximate length of exposure is then set on the camera control, based on experimental data or the manufacturer's data.

In fluorescence microscopy, while these calculations, mental or otherwise, are proceeding, block off the light to avoid fading the specimen.

Automatic electronic compensation for reciprocity failure is provided in some models; the better ones have a choice of several settings for use according to the film and the estimated length of the exposure. If there is only a single correction provided, it may not be appropriate to the film/developer combination in use, and calibration by the user is essential, followed if necessary by the setting of a film speed rating appropriate to the exposure time. The nature of the correction applied by the system should be ascertained from the manufacturer, and compared with the reciprocity failure curve of the film type in use.

Automatic correction for reciprocity failure uses the formula

$$T_c = (T_m)^p$$

where T_c is the corrected time, T_m is the uncorrected time, and p is a constant for which values are set by the selector switch. It would be helpful if manufacturers indicated the actual values of p on the selector switch; advanced instruments with digital entry could even allow the desired value of p to be entered. Such an arrangement would encourage film manufacturers to quote appropriate values of p (see Rost, 1992, for examples) that could then be applied to any equipment. Typical values of p are about 1·25 to 1·45, but we have noted values as low as 1·1 for film resistant to reciprocity failure, and as high as 1·8 for film very subject to reciprocity failure.

Bracketing

Film has a limited tolerance for incorrect exposure. This tolerance is known as the exposure latitude of the film. It is greatest in black-and-white (B&W) film, rather less in colour negative film, and least in colour transparency (diapositive) film and high-contrast B&W film. Examples of the effects of incorrect exposure of colour transparency film are shown in Plate 1.

A discussion of situations in which bracketing is advisable or essential, and some guide to its implementation, are given in Chapter 3. The special requirements for bracketing in fluorescence microscopy are described in Chapter 11.

17
Digital, confocal and video techniques

The now classical techniques for image capture and storage are drawing (see Chapter 19) and photography, the latter employing emulsions of silver halides. Comparatively recently, electronic methods have become available, and their use is expanding rapidly. They are the subject of this chapter. The technology of electronic image acquisition, processing and storage is undergoing unprecedented change and development. In this chapter, no more than general principles have been outlined; anything more would be outmoded shortly after publication of the work.

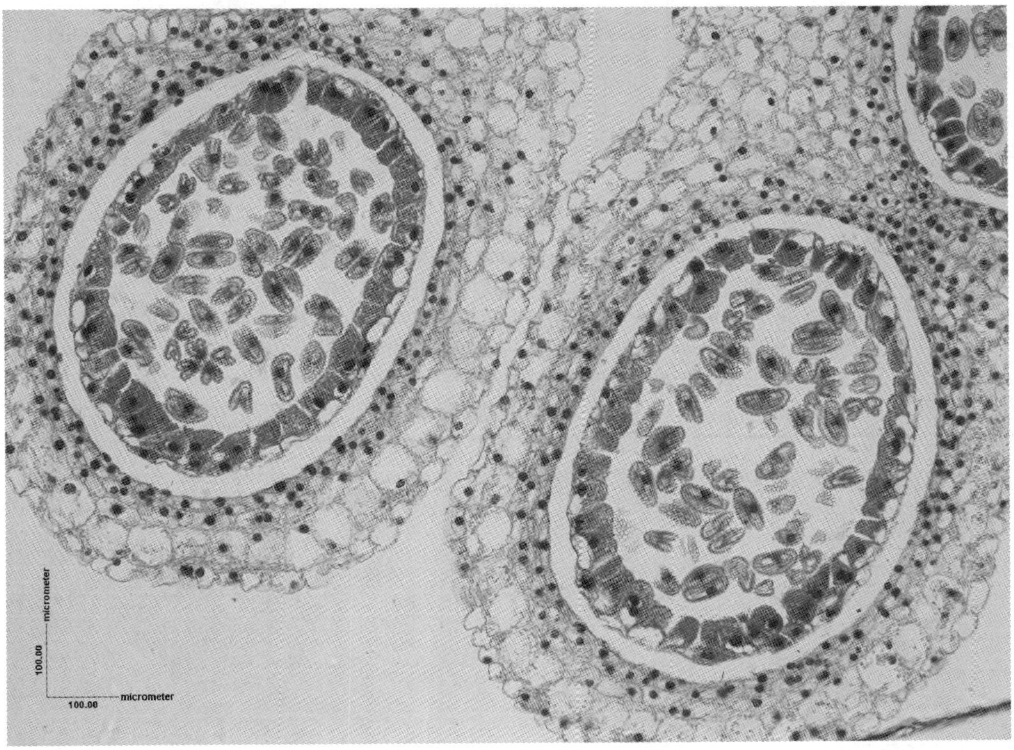

Fig 17.1. Section of part of a lily flower, photographed with a digital camera. *Lilium* anther transverse section, trans-illumination brightfield, Zeiss *Axiotech* microscope, Kontron Elektronic (now Jenoptik) *ProgRes 3008* digital camera with 0·63× television adapter. Planapo 10× objective, NA 0·45. Field size 1·4 mm × 1·0 mm. Scale bar inserted with KS image analysis software. Image 1450×1996 pixels (note that the full resolution is not apparent in this reproduction; but see Figs 17.3 and 17.4). File size (TIFF format) 2·8 Mb.

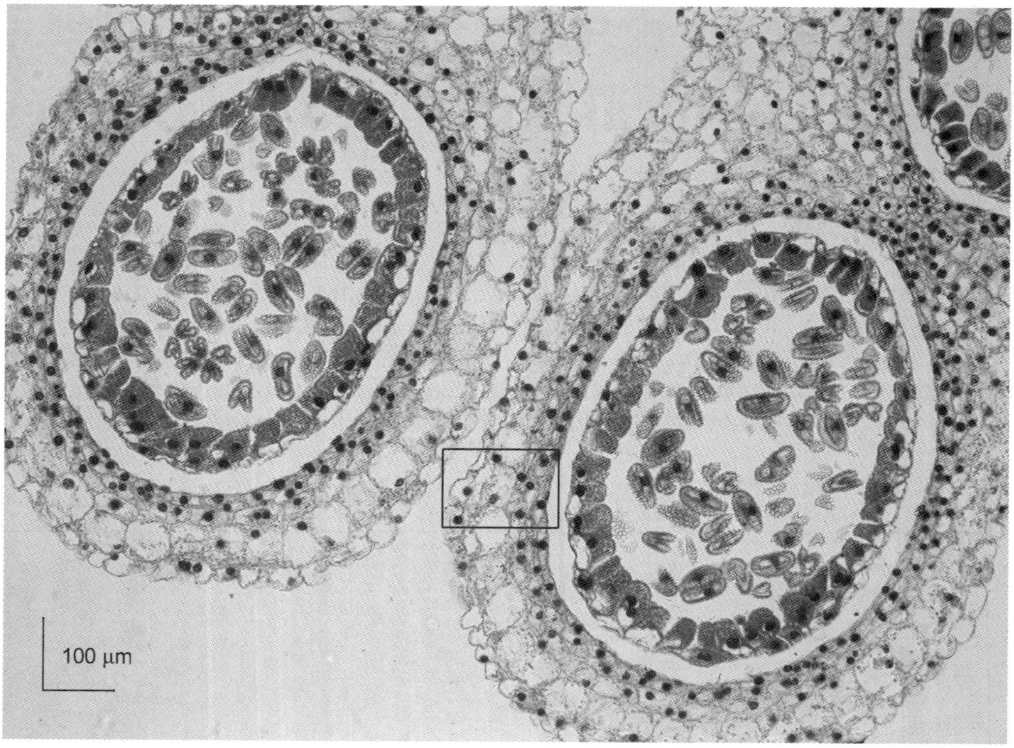

Fig 17.2. *Lilium* anther transverse section, same original photograph as Fig 17.1. The picture has been modified, using *Photoshop* software. The changes are: removal of the edge of the coverslip (bottom right); increase in contrast; insertion of scale bars and lettering; and insertion of the rectangle, which indicates the area reproduced in Fig 17.3. Image size 1521×2094 pixels. File size (*Photoshop* format) 3·0 Mb.

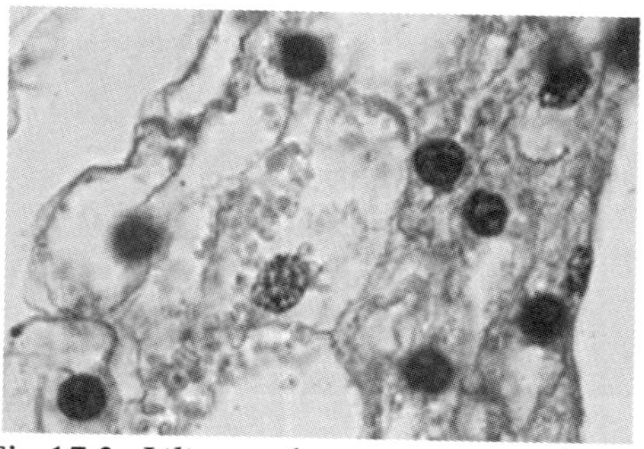

Fig 17.3. *Lilium* anther transverse section (detail), same original photograph as Fig 17.1, enlarged 4× to show the detail that is obtainable. Image size 472×702 pixels. File size (*Photoshop* format) 326 kb.

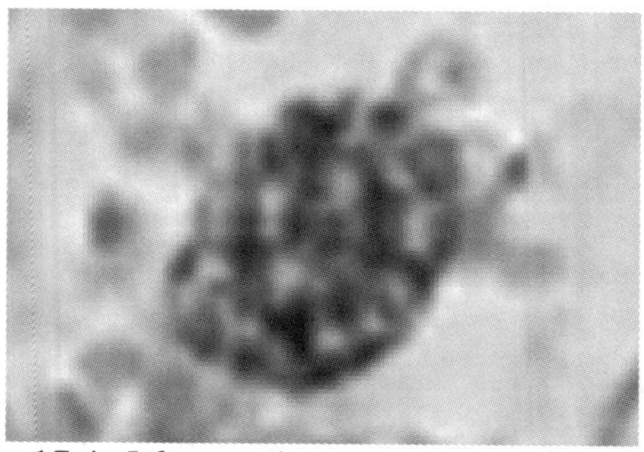

Fig 17.4. *Lilium* anther transverse section (detail), same original photograph as Fig 17.1, enlarged 20× to show the individual pixels. The area contains the nucleus shown in the centre of Fig 17.3.

Definitions/Glossary

Some of these definitions refer specifically to usage in relation to microscopy. (For more definitions, see Inoué & Spring, 1997.)

bit: a contraction of 'binary digit', the smallest unit of information using the binary system.

bit depth: the number of *bits* per *pixel*. This determines the range of tones and colours which can be represented.

byte: a unit of stored data, corresponding to a written or spoken word, made up of a number of *bits* (typically 8, 16 or 32 bits).

C-mount: a standard mount for lens on camera, originally for 16 mm film cameras, now used by most video cameras. The male (lens) thread has a diameter of 1 inch (25·4 mm) and a pitch of 32 threads/inch (about 0·79 mm).

CCD: a light-sensitive semiconductor chip used for detecting images in digital cameras (still and video). See text.

CMYK colour: colours expressed in terms of three primary colours, namely cyan, magenta, yellow, and black. These colours are used for printing.

compression: reducing the amount of storage space required by a *digital image*.

convolution: adjustment process for a *digital image* in which the value of each *pixel* is determined from its initial value and that of surrounding pixels according to a mathematical algorithm.

digital image: an image converted into an electronic signal, which is displayed in a *pixel* array. A digital record of an image that has been divided into pixels (or *voxels*) and the pixels stored digitally.

frame (video or ciné): a single image from a video or film series.

frame grabber: a computer system for isolating and recording a single video frame as a still image.

GIF: the standard format for *digital images* on the Internet.

JPEG: a standard form of *compression* for *digital images*, to reduce the amount of digital storage space required.

kilobyte (kb): 1024 *bytes* (2^{10} bytes). A common unit of electronic storage requirement or capacity. See *byte*.

megabyte (Mb): 1024 *kilobytes*, or approximately one million *bytes* (actually 2^{20} bytes). A common unit of electronic storage requirement or capacity. See *byte*.

PICT: a standard format for storage of digital images, enabling images to be exchanged between different types of software.

pixel: one element of a two-dimensional picture (*pix-* for picture, *-el* for element). A single, finite-sized element of a digitised image. A pixel may be square or rectangular. Pixels are defined by their X and Y coordinates, grey level (luminance) or luminance in each of three primary colours; these data are stored as binary numbers.

RGB colour: colours expressed in terms of three primary colours, namely red, green and blue; these are the colours used in computer monitors (cf *CMYK*).

TIFF: a standard format for storage of *digital images*, enabling images to be exchanged between different types of software.

voxel: an element (corresponding to a *pixel*) in a three-dimensional image.

Digital imaging

Digital images

Digital 'images' (Figs 17.1–17.4, 17.6, 17.8) are built up from a large number of small areas of equal size, known as *pixels* (*pix-* for picture, *-el* for element). Pixels (Fig 17.4) are usually square but may be rectangular. Black-and-white (B&W) pixels are defined by their horizontal and vertical (*X* and *Y*) coordinates, and their luminance (grey level); these data are stored as binary numbers. For colour pixels, the luminance is specified for each of three primary colours, either red, blue and green (the RBG system) or cyan, magenta, yellow and black (the CMYK system). These data are stored and processed as binary numbers, using standard computer technology. The images can be displayed on a computer monitor, and printed (in B&W or colour) with a digital printer.

Comparison: digital photography versus silver photography

To change from silver to digital image processing involves a very considerable investment of resources, both money and time. Therefore, many potential users are holding back before making major changes. Will it be cheaper next year? Hardware and software is under constant review; cameras, computers, printers and software have all been subject to price reduction or at least more is on offer for your money. However, increased efficiency may justify immediate action.

The main *advantages* of digital photography are:

- No need for a darkroom.
- No messy and toxic chemicals.
- Image available immediately, without delay for chemical development, fixation, washing and drying.
- Direct entry to computer for image enhancement, editing, labelling and/or analysis.
- Wide range of spectral sensitivity (including the infrared).
- High efficiency of photon capture (potentially greater sensitivity than photographic film).
- Distribution by Internet is cheap and easy (prints are not necessary).

The main *disadvantages* of digital photography are:

- At present, the resolution of the picture is much less than can be obtained on film (but does it really matter?).
- The dynamic range of linear response is typically smaller (100:1) than film, depending on the signal-to-noise ratio.
- Photographic film is the most economical storage medium (in terms of cost and space per bit of information), and is also the most reliable.
- A new dedicated computer almost certainly will be required, and possibly duplicated workstations.
- Computer breakdown, although rare, is a possibility.
- High initial capital investment in a camera.
- Slow image capture time, and possibly retrieval time, for detailed images.
- Limited sensitivity range of current commercial cameras (ISO equivalent 100 to 800) compared to film (25 to 3200).

Acquisition of data

Digital photomicrographic images are generally acquired in the following ways:

- Direct photography using a digital camera on the microscope.
- Video photography combined with a computer 'frame grabber'.
- Direct digital imaging using a confocal scanning microscope.
- Digital scanning of an existing photograph.

These four methods are described below.

Digital photography

Compared to the silver photography described in other chapters, digital photography differs in the following ways. The camera is a digital one, employing a charge-coupled device (CCD) as the light-sensitive device. The optical image is represented by a 'digital image', which is an electronic description of the image. The digital image is read from the CCD by a computer, and all subsequent image processing is carried out by computer. The digital image is stored on normal computer storage devices, such as the computer's hard disc, exchangeable floppy disc or hard discs (such as *Zip* and *Jaz* discs) or CDs. A print ('hard copy'), if required, is made by a computer printer. The image may be in B&W or colour.

Charge-coupled devices

A CCD is a solid-state photometric device on a semiconductor chip. The light-sensitive region is divided into rows and columns of small areas, each determining one pixel of the image. The CCD of a video camera currently (1999) contains typically 750×580 pixels, covering an area of the order of 8 mm × 6 mm. Still cameras may have a larger number of pixels: at the present time, at least 1 million pixels (eg 1280×960 pixels) is regarded as the minimum for a good-quality CCD camera.

Photons striking the pixels cause an electric charge to accumulate at a rate proportional to the intensity of the light. At the end of the exposure the amount of the charge on each pixel is read out, a row at a time, as a video frame or still.

The sensitivity and dynamic range of a CCD is dependent upon the signal-to-noise ratio (S/N), which in turn depends upon the design of the CCD and its temperature. A typical consumer-grade video CCD can be expected to have a dynamic range of about 100:1 (8 bits). A higher dynamic range (eg 1000:1, or 10 bits, or a density range of 3·0 density units) is obtainable by cooling the CCD. The output signal (image) is corrupted by electrical 'noise' (see next paragraph). CCD devices are particularly sensitive to infrared, which may lead to incorrect exposure (Richardson, 1997).

Image quality

Image quality is determined by two main factors: the total number and shape of the pixels making up the image, and the bit depth (the number of bits per pixel). The latter is in practical terms dictated by the S/N ratio of the device. A further factor is the width of the gaps between the sensing elements of the CCD. In sensor/image shift cameras, the concept of pixel-limited resolution no longer applies to the sensing device, only to its output.

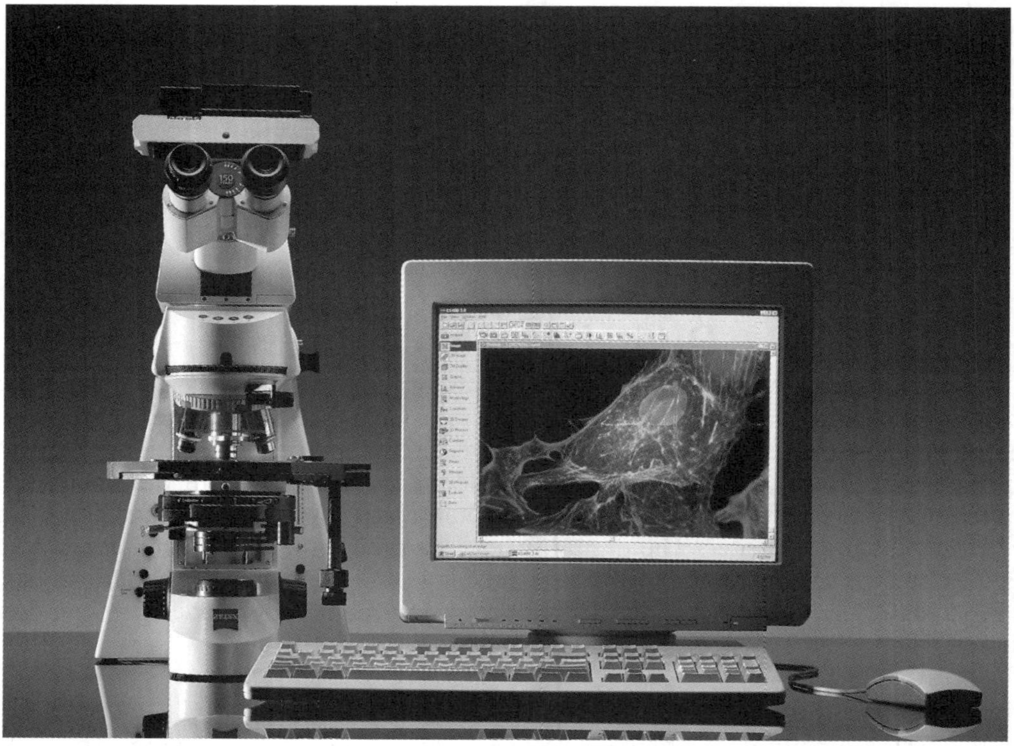

Fig 17.5. Zeiss *Axioskop 2* microscope with cooled digital camera, Zeiss *KS400* image analysis software, monitor and keyboard with mouse. Photograph courtesy Carl Zeiss Pty Ltd, Sydney.

Noise is mainly thermal, ie associated with the CCD not being at absolute zero temperature. Thermal noise can be reduced by cooling the CCD, a procedure carried out by a Peltier cooling device (particularly in astronomical CCD cameras, where high sensitivity is paramount). Peltier cooling devices make use of the fact that an electric current passing in a particular direction through the junction of two metals will cause heat to flow outwards from the junction. Peltier cooling devices are relatively small and highly reliable.

Sensor/image shift cameras, eg the Jenoptik *ProgRes 3008*, move the sensor during imaging to match the image resolution. The concept of pixel-limited resolution no longer applies.

Digital photomicrography

As in conventional (silver) photography, one has the option of either purchasing an excellent (but expensive) dedicated digital photomicrographic camera, or attaching a digital single-lens-reflex (SLR) or a large-format camera with digital back using the arrangements described in Chapter 4. A dedicated digital photomicrographic camera, such as the Jenoptik *ProgRes 3008* or the Leica *DC-100*, can be expected to be operated in essentially the same way as the cameras descibed in Chapter 14. Of course, there is no film to load! The ISO speed rating range will be about 100–800 (rather than the usual 25 to 3200). The CCD serves as its own exposure metering device, allowing very sophisticated assessment of the exposure. The image will be displayed on a monitor, and stored on a digital storage device. The process of taking photomicrographs is the same as that described in Chapters 3 and 15.

Confocal microscopy

Confocal scanning

The laser-scanning confocal microscope (LSCM) is a twentieth-century invention, depending on the use of a laser and computers. It is probably the greatest advance in microscopy since the advent of electron microscopy.

We will not here attempt to describe laser-scanning confocal microscopy in detail; to do so would double the size of this book, at least! Microscopists with access to an LSCM will need to obtain one or two of the specialist works on the subject (eg Corle & Kino, 1996; Gu, 1996; Pawley, 1995). Here, we will confine ourselves to describing the basic principles, and giving some indication of when to use an LSCM.

The use of confocal microscopy is advantageous in two main circumstances: for use with thick specimens (particularly if three-dimensional data are required), and when the highest resolution is needed. Confocal microscopy is possible using transmitted or reflected light, but is most commonly applied to fluorescence microscopy (Figs 17.6, 17.9), for which it offers substantial advantages.

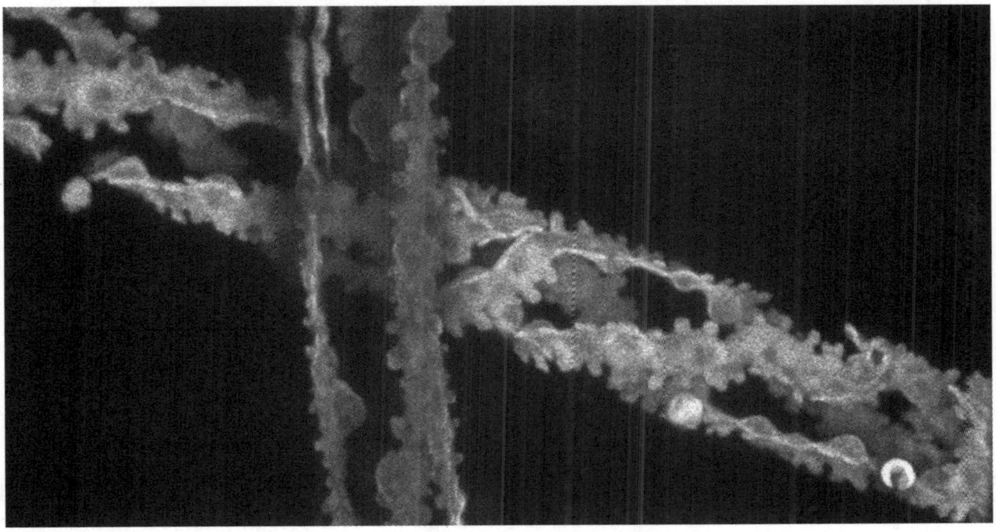

Fig 17.6. Photomicrograph taken with a confocal fluorescence microscope. Living *Spirogyra* sp, a fresh-water alga. Compare with Fig 4.5, taken almost 50 years earlier! Fifteen optical sections were taken with a depth (z) step size of 0·7 μm, each individual section having extremely limited depth of field. The image presented here is a projection of the maximum pixel value of each optical section, the result being a vastly improved depth of field. Zeiss *Axiophot* microscope with Bio-Rad *MRC 600* confocal system. Field size 55 μm × 110 μm. Zeiss Plan 40× objective, NA 0·65. Epi-illumination fluorescence, 488 nm excitation. Reproduced by kind permission of Jenny Norman, Macquarie University.

In a confocal microscope, both the area of illumination and the area from which measurement is made are confined to a single spot (Fig 17.7); the illuminating laser (or other point source) and a pinhole in the emission-measuring system are focused on the same spot in the object plane, and the specimen is moved mechanically in raster fashion with respect to the spot.

A confocal microscope possesses superior imaging capabilities compared to a normal microscope. For a given NA, the resolution of the system can be greater by a factor of 1·4 compared to conventional microscopy. Moreover, the technique lends itself particularly to fluorescence microscopy. Firstly, the resolution of the scanning system is dependent on the excitation wavelength, rather than the emission wavelength as in a conventional fluorescence microscope, and therefore greater resolution is obtainable. Secondly, the confocal fluorescence microscope possesses a unique depth-discriminating property, whereby the detector does not accept all the light from out-of-focus planes and so these are imaged less strongly than the in-focus plane. In consequence, background fluorescence may be sharply reduced, and it is possible to obtain three-dimensional data by stereoscopic imaging or by building up a series of optical sections.

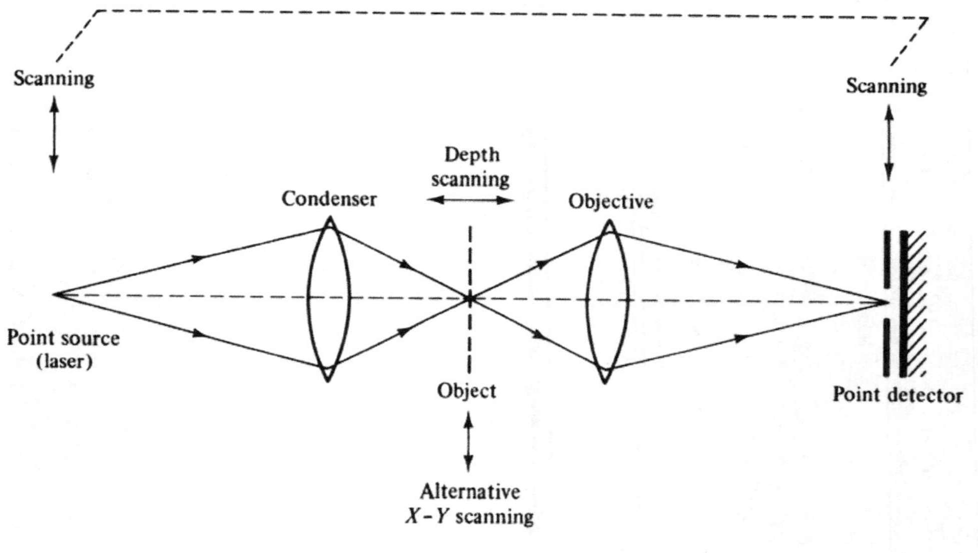

Fig 17.7. Schematic diagram of a confocal fluorescence microscope. A point source is imaged onto the specimen, and the same point is imaged onto the detector. In practice, fluorescence epi-illumination is most commonly employed. Reproduced from Rost (1991).

Two-photon fluorescence microscopy, as its name suggests, involves the excitation of the specimen by low-energy photons absorbed in pairs. The specimen is excited by short bursts of very intense light of a relatively long wavelength, such that simultaneous absorption of two photons is required to produce enough energy for excitation.

Three-dimensional information can be built up by multiple images at different focusing levels. Such data can be presented as stereo pairs. Anaglyphs (see Chapter 13) can conveniently be made automatically from digital images and displayed on a colour monitor.

Digital (computer) processing

Scanning

Given existing photographic prints or negatives, conversion to a digital image is required before digital processing can be commenced. This is achieved by a scanner. These are designed to accept prints, negatives and transparencies, or all of these. A specially high resolution is required for satisfactory scanning of 35 mm negatives and transparencies. Polaroid 4×5 inch print and negative films are a useful complement to the 'digital darkroom'.

Digital processing: image analysis, editing. The 'digital darkroom'

The standard software for general image editing is Adobe *Photoshop*. This software accepts digital images from storage media or from a scanner. It is possible to do almost anything with an image, using *Photoshop* or similar software.

In relation to scientific photography, the following procedures are legitimate:

- **Production of a print or copy** from a negative, transparency, or Polaroid print. An original can be scanned in, adjusted as necessary (see below) and printed on a digital printer to near photographic quality. Superior prints from digital images can be made on dye-sublimation printers, but they cost some 20 times as much. Printing from a negative requires digital inversion. A digital image can also be printed as a transparency. For small numbers of prints these procedures are much easier and quicker than corresponding photographic techniques, and do not require any messy chemicals or a darkroom.
- **Adjustment of brightness and contrast**. These procedures are analogous, in silver-photographic terms, to altering the exposure during printing and to choosing the grade of paper. However, the adjustments can be much more sophisticated using *Photoshop*, and can be applied equally to B&W and colour images.
- **Removal of a colour cast** (eg due to wrong lamp current or an unsuitable blue filter).
- **Enlargement or reduction** of the picture to any desired size.
- **Cropping** of the image, to select the desired area.
- **Assembly of two or more images** into a single plate. This may include isolation and rearrangement of portions of a photomicrograph, as in a karyogram (see Fig 17.8)
- **Superimposition** of lettering, a scale bar, arrows, etc.

The following procedures may have a place in scientific photography:

- Sharpening of the image
- Conversion of B&W to false colour to bring out specific detail.
- Isolating the picture by addition of a border, either a line or an area (Fig 5.1).

The following additional procedures are not appropriate for scientific photography, but may be of value in the production of teaching material:

- Removal of artefacts (Fig 17.2).
- Fading-out of less relevant portions of the picture to emphasise the main feature.
- Removal of unwanted objects from the periphery of the picture (Figs17.2).
- Toning a B&W image to monochrome colour.
- Hand-colouring a B&W image.
- Replacement of the background by a more appropriate tone or colour.
- Conversion to a diagram.

Photoshop and similar software have many other capabilities, which can be applied to photomicrographs for artistic purposes (see the cover).

Provided that the publisher is suitably equipped, photographs and diagrams may be submitted for publication on a floppy or *Zip* disc.

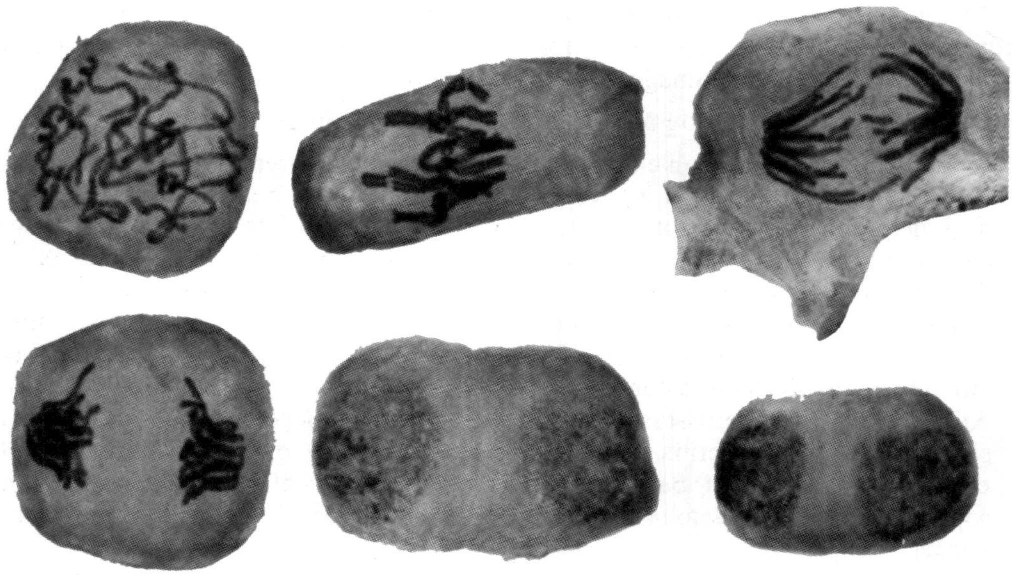

Fig 17.8. Dividing cells from Plate 16, cut out and rearranged in sequence using Adobe *Photoshop* software. The original photograph was scanned to produce a digital 'image' in a Macintosh computer. Images of individual cells were electronically copied, trimmed to their outlines, rotated as necessary, and 'pasted' into the required positions.

Image processing

Image processing involves calculating new values for each pixel, using some algorithm (ie a mathematical process). These processes are invaluable for adjusting overall brightness and contrast, and for correcting colour casts. Detail that is present in the image but hard to see can be made more visible by sharpening. Of course, the process of sharpening is unable to reveal detail not present in the original image.

Convolution processes change pixel values on the basis of the values of the original pixel and of its neighbours, according to some mathematical formula. Examples are sharpening, smoothing, and finding edges. The relative influence of neighbouring pixels is determined by a numerical matrix known as a *convolution mask* or *kernel* (for examples see Davies & Fennessy, 1998, and the instruction manual for NIH *Image*, see next page).

Point processes change pixel values without regard to the values of neighbouring pixels. A *mapping function* expresses the mathematical relationship between the pixel brightnesses of input and output images. Examples are changes in brightness and contrast, colour correction, and inversion (conversion from negative to positive image or vice versa).

Monitor

A monitor is a device which displays a digital or video image from a computer, digital camera or video camera. It resembles a television set, but has no tuner or receiver for television broadcasts. For viewing images, a screen measuring (across the diagonal) at least 40 cm (16 inches) is desirable. The diagonal of the actual picture measures less than the nominal size of the monitor. The colours displayed on different monitor screens are notoriously inconsistent.

Digital storage

Images are stored in a variety of electronic formats. The standard ones, by means of which data stored by software of one kind can be read by software of another kind, include GIF (standard for the Internet), JPEG, PICT and TIFF. To save space, images are commonly compressed. Unfortunately this means that some data are discarded during compression, degrading the image somewhat. If you are doing quantitative image analysis, you should not use PICT, which carefully records the colour of each pixel, with less attention to the actual pixel value. Therefore, in PICT files there is no guarantee that the pixel values will remain fixed. On the other hand, TIFF is a machine- and system-independent image standard that avoids this problem.

Magnetic discs of various kinds are used for initial storage, especially during the editing process. The computer's own hard disc is a typical starting point, but these soon fill up and images must be transferred to longer-term storage. Floppy disks have storage space (1·4 Mb) at most for only a few B&W images, not enough for colour unless much compressed. *Zip* discs (storage capacity 98 Mb) are currently widely used. There are others with even higher storage capacity, and doubtless these will be used increasingly. Magnetic discs (floppy, *Zip*, etc) are susceptible to corruption, and may suddenly become unreadable; backup is essential. For long-term storage, the best by far at present are optical discs (photo CDs). For further details, see Cox (1995).

Hard copies (prints and transparencies)

Software such as Adobe *Photoshop* can be used for the assembly of plates for publication (see Fig 17.8). The best printouts of images are currently given by dye-sublimation printers and ink-jet printers. At at the time of writing, the latter use inks which are not permanent, and give an image life said to be about two years under good conditions. Laser-printer printouts on archival-quality paper are of archival quality, because they use carbon particles to form the image, but printing is slow and pictures can be printed only as half-tones or using dithering (see Cox, 1995).

Conversion from digital file to film image is comparatively expensive, one commercial transparency costing almost as much as photography with a 36 exposure film.

Image analysis

Image analysis is outside the scope of this book. We mention only that digital images lend themselves immediately to computer entry, for all kinds of analysis such as counting objects, determining areas, etc. A starting point might be the public domain NIH *Image* program (developed at the US National Institutes of Health) available on the Internet at http://rsb.info.nih.gov/nih-image/

Noise

Noise is the term for any unwanted elements in an electronic signal, including digital and video images. Noise may be due to thermal effects, or to electrical interference from outside, or to defects in the equipment.

Video microscopy

Photography of moving objects was for many years carried out using ciné (movie film) techniques. The first generation of video cameras were derived from photomultiplier tubes, and were bulky and expensive. The development of video cameras using CCD sensors, together with advances in video recording and computer processing and storage technology, has made video technique more easily applicable and more powerful. Video systems are also applicable to the observation and recording of dim light (as in video intensification fluorescence microscopy, for which see Chapter 11), and invisible wavelengths (infrared and ultraviolet, see Chapter 12).

Attaching a video camera (previously called CCTV camera, closed circuit television camera) to the microscope has particular advantages for recording of moving or living material. Controlled electronic enhancement of intensity and contrast of a less than perfect microscope image is relatively simple. The moving image can be recorded cheaply on videotape or optical disc, in real time or time lapse. Through a frame-grabbing card in a computer, the full range of digitised computer image processing can be applied to the video image, including printouts of individual frames. Moreover, video techniques can advantageously be applied to the examination of images at low light levels (as in video intensification fluorescence microscopy (see Chapter 11), or using wavelengths of light invisible to the eye, eg infrared and ultraviolet (see Chapter 12).

The technique of video microscopy has been comprehensively described by Inoué & Spring (1997). We give here only a summary of the basics.

Practicalities

Video cameras are readily attached to trinocular microscopes, in much the same way as conventional cameras. The standard video camera lens fitting is C-mount (we wish that still cameras were as uniform in their lens fittings!). On some microscopes, a video port with a C-mount is built-in. Otherwise, an adapter, incorporating a relay lens, is required. For video recording, the following is the minimum requirement:

- A video camera, fitted to a suitable port on the microscope (eg replacing the normal photomicrographic camera).
- A video monitor to display the output of the camera.
- A video recorder to record the output of the camera.

The recorder may be replaced by a computer, in which case a separate video monitor for the camera may not be required.

In order to keep the brightness of the optical image within the dynamic range of the video camera, some system for regulating the intensity of the light is required. In many cases, the current/voltage control for the lamp is all that is needed. However, for colour work this is unsuitable (because the colour temperature will vary too). A pair of polarising filters, one rotatable, is suitable in many applications. For fluorescence, a modern arc-lamp system with variable output is best. Aperture and field diaphragms must of course not be used for this purpose! Alternatively, some cameras have an *auto iris*, an iris diaphragm that is automatically varied to maintain constant brightness of the image on the CCD. A monitor is required for viewing; this may or may not be part of a computer system.

Video (television) cameras

In a conventional television camera, an optical image is projected onto a photocathode and scanned by an electron beam. The output of the camera is an electrical signal proportional to the intensity of the optical image at the point being scanned at the moment. The picture is scanned in horizontal lines, either 625 or 525 lines in the full height of the picture. Alternate lines are scanned in successive frames, so that the complete image is scanned over two successive frames. Frames are obtained either 50 or 60 times per second, depending on the frequency of the local electricity supply (usually 50 Hz, except in the USA and some other countries which use 60 Hz). The output from the camera includes also synchronisation pulses to keep the receiver in synchrony. Modern miniature video cameras use a CCD sensor.

Video recording and frame-grabbing

The video images can be recorded on videotape, captured by a computer, or photographed from the monitor screen. Recording on videotape with a standard video recorder (VCR) requires the least expensive equipment, and the greatest storage capacity. Finding a desired sequence, using the fast-forward mode, is relatively simple. A *jog-shuttle control*, available in video editing decks and some VCRs, enables examination of individual frames and of slowing down or speeding up playback. Copying tapes involves some loss of information.

Digital recording requires expensive equipment, and provides less storage. However, high image quality can be obtained, which is not degraded by subsequent copying and image processing. Compression, to obtain longer recording times, does lead to loss of image quality, but this may concern only the background and therefore be insignificant. Digital frame-grabbing, using a computer, enables stills to be extracted from a video sequence.

Photography from monitor screen

Photographs can be taken from the monitor screen. Resolution is impaired (compared with direct photography) but the exposure is determined only by the brightness of the monitor and therefore the exposure is short and consistent.

Conventional practice is to set up a camera on a tripod on the floor in front of the screen, in a darkened room (to minimise reflections from the screen). When using a 35 mm SLR camera, a lens of about 150–200 mm focal length is convenient as it allows the camera and its tripod to be sufficiently far away from the screen to leave the area in front clear, and also to avoid distortion due to photographing a curved screen from too close. Screens may be designed to be viewed from a certain distance; in such case the camera lens should be at that distance from the screen.

Almost any B&W or colour film of normal contrast can be used. The shutter speed, about $^1/_8$ to 2 seconds, should be long enough to cover several frames of video, otherwise the raster pattern will appear. This problem is particularly apparent with cameras with focal plane shutters (as in most SLR cameras, see Chapter 4), which record a diagonal stripe if a short exposure is used. The brightness setting of the monitor should be noted; the brightness setting, once set to a suitable level, will rarely need be changed, and the exposure required for the camera will also remain constant (for the same lens aperture and film speed). If it is possible to have the computer display a standard tone of grey, this is a helpful basis for exposure measurement. Such grey display can be achieved with a variety of software, including both graphics and word-processing programs. It is preferable not to use the 'auto' setting of a camera shutter, since this may inappropriately vary the exposure from one experiment to the next.

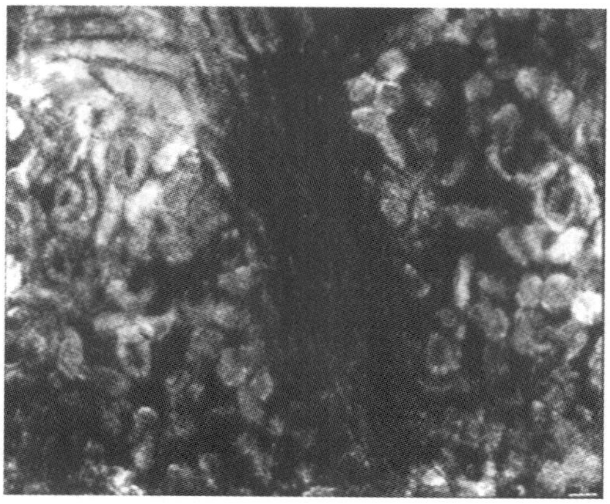

Fig 17.9. Photography from a monitor screen. Surface of leaf of *Eucalyptus* sp, confocal fluorescence microscopy, excitation 488 nm, emission barrier filter LP600, field size 400 µm × 500 µm. Saroastro laser scanning confocal microscope, objective 40× water immersion. Photograph taken with Pentax 6×7 camera, *Macro-Takumar* 135 mm *f*/4 lens, Fuji *Velvia* film (used because colour pictures were required).

Drawing by tracing from monitor screen

If a drawing or diagram is required, it may be convenient to reproduce the image from a video or computer screen by using tracing paper (see Chapter 19 for hints on drawing).

Further reading

If you are contemplating entering this field and have no close contact with experienced colleagues, we recommend that you begin by browsing the numerous Web sites on the Internet which are related to your particular interest. Useful starting points might be the sites of the (British) Royal Microscopical Society (http://www.rms.org.uk/index.html) and the Microscopical Society of America (htttp://www.msa.microscopy.com). Some of the commonest terms which will be encountered are defined in the Box. Invaluable references include Inoué & Spring's (1997) book on video microscopy, and the compendium on confocal microscopy edited by Pawley (1995), which extend much of the subject matter of this chapter (not only video and confocal microscopy). Other particularly useful works include those of Corle & Kino (1995), Davies & Fennessy (1998), Ray (1994b), and Sluder & Wolf (1998).

Digital techniques used for this book

Digital methods were used extensively in the production of this book. Some images were captured digitally (Figs 17.1–17.4, 17.6). Others were scanned in and modified digitally (Figs 5.1, 5.2, 17.8). Line drawings were either drawn by hand, scanned in, and edited in Adobe *Photoshop*, or created directly using *Claris Office* or *Photoshop*. Image processing was carried out on an Apple *Power Macintosh*, with 128 Mb of RAM. The entire text was typed on computers, edited, line drawings added, and the whole printed out as camera-ready text using an Epson ink-jet printer.

Part V
Materials and processing

Chapter 18 describes the purely photographic side of the business, discussing film types and processing techniques, extending the information given in Chapter 1.

Chapter 19 describes the production of drawings as alternatives to photographs. Equipment, materials and techniques are described briefly, with particular emphasis on modern mechanical aids. No previous knowledge or experience in drawing is required.

- Aims: to describe the materials of 'silver' photography, and to offer some helpful suggestions on processing. To describe how to use drawing attachments to produce ordinary or archival drawings.

- Prerequisite knowledge: Chapter 18 assumes the subject matter of Chapters 1 and 3. It is not necessary to have read Parts II–IV. Chapter 19 assumes the subject matter of Chapters 1 and 2, but no previous knowledge or experience in drawing is required.

- Exercises: see Appendix A3.

- Further information: see sections entitled Further reading, at ends of chapters.

18 Photographic materials and processing

Photography is essentially a process used to obtain a permanent record of an optical image that may be produced by a camera lens, microscope, telescope, or other optical device. Photography had its origin in 1727 when the German chemist Johann Schulze discovered that silver nitrate darkened when exposed to light. The speed of this reaction was too slow for practical use, but it was found that a more rapid reaction was obtained with silver halides (silver chloride, bromide, and iodide). Under the influence of light, the halide is oxidised, and the silver ions are reduced to metallic silver. The phrase *silver photography* is sometimes used to distinguish the photographic processes discussed in this chapter from other recording processes such as xerography (used in photocopiers) and digital (electronic) photography.

The basic processes involved in obtaining a black-and-white (B&W) photographic print are:

1. Film is *exposed* to light in the form of an optical image.
2. The light acts on a photosensitive *emulsion* to produce a *latent image.*
3. The latent image is *developed* to form a visible image that is negative, ie the tones are reversed.
4. The film is *fixed* to prevent further alteration by light.
5. Photographic *paper* is exposed to an optical image of the negative.
6. Steps 2–4 are repeated, producing a *positive* image on the paper.

Positive transparencies, and colour prints from these, are produced by *reversal processing*, in which all processes take place on the original film. Colour images are produced by use of three separate layers sensitive to different parts of the spectrum.

Black-and-white photographic materials

By 'photographic materials' we refer mainly to *film*, on which initial photographs are taken, and *paper*, on which prints are made. Associated with these are various chemicals, used for processing the film and paper.

The actual photosensitive material that reacts to light is called the *photographic emulsion*. This consists of crystals of silver halide suspended in gelatine, coated as a thin layer onto a support, which may be a transparent film, glass, or an opaque material such as paper.

Photographic film consists basically of three layers (Fig 18.1): the photographic emulsion that is sensitive to light; the support or base; and the backing, which is a light-absorbing layer to prevent unwanted reflections, and which is removed during processing of the film. The emulsion consists of minute crystals of silver halide suspended in a gelatine matrix. It contains silver halides (*halide* is a generic word encompassing chloride, bromide and iodide), which, under the action of light, are reduced to metallic silver. If the emulsion is exposed to light for long enough, it will go black due to the formation of silver. However, if the emulsion is exposed to a small amount of light, the amount of silver produced is not enough to be visible. The quantity of metallic silver can be very greatly increased by chemical treatment known as *development*. This converts what is known as a *latent* (ie as yet invisible) *image* to a visible image. To prevent further action of light, unreduced silver salts are removed by a chemical process called *fixation*, and the remaining chemicals (other than silver) are removed by washing.

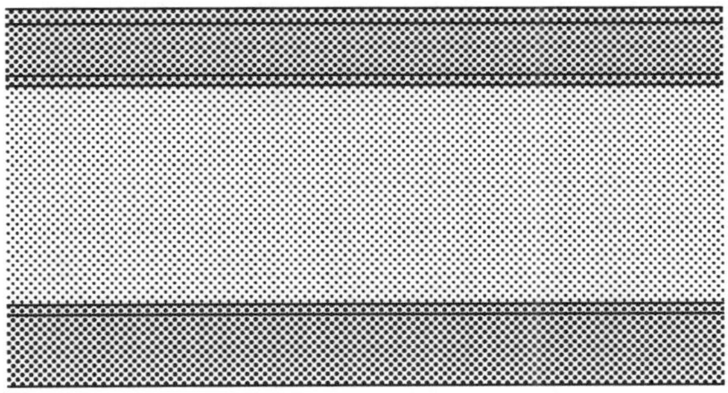

Fig 18.1. Section of a typical black-and-white film. The film base is usually cellulose triacetate; the other layers are mainly gelatine. The gelatine supercoat protects against abrasion. The emulsion is the photosensitive layer. The subbing layers, of gelatine and cellulose, promote adhesion between the layers. The backing prevents unwanted reflections and equalises the curling effect of the gelatine layers.

The positive–negative process. If light in the form of an image is allowed to shine on film, the processes of exposure and development lead to the production of a B&W image. In this image, regions in which the light was brightest become blackest, and the dark regions remain clear. Therefore, the photographic image produced is a *negative image*, in which the tones of the original are reversed (Fig 18.2b). If light is shone through the negative image and focused onto another photographic emulsion, a repetition of the photographic process reverses the tones of the negative image to make a positive image once more (Fig 18.2c). This is the basic negative–positive process, invented by Fox Talbot.

Photographic paper consists of a layer of photographic emulsion on a sheet of paper, that is usually coated with a resin to make it waterproof. Images from photographic negatives are produced on such paper to make a positive print.

Exposure

The total amount of light that falls on a given area of the emulsion is determined by two factors: the intensity of the light, and the length of the exposure. The exposure is actually the total number of photons per unit area of the emulsion; this number is the product of the intensity (photons per second per unit area), and the duration of exposure (in seconds). The proportion of photons that result in the production of a silver grain is the *quantum efficiency*, which depends on the sensitivity of the emulsion and on the wavelength of the light.

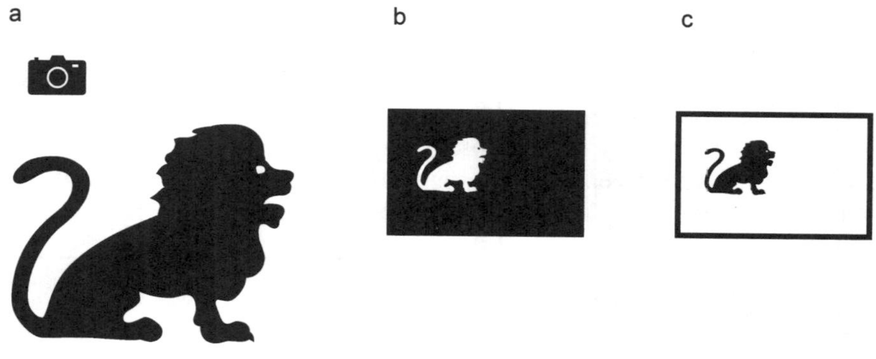

Fig 18.2. Diagram illustrating (a) original (positive), (b) negative, and (c) positive print.

Sensitivity of emulsions and density of images

The transmission of light through a developed image on film depends upon the amount of blackened silver grains. The proportion of light transmitted is called the transmittance (T), and its reciprocal the opacity ($1/T$, or T^{-1}). However, it is easier to deal with the logarithm of the opacity, known as *density*. Density (D) is defined as

$$D = \log \text{opacity} = \log (1/T) = -\log T$$

The *characteristic curve* (Fig 18.3) of a film is a representation of the response of that film to various amounts of exposure. It is a plot of density (on the Y or vertical axis) against the logarithm of the photographic exposure (on the X or horizontal axis), and has variously been called the H & D curve (after Hurter and Driffield, who first plotted these curves in 1890), the D–log E curve, and currently the D–log H curve. H is the physicist's description of photographic exposure, defined as $E \times t$, illuminance (E, ie light intensity incident on the emulsion) multiplied by the duration of the exposure (t). As actual illuminance values may be difficult to measure, relative illuminance values are often implied. For a negative film, the D–log H curve appears as in Fig 18.3. In a single photographic 'exposure' through the microscope, t is unchanged, but the value of E varies considerably, because different areas of the specimen transmit or (reflect) very different illumination intensities.

Below the threshold, exposure increments do not affect the resulting density. Here, the density is described as *base plus fog*, or D_{min}. Fog is due to the development of unexposed grains and the lack of 100% transparency of the supporting film. On the curve, the point corresponding to the first perceptible increase in density is called the *threshold*. The need to overcome this threshold is the basis of the pre-exposure technique (see below, Emulsion speed). The *toe* of the curve shows increasing density with exposure, and in pictorial photography bears the shadow detail of the scene. In the straight-line portion of the curve, density differences in the negative correspond proportionally to differences in brightness in the original image. The straight-line portion represents the middle densities of a photograph, and normally the exposure given to the photomicrograph should be chosen so that all the detail in the microscope image lies on this portion of the curve. Towards the shoulder, a given increase in exposure produces relatively less increase in density, the film reaching its maximum density at the *shoulder* of the curve. In pictorial photography, this region below the shoulder carries the highlights of the scene.

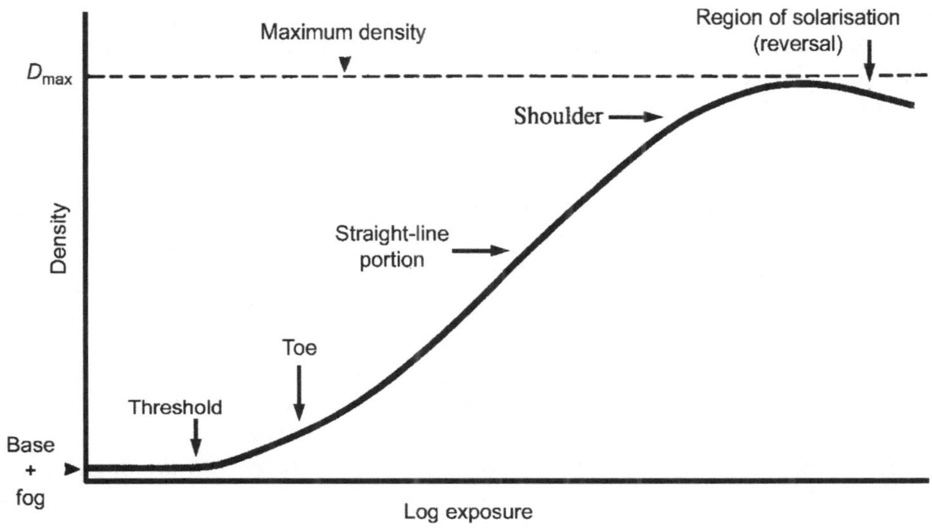

Fig 18.3. Characteristic curve, *D*-log *H*, of a monochrome (B&W) negative.

In a sunlit pictorial scene, the value of *E* might vary between 1 and 1000, a range of figures that will not fit on the straight line portion. Some of the scene is 'lost', in that detail in the shadows or detail in the highlights is not distinguished as a density variation. In a brightfield photomicrograph the range of values for *E* is very much compressed, for intense staining of the specimen is rigorously avoided. A consequence is a very much greater tolerance of the film for incorrect exposure. Different exposures will give darker or lighter negatives, but the contrast, the difference between the densities of the darkest and lightest portions of the negative, will be constant. Negatives darker or lighter will print equally well, a phenomenon quite unusual in pictorial photography. On the other hand, in some techniques such as darkground, fluorescence and polarisation, intensity variation even greater than 1:1000 may unavoidably occur. Such contrasty images are difficult to handle photographically, for some of the values of *E* will lie outside the straight line region.

In many modern films, the straight line portion is absent, because there is a tendency to extend the toe region greatly. In a number of these films, the characteristic curve may not even show a shoulder, because densities in this region approach 4 or more, a density that is much too high for detail to be reproduced on paper. Theoretically, photomicrographs taken on such film will show tonal differences in the final prints depending on which part of the toe the camera exposure lies.

Gamma, average gradient, and contrast index

The slope of the straight line portion of the characteristic curve (Fig 18.3) is a measure of the contrast or gamma (γ) of the emulsion. Gamma (a Greek letter, corresponding to '*g*') is a measure of the increase in density resulting from unit increase in log *H* (log illuminance, or log photographic exposure). Gamma can also be regarded as the ratio of the contrast in the photographic image to that of the original subject. It is defined as the tangent of the angle that the straight line portion of the characteristic curve makes with the horizontal axis. For a pictorial film, gamma usually has a value somewhat less than 1·0, typically about 0·8. Films designated for copying of line originals, material such as the text on this page in which only B&W (without halftones) are relevant, have a gamma value nearer 5.

The characteristic curve is altered by a change in developer and/or development time, so that each film has a series or *family* of characteristic curves for a developer. A technical brochure for a particular film will typically have two diagrams, one showing a family of *D*–log *H* curves with different development times in a named developer, and the other a curve of development time against gamma. Increasing development times produce an increase in the slope of the curve, ie an increase in gamma or contrast. This is more than dull theory, for it is a very practical way for the photomicrographer to increase recorded contrasts. During development, by adjusting the development process, emulsion contrast is adapted to complement the contrast range of the specimen.

Perhaps more useful than gamma is the concept of *average gradient*, $\bar{G}$, or *G*-bar. Two points are chosen on the characteristic curve, one at $D = 0{\cdot}1$ above fog, the other at $D = 1{\cdot}50$ or $1{\cdot}60$; the slope of the line drawn between the two points is an average gradient for the range of exposures selected. Some film manufacturers will indicate development instructions (time and temperature) to achieve a certain $\bar{G}$ value.

As stated above, the characteristic curves of many modern emulsions have a very long extended toe region, meeting the shoulder without an identifiable straight-line portion. For such films, *Contrast Index* (CI) is used. The slope is measured of a line drawn between points on the characteristic curve, points that identify the exposure range of the most significant subject matter. It is a measure of the average gradient of the most useful part of the curve. A CI of 0·6 is considered to give to a pictorial daylight scene a negative that prints on a Grade 2 (normal) paper.

Gamma, average gradient, and Contrast Index are all concepts relating to the effect of development on a film. Different developers or changed development times will lead to variation in gamma, $\bar{G}$, and CI. Contrast in the negative is a related but different consideration, for negative contrast depends also on the subject tonal range and the actual exposures that are given to the emulsion, ie where the exposure range lies on the *D*–log *H* curve.

Emulsion speed

Speed or *sensitivity* refers to the capacity of the film to record light; the faster or more sensitive the film, the weaker is the light with which a photograph can be taken in a given exposure time, or alternatively the shorter is the exposure required for a given intensity of light. The numerical value for film speed rating is called the Exposure Index (EI). Manufacturers' exposure indices are now usually given in the ISO (International Organization for Standardization) system, which is similar to a combination of two systems previously used, ASA (American Standards Association) and DIN (Deutsches

Industrie Norm). In the ASA system, the number is directly proportional to the speed; so that a film rated at 64 ASA is twice as sensitive as one rated at 32 ASA. The DIN system uses a logarithmic scale; an increase of 3 DIN degrees represents an increase in sensitivity by a factor of 2. The ISO rating has an arithmetic rating (similar to the ASA) followed by a logarithmic rating expressed in degrees, similar to the DIN system; however, the ISO rating is based on criteria that differ slightly from those of the ASA and DIN. An ISO rating of 100/21° is one-quarter the speed of ISO 400/27° (see Table 18.1).

Emulsion ISO rating is defined using daylight as the radiation source, an exposure between 1/1000th and 1 second, and prescribed development conditions with a developer not commercially available. Based on a density 0.1 above D_{min} on the *D*-log *H* curve, the ASA component (the arithmetic component of the ISO rating) is defined as $0{\cdot}8/E$, where *E* is the exposure in metre-candle-seconds. Since these standard conditions are seldom met in photomicrography, it is reasonable to expect to employ a different EI rating on the camera unit. It is important to note that, when setting the speed rating on a camera or exposure meter, the photographer is not necessarily bound by the ISO rating given on the film packet, but is entitled to set any EI chosen as the most appropriate to the prevailing circumstances. However, in some camera systems, the DX barcode (on the film cassette) determines the speed rating set, and any required adjustment must be made by a compensation adjustment.

In photography, a factor of 2 in exposure or sensitivity is referred to as one stop, this being the usual relationship between successive graduations of camera dials for setting lens aperture. Multiples or fractions of a stop are in geometric proportion, ie 2 stops corresponds to a ratio of 1:4, $^1/_2$ stop corresponds to 1:1·4, and $^1/_3$ stop and $^2/_3$ stop to 1:1·26 and 1:1·59, respectively.

Table 18.1. Comparison of film speed scales: ISO arithmetic and logarithmic, ASA and DIN

ISO arith	ISO log	ISO arith	ISO log	ISO arith	ISO log
ASA	DIN	ASA	DIN	ASA	DIN
6	8°				
8	10°	80	20°	800	30°
10	11°	100	21°	1000	31°
12	12°	125	22°	1200	32°
16	13°	160	23°	1600	33°
20	14°	200	24°	2000	34°
25	15°	250	25°	2500	35°
32	16°	320	26°	3200	36°
40	17°	400	27°	4000	37°
50	18°	500	28°	5000	38°
64	19°	640	29°	6400	39°

The sensitivity of the film is affected by several factors. The ISO rating quoted by the manufacturer refers to exposures of about 1/100 second; at the much longer exposures required for DIC, phase-contrast or fluorescence photomicrography (from tens of seconds to many minutes) the sensitivity is appreciably less, enough to invalidate calculated exposures. The speed at which film should be rated is also affected by variations in development; and underexposure can to some extent be compensated for by prolonging the development time (see below, Push processing). Sensitivity to very weak light can be increased by prior controlled exposure to weak light. The film is given a small uniform pre-exposure to take it over its threshold, thereby increasing its sensitivity to dim light. This method was applied to fluorescence photomicrography by van der Ploeg, Bosman & van Duijn (1976). Another technique is hypersensitisation (used by astronomers) in which the film is baked in an atmosphere of hydrogen before exposure.

Reciprocity failure

All photographic material is subject to an effect known as reciprocity-law failure, reciprocity failure, or the Schwarzschild effect. The reciprocity law states that for constant image density, the required exposure time is inversely proportional to the light intensity, ie there is a reciprocal relationship between light intensity and the required exposure time. Thus the same image density can be obtained by doubling the exposure and halving the light intensity, or vice versa. The reciprocity law does not hold under conditions involving very long or very short exposures, where the emulsion is less sensitive. Reciprocity failure can be explained in practical terms as follows. A particular number of photons (say a million) falling on a photosensitive surface (photographic emulsion) during a period of 1/100 second have more effect on the emulsion than the same number of photons falling on the emulsion during 100 seconds. At the other extreme, the same million photons falling on the emulsion during a very short period (say 1 ms) would again give less effect, manifested as lower density of the photographic image. In other words, if the light is very weak, increasing the exposure time in inverse proportion to the light intensity is insufficient; an additional increase in exposure is needed to compensate for loss of emulsion sensitivity in dim light. The range of exposure times during which greatest sensitivity exists varies according to the type of emulsion, as does the degree of reciprocity failure outside that range. There is of course still an inverse relationship between the intensity of the light and the required exposure time; the relationship takes the form

$$\log(\text{exposure time}) = \frac{p}{\log(\text{light intensity})}$$

where p has a value greater than 1 instead of exactly 1. For exposures of the order of 10 to 100 seconds, p typically has a value of about 1·2 to 1·5 (see Rost, 1992, for examples). A practical study of films was described by Dragesco (1988). In many of the more modern and expensive photomicrographic systems, electronic compensation (correction) for reciprocity failure can be dialled into the automatic exposure determination (see Chapter 16). This is a very useful facility.

Detail, sharpness, etc

The ability of a photograph to reproduce the fine details of an object is quite difficult to quantify. It seems impossible to have a single simple quantitative measure of this characteristic. There are several quantitative measures, some of which are described below. However, photographers usually prefer to employ more qualitative or descriptive words in their assessment of emulsions or photographs, accepting that there will always be difficulty in making comparative judgements. The three main headings under which the resolution of detail can be considered are: grain or granularity, resolution, and sharpness or acutance.

Grain, graininess, rms granularity

The discrete image-forming components of a negative, the silver molecules that are formed after development, are so small that a microscope is required to show them. What can be recognised, however, even with moderate (4× to 10×) enlargement of the negative, is an apparent clumping of the separate silver molecules into 'grains' (Fig 18.4). The word *graininess* describes a subjective appraisal of the appearance of irregularities in the print or film. The more rigorously defined *granularity* uses for its basis the statistical variation of microdensities in an emulsion. Measurements are made of deviations from the mean of a film density averaging 1·0, the measured areas having a diameter of 48 µm. The statistical computation involves standard deviations, derived from 'root mean squares' (rms) of the density variations, and hence technical descriptions refer to *rms granularity*.

Fast films generally have a coarser grain structure than slow films and are therefore unable to record details as fine as can be recorded with a slower film. For scientific and technical purposes, one usually makes use of a fine-grain film whenever possible. In difficult circumstances, including fluorescence photomicrography, in which fast films are essential to capture weak, fleeting images, some graininess is usually inevitable and quite acceptable. In any case, the resolution of the film (see below) is seldom, if ever, limiting to the resolution achieved by the whole imaging (microscope) system.

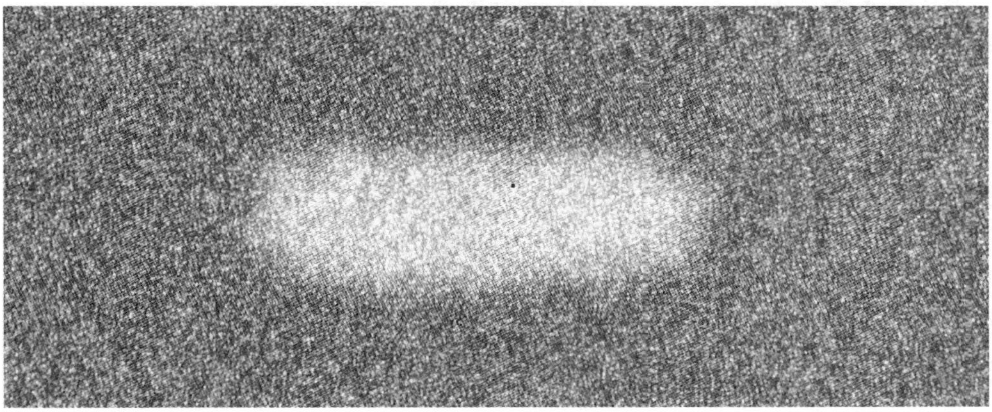

Fig 18.4. Print enlarged (as a photomicrograph) from part of a negative, to show graininess. This is a 250× enlargement from the negative from which Fig 2.10 was printed. It shows the '–' in '160/–' on the objective. Note the edge effect, the faint dark halo surrounding the dark object (cf Fig 18.5). Field size 0·5 mm × 0·2 mm (500 µm × 200 µm).

Resolution

The resolving power of a photographic emulsion is limited by the size of the clumped grains of silver (see Fig 18.4). The resolving power of the film is usually expressed as the numbers of line pairs per millimetre (LP/mm) of paired white and black bars that can be separately identified in the processed emulsion (Fig 6.6). Larger line-pair numbers indicate better resolving power. On the other hand, microscopists are used to a different appraisal of resolving power (minimum resolved distance, see Chapter 6), in which smaller numbers are sought after, representing finer and finer distances *in the specimen* that can be separated as detail in the image.

Film resolving power is often quoted for high- and low-contrast images, with CI 1000:1 and 1·6:1, the latter figure probably being more realistic for microscope work. Among the commoner Kodak films, the resolving power varies from 320/25 LP/mm (ie 320 LP/mm for 1000:1 contrast images, 25 LP/mm for 1·6:1 contrast images) for *Technical Pan*, to 100/32 line pairs/mm for *Tri-X*. *T-Max* 100 has a resolving power of 200/63 LP/mm, together with very low rms granularity, and is representative of the newer general-purpose films that have been introduced this decade, not only by Kodak.

Because microscope images are always the result of enlargement by the objective and then by the eyepiece or projective, the detail that needs to be captured in the film plane is typically much less demanding of the emulsion than might at first sight seem to be required. For example, if, using a 100× objective of high quality, the microscope resolves 0·2 μm (close to the best that it can possibly achieve), and there is a magnification of 330× on the film plane (a typical figure with a 35 mm camera), the resolution required of the film is 330 × 0·2 μm = 0·07 mm, which equates to less than 15 LP/mm. This is well within the capacity of a 400/27° ISO film, even with low-contrast images.

Sharpness, acutance

Sharpness refers to the ability of the photographic system to reproduce abrupt density changes in the image. *Acutance* (Fig 18.5) is a related, mathematically defined, expression relating to the curve gradients and the densities involved at the boundary of an opaque object.

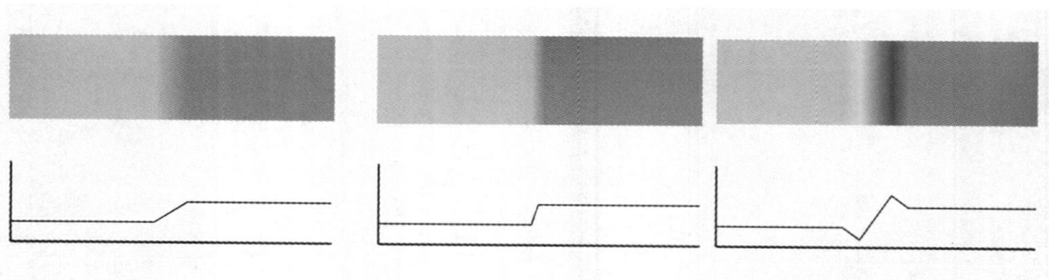

Fig 18.5. Diagram illustrating acutance. The upper row shows the density increase at the edge of a darker image. The bottom row shows (diagrammatically) corresponding density changes. Left, low acutance (gradual transition from light to dark). Middle, high acutance (rapid transition from light to dark). Right, edge effect (as in Fig 18.4), in which the edge is first over-light, then over-dark, before reaching the definitive level of dark grey.

Definition

Photographic *definition* is a descriptive phrase, frequently encountered, that in a sense tries to encapsulate the loose meanings of graininess/detail/sharpness combined into one set of words. It is probably no more successful than any of the other single quantitative measures of granularity/resolution/acutance/modulation-transfer-function. Therefore, subjective appraisal still persists, even in the eyes of acknowledged and experienced practitioners of the science of photography, as much as it does in the entirely artistic pursuits.

Speed and sharpness

In general, the faster the film, the coarser is the grain, and the lower is the contrast; the slower the film, the less is the grain, and the higher is the contrast. In faster films, the developed silver grains are larger, and more variable in size. Both overexposure and overdevelopment tend to increase grain size.

Chromogenic film

Chromogenic film is film in which the final image is formed by a deposit of organic dyes. The dye replaces the silver, which is removed by a bleach-fixer during processing, leaving the dye behind to form the image on the film. Chromogenic B&W film is similar to colour negative film, but with only a single dye layer. The current chromogenic B&W films are Ilford's *XP2* and Kodak's *T400CN* films, both rated at 400/27° ISO. These films can be developed in the standard C-41 colour negative process and all compatible processes, but for optimal results *XP2* should be processed in Ilford's *XP2* developer. Negatives processed in C-41 or equivalent have a brownish colour. The choice of paper contrast for printing may be different than with other monochrome films. Chromogenic film can also be processed as a conventional B&W film, or reversal-processed to a transparency (with the colour E-6 process; reduce the speed rating to ISO 100–200 or push-process). Because of their ease of commercial processing, potential high speed, wide latitude, capability to cope with a high-contrast subject, and comparatively fine grain, these chromogenic films may be preferred to conventional B&W films for difficult circumstances such as fluorescence photomicrography.

Special-purpose B&W films

Infrared film

Special films are available with extended sensitivity in the far red and infrared. Silver halide emulsions are basically sensitive only to the high-energy (blue) end of the spectrum: the construction of red-sensitive (panchromatic) films require the addition of an organic dye that absorbs red light and transfers the photon energy to the silver halide. Photography using infrared film is described in Chapter 12. Film with extended red sensitivity is required for good reproduction of any red stain.

Polaroid film

Polaroid film is characterised by the possibility of very quick ('instant') processing. More or less immediate processing and the fact that specialised processing facilities are not required, neither personnel nor darkrooms, transforms comparatively expensive photographic material into economical photography. Polaroid is the material of choice in situations where quick results are essential, of prints up to 4 inches × 5 inches (9 cm × 12 cm) in size or of 35 mm transparencies, B&W or colour. Polaroid negative–positive film in the 4×5 inch format is large enough to be scanned into a computer using a relatively inexpensive scanner. The studio, fashion or architectural photographer will use Polaroid film to get rapid appraisal of composition, lighting or exposure, or the functioning of complicated equipment such as multiple flashes, prior to the use of more conventional film for later processing. There is a possible inference here that Polaroid films might be useful only because of their rapid processing, and that they are of lesser photographic quality than the conventional negative films; this is not true of the larger-format Polaroid films.

Choosing B&W films

The usual aim of photomicrography is to reproduce, in the final print, the full tonal range that is present in the microscope image, from very light to very dark. Therefore, a fine-grain high-resolution emulsion is the normal choice. Films of medium contrast such as Ilford *Pan F* or Kodak *Panatomic X* are therefore highly recommended. The Kodak *T-max* and Ilford *Delta* ranges of films, although rather more expensive, very definitely have finer grains than earlier films of equivalent ISO rating. However, since most material used for biological photomicrography tends to have a lesser contrast range than a typical photographic scene, some slight increase in development time, say 20%, is usually recommended to increase the negative contrast. For some specialised purposes, such as recording chromosomes, film with inherently high contrast (eg Kodak *Technical Pan*) processed in a medium contrast developer is preferred, but high contrast is not usually necessary nor desirable for photomicrography. On the contrary, techniques of microscopy that produce images of high contrast, such as darkground and polarisation, tend to require film and processing procedures that give lower contrast.

B&W films of very high contrast, such as lithographic film, have the advantage of extremely high resolution and of ultrafine grain-size. However, because of their excessive contrast, such films are seldom useable for normal histological photomicrography. If very soft-working developers can be employed, then the high-contrast, ultrafine-grain films may well be favoured. Kodak *Technical Pan* is one such film, in which the contrast range can be regulated by the choice of different combinations of developer, developer dilution, and development times.

Co-authors Fred and Ron have agreed to differ on the importance traditionally placed on fine grain film for B&W photomicrography. Ron suggests that fine grain is always to be preferred; Fred suggests that the emphasis on fine grain is overdone.

Having said all this, the point must be made that for general use, any general-purpose medium-speed film is perfectly satisfactory for the majority of photomicrographic work. The only significant exceptions are in fluorescence photomicrography, and in photography of moving specimens, for which a faster film (say 400/27° ISO) is commonly necessary. Choosing the film is less important than knowing how to obtain the desired results with it. Anyone new to B&W photography is advised to choose any general-purpose medium-speed (say 50/18° to 125/22° ISO) B&W film, taking into account cost and availability. It is then important to stick with the same film long enough to build up experience of the results obtainable under various conditions of exposure, development and printing.

Colour films and paper

Colour film

Colour film is more complicated than B&W film, as one might imagine. The essential difference is that there are three emulsion layers, each designed to record light of a different colour (see Fig 18.6). It must be explained first that a simple emulsion is sensitive only to blue light; by addition of sensitiser chemicals, it can be made sensitive to longer wavelengths too. In colour film, the outermost layer of emulsion is sensitive to blue light only. The next layer is a yellow filter, to remove any blue light not absorbed by the emulsion; the yellow dye is removed during development. The next layer is sensitive to blue and green, but since blue light has been removed, records only green. The bottom layer of emulsion is sensitive to blue and red, but records only red. During development, the latent image of each layer is developed and converted from a silver image to a coloured image. The surface coating commonly incorporates a filter to block ultraviolet light. Colour negative film normally incorporates a yellowish or brownish filter known as the 'mask'.

Each emulsion layer of colour film is subject to reciprocity failure, their sensitivity decreasing in long exposures. Unequal reciprocity failures in the three layers produces a progressive change in colour balance with lengthening exposures.

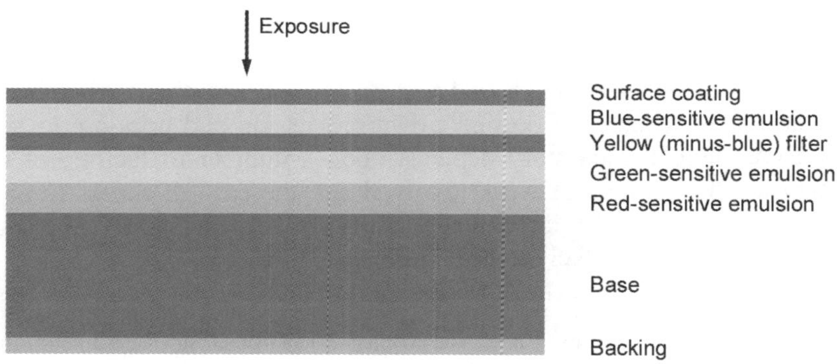

Fig 18.6. Magnified cross-section of a typical colour film.

Reversal processing

As an alternative to printing from a colour negative onto colour paper, the image may be reversed directly on the film, by a process usually involving exposure to light followed by a second development. This gives a coloured, positive image on a transparent base, resulting in a colour transparency or diapositive. There are therefore two basic kinds of colour film on the market: negative ('print') and positive ('slide', reversal) films. The processing methods are different. At the present time, colour negative film is processed by a method best known by its Kodak designation C-41. Colour positive films are usually processed by the E-6 process (again, this is the Kodak designation). However, *Kodachrome* requires a special process, currently K-14.

Choosing colour film

Colour negative film is relatively uncritical: any general-purpose or high-contrast colour negative film should be satisfactory. Colour reversal (transparency) film is another story: the film needs to be chosen with care, particularly for brightfield microscopy of sections stained with Eosin, and for fluorescence microscopy. For brightfield work, one of the films giving more saturated colours is best: we prefer Fuji *Velvia*. Fluorescence microscopy usually requires a relatively fast film resistant to reciprocity failure.

Colour paper

Corresponding to the two basic types of colour film (negative and positive), there are two basic types of photographic paper. Negative paper is similar to colour negative film, but on an opaque white base, and is processed using the same chemicals. Positive or reversal paper is also similar to reversal film, but on an opaque white base, and requires special processing. At the present time, colour papers of different contrasts are not available.

Processing and printing

Detailed descriptions of the techniques of photographic processing (developing and printing) are to be found in many photographic textbooks. To duplicate these descriptions here would require more space than we have available. We therefore discuss only those points that, in our experience, are of particular interest to the microscopist.

To do it oneself, or send the work out?

The decision as to whether to do one's own processing and printing, or to send the work out to a commercial laboratory depends upon a number of factors, of which the most important are the volume of work involved and the ease of access to commercial laboratories. In a major city of a developed country, eg here in Sydney, the situation (at least for the 35 mm format) is likely to be as follows:

Film:

- Conventional B&W negatives: these are so easy to process, and require such minimal equipment, that it is almost certainly best to do it oneself.
- Colour negatives and monochrome chromogenic film: the automated C-41 process is widely available in mini-labs, and so cheap, that there is unlikely to be any point in doing it oneself.
- Colour transparencies, E-6 process: a small laboratory is unlikely to be able to compete with commercial processing using automated equipment.
- Colour transparencies, *Kodachrome*: the film must be sent to Kodak or one of a very few commercial laboratories.

Prints:

- B&W prints: these, in modest sizes, are not difficult to make oneself, and one can print each negative exactly to one's own requirements. However, some expensive equipment (particularly the enlarger) and dedicated darkroom space are required. It is becoming more and more difficult to have B&W printing done commercially. Few mini-labs can produce true B&W prints from chromogenic film.

- Colour prints from negatives, either small or standard enlargements, are usually adequately handled by the local mini-lab. The laboratory may need some polite guidance about the required print (darker, lighter, appropriate background colour).
- Colour prints from transparencies: direct printing from transparencies is only worthwhile if the highest quality print is required, in which case a professional laboratory will do the best job (at a price). For general use, particularly for theses, it is very much more economical to re-photograph the transparencies onto colour negative film and have prints made from those (assuming that the original material is not available to re-photograph on colour negative film).
- In all cases, the use of digital printing (see Chapter 17) should be considered.

Processing B&W films

With the advent of efficient and cheap colour-processing laboratories for 'amateur' photography, it has become difficult to have B&W film processed commercially. Most microscope users have some laboratory training, and, in the absence of a specialist photographic processing laboratory, should be encouraged to do their own processing.

Be aware of the dangers to yourself, and to the environment, of chemicals that are in the darkroom. Some individuals are susceptible to dermatitis from developers, and should keep their fingers out of the solutions (wearing gloves, and using print tongs). The fixative fumes will cause corrosion of metals (eg enlargers) in the darkroom, and the fumes are blamed for the asthmatic condition of many an old darkroom campaigner. Silver recovery from the fixative before disposal is now demanded by most urban water authorities. The water flow and wastage from washing processes is another matter that should be kept under scrutiny. Good ventilation is essential, and needs careful planning before some odd unused corner of a building is converted into a darkroom.

Development

Development essentially involves the selective reduction of exposed silver halides to metallic silver, which is deposited as silver grains. The process of development increases the effective sensitivity of the film by an enormous factor, estimated to be one thousand million times. As a chemical process, development progress is dependent on time and temperature; charts and tables that give the appropriate time to achieve the required gamma at a given temperature of developer are available from film and chemical manufacturers.

Co-author Ron's preference for a routine developer is Ilford *ID11* (identical in composition with Kodak *D76*), used without dilution, with a somewhat longer than recommended development time, and with replenisher added as required. Co-author Fred's favourite developer is Ilford's *Microphen*, in 1 + 3 dilution, with suitably increased development time, discarded after developing one film. In employing our preferred (and different!) developers, we do not imply that all other developers are inferior. Indeed, our different choices serve to illustrate the versatility of the photographic process. Ilford *ID11* and *Microphen* are quite conventional choices, and there are many equivalents.

Developer replenishment. One-shot developers (use once and discard) are preferable. Otherwise, some economy can be effected by using a replenisher (eg Ilford *ID11R*). The replenisher contains concentrates that replace chemicals depleted from the developer. The small volume of developer lost during processing is replaced from time to time with sufficient replenisher solution to maintain a constant volume of developer stock.

Special processing

It is best to choose a film, and a development procedure for that film, that will give the appropriate compromise between speed, grain and contrast. Occasionally, a deliberate variation in development procedure may be required, eg for correction of exposure error.

The contrast of a photograph can be controlled to some extent by choosing the various parameters of the development process: the chemicals of the developer, its dilution, its temperature, and the development time.

Push processing is a procedure in which the film is underexposed and developed for a longer time to compensate for this underexposure (Table 18.2). This strengthens what would otherwise have been a very pale negative, and allows the speed rating of a film to be increased. Push-processed B&W films give negatives that have increased contrast and a larger grain size than film processed normally. Some detail will be lost, due both to overall reduction of image quality (increased graininess) and to underexposure in the darker regions of the microscope image. Although pushing does produce a more acceptable negative than would be obtained by underexposure alone, the film does not really undergo a speed increase. Since the ISO speed rating of negative film is based on the minimal exposure required to produce an acceptable photograph, underexposing the film will excessively underexpose the areas corresponding to darker areas of the optical image. Overdeveloping the negative will darken the areas that were adequately exposed, but will not develop the excessively underexposed areas and it is for this reason that negative film cannot have its true sensitivity increased, and also why contrast is increased. As a rule of thumb, the required increase in development time for push-processing is an increase of 50% for the first stop, and an additional 25% of the basic development time for each additional stop.

Push processing enables an EI to be achieved that is much higher than the ISO rating of available films, allowing acceptable photographs to be taken under conditions that would otherwise be impossible. Instructions are provided by Kodak for pushing their *T-max P3200* film to a speed rating (EI) of 25 000/45°. However, a normally processed film of a high ISO rating is always better than a slower film push-processed to the higher rating. There is little point in choosing and then pushing an ISO 100/21° film to 400/27° when there exist several films of the higher rating.

Table 18.2. Push-processing development times

Push-processing development times for B&W film normally rated at 100/21° ISO and requiring 8 minutes development. A similar table is easily constructed, in proportion, for other speeds and development times.

Speed rating set on camera ISO	Development	Development time (minutes)	
100/21°	Standard	8	(standard)
200/24°	Pushed 1 stop	12	(1·5×)
400/27°	Pushed 2 stops	14	(1·75×)
800/30°	Pushed 3 stops	16	(2·0×)
1600/33°	Pushed 4 stops	18	(2·25×)

Pull processing implies a deliberate underdevelopment of film, possibly to reduce contrast or as an attempted correction for unintentional overexposure.

Film intensification is a process to increase the density of the image. The silver of the negative is either augmented or replaced by another metal to give increased density. Where there is no silver image, intensifiers cannot produce one!

Reducing removes some of the silver. This process can be applied either uniformly over the emulsion (increasing contrast), or more vigorously over darker parts of the negative (promoting highlight detail).

Fixation

The solution that stabilises the exposed emulsion against further exposure to light is called a fixative. Sodium thiosulphate solution ($Na_2S_2O_3$, the incorrect name 'hypo' still persists) is the traditional solvent of unexposed silver halides. Ammonium thiosulphate is a more modern and fast-acting fixative. Prior to transferring the film into fixative, the film should be rinsed vigorously in water (avoiding temperature changes throughout these darkroom processes), and then the action of the developing agent checked by changing the conditions from alkaline to acid. For this purpose, a stop bath of 2% (by volume) acetic acid solution is often used, or the fixative acidified.

Fixative baths inevitably become contaminated with developer products and silver thiosulphate compounds, all of which will lead to discoloration of the film or paper with prolonged exposure to light. It is a safer procedure to employ a two-bath fixation process, in which the second bath is a fresh fixative solution. As the first bath becomes sluggish and more soapy to the feel (from the developer), it is replaced by the second bath, and fresh fixative is made up to take its place. By this means, the final fixation should always be in a fresh fixative solution.

The fixative when depleted is comparatively rich in silver salts. In large processing laboratories, it is an economical proposition to arrange for silver recovery; in smaller laboratories, some thought should be given to protection of the waterways into which the waste silver will find its way. Arrange for proper waste disposal. As mentioned above, recovery of silver from the fixative before disposal is now demanded by most urban water authorities.

Silver iodide is present in fast films; when carried over to the fixative, the iodide inhibits the solution of silver bromide. For this reason it is not wise to use the same fixative bath for processing both film and paper. Avoid overlong fixation times, for fixative byproducts then become more difficult to remove with subsequent washing.

Washing

Washing is the removal of all chemicals from the emulsion and its support that will impair the long-term stability of the photograph. The usual washing times for film are of the order of 20 minutes, depending on the temperature and the efficiency of the circulation of the water in the washing device. A final rinse in a photographic-quality wetting agent is a wise precaution against drying marks on the film. Any sediment that has found its way onto the film must be completely removed before drying; once the film has dried, the sediment is almost impossible to displace, ruining good negatives. If sediment problems persist, it may become necessary to install a particle filter in the water supply.

Drying

Drying of films is best carried out in a drying cabinet, in which the film can be gently dried by circulating warm, dry, dust-free air. A commercial drying cabinet is fine, but expensive. Failing that, the film can be hung to dry in any region where the air is dust-free and not too humid. A weight clipped to the bottom of a drying film will keep it straight and discourage it from rubbing against other films.

B&W printing

The enlarger

If B&W photomicrography is to be attempted, most users will opt for 35 mm negative film. It follows that enlargement is involved to get working size prints, often described as *postcard size*, approximating to 100 mm × 150 mm. In those laboratories where economies are being enforced, there is a great temptation to economise most in the selection of darkroom equipment. However, the optical quality of the enlarging lens should not be such as to degrade the results of expensive cameras and microscopes. Even in the most expensive of enlargers there can be deficiencies of field curvature that demand closing down of the lens aperture. Generally, an enlarging lens has best resolving power when closed down 1 to 2 stops, but this setting seldom gives edge-to-edge sharpness for critical printing.

An autofocusing enlarger is a very considerable help whenever publication of plates with more than one photograph is to be undertaken, enabling rapid setting of the projected image to exactly the right size. In universities, there may be a need for finished prints that are to be bound into a thesis. A substantial and heavy printing easel is required, with masking arms that can be set to give wide borders to the prints as specified by the examining body.

Indicator stop baths

To prolong the life of the first fixative, it is helpful to remove surplus developer by taking the prints through an acidified stop bath. There are several indicator stop baths sold commercially as liquid concentrates. These, after the recommended dilution, show a yellow colour when the stop bath is fresh, changing to a purple colour when the stop bath is exhausted. Although the yellow/purple colours are masked in the yellow light of a darkroom, a change from light to dark of the stop bath is readily perceived.

B&W photographic papers

Contrast: graded papers

Historically, there have been six contrast grades, from the softest (No. 0) to the hardest or most contrasty (No. 5). A negative ideally would be produced that printed on a 'normal' (No. 2) paper, but a soft negative or image could be corrected by printing on a contrasty paper, and a hard image could be corrected by printing on a soft paper. This gives to the darkroom operator very considerable control over the contrast of the finished print, modifying deficiencies of the original specimen or mistakes of exposure in the camera. The use of the word *normal* for No. 2 grade paper should not be taken to mean that other grades are *abnormal*. When matched to the right negative, all grades produce high-quality prints, and are capable of producing the full range of intensities from black to white.

Contrast: variable grade papers

It is an expensive investment to build up stocks of six different grades of paper. Helpfully, graded papers have been augmented by papers with a mixture of emulsions giving high contrast (sensitive to blue light) and low contrast (sensitive to green light). If the enlarger light is filtered yellow (ie blue light is removed), the blue-sensitive emulsion is not activated, and low contrast results from the green-sensitive emulsion. Conversely, light from a magenta filter (ie a filter blocking green) activates only the blue-sensitive emulsion and leads to high contrast. In white light the emulsions produce 'normal' contrast. Up to 12 filters, from yellow (No. 0) to magenta (No. 5) and the half grades in between make up a set for one brand of enlarging papers, although five or six is often sufficient for a darkroom. The choice of the best filter for a particular negative may still be problematic, but only one box of paper suffices to give a very full contrast range.

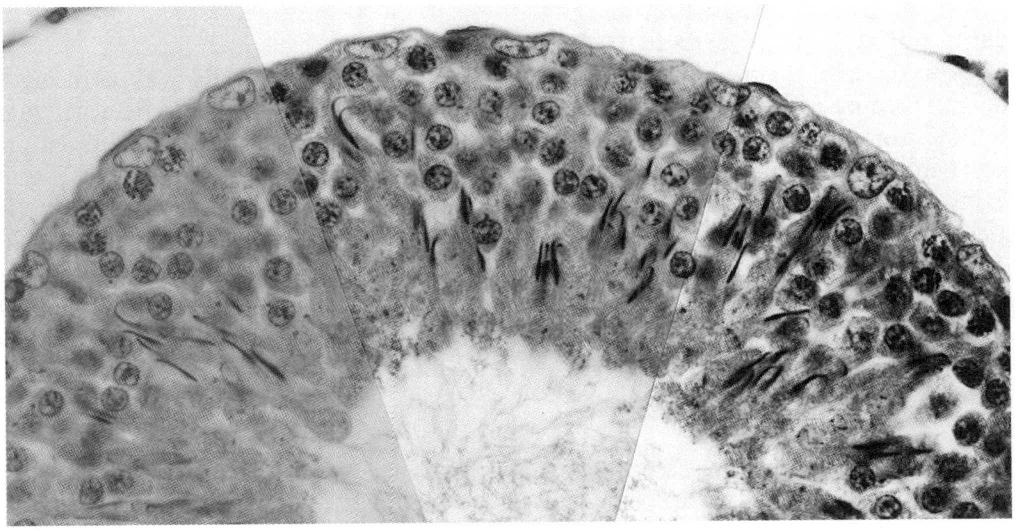

Fig 18.7. Control of contrast through printing. From left to right, *soft*, *normal* and *hard* prints of a section through mammalian testis, using paper of grades 1, 3 and 5, respectively. Field size 120 μm × 250 μm. The most contrasty print (right) might usually be chosen, but note the absence of detail in sperm tails in the lower centre of the field. Because of the detail that is present both in the darkest regions of the print (the nuclei) and in the lightest regions of the print (sperm tails), this is a very difficult negative to print satisfactorily. It is a good example of an instance in which some other technique, eg darkground or DIC, might be considered for better overall rendition.

Choosing the right contrast grade

The matching of paper contrast to negative is a skill requiring practice and a discerning eye. The most common tendency of photographers untrained in scientific photography is to produce an enlargement with too much contrast. Although the pictorial photographer would reject as far too unimaginative the advice that follows, for scientific work, especially photomicrography, the perfect print contains no blacks and no whites, meaning that wherever there is detail or information in the negative, that detail will be lost if it the area is printed black (or, alternatively, white). The lightest tone of a photomicrograph, ie the clear background of a brightfield picture, or the halo of a phase-contrast image, should appear just off-white, a very light grey. This off-white is most easily judged against the fully white, masked edge of the print. A darkground image will have true blacks, but only in the background, not where there is dark detail showing in the microscope image. The perfect print of a well-stained brightfield image will range from just off-white to something short of completely black.

If photographic prints are to be re-photographed, as for a composite plate of micrographs, remember that more contrast will be introduced by the photographic copying process; to allow for this, prints intended for copying should have more grey in the light tones, and less black in the dark tones, ie be softer than the 'ideal print'. Prints meant to be viewed from some distance, eg posters and exhibition prints, may look better if the contrast is somewhat greater than normal.

Resin-coated paper versus fibre-base paper

Most modern darkroom papers are plastic- or resin-coated (RC) as a means of reducing wetting of the paper, thereby enabling every processing stage to be accelerated. The time from enlarger easel to developed, fixed, washed, light-stabilised and dried print takes 4 minutes rather than 2 hours. A further considerable advantage is that drying and glazing (getting a gloss finish to the print) does not need special equipment, and the RC papers are resistant to curling. A disadvantage is that RC papers are less easy to retouch.

Premium-quality photographic paper as sold by various manufacturers is still on fibre-base paper. Once the paper fibres have been wetted, especially after fixation, the complete extraction of chemicals that have been adsorbed onto the paper fibres is prolonged, possibly lasting several hours with the thicker papers.

Paper surface

Photographic papers are sold in a variety of surface textures, gloss, semi-matt, matt, silk, velvet stipple, etc. The deepest black that is obtainable on a print is largely affected by the surface characteristics of the paper, but is also affected by the emulsion itself. A rough or matt surface does not give the same maximum reflection density as a glossy surface, and therefore restricts the total contrast range of the print, a fact well known in the superior quality of the illustrations in glossy magazines. It would seem from the above that glossy prints ought to be specified for all scientific photography, especially that which is to be submitted for publication. This advice should be accepted with caution.

If glossy paper is selected, and the finished print dried rather than glazed, the deepest blacks are not as good as with a glossy finish, but the contrast range more closely approaches the quality that publication processes can achieve. The prints themselves are much more easy to produce, the surface can be written on (for inclusion in the laboratory notebook), and the surface will more readily accept *Letraset* or similar labelling.

Photographs with considerable black content (eg fluorescence), if glazed, present very real problems in the copying process, for the reflections of the camera and its lens are photographed together with the original print. Glossy photographs also need very careful display lighting if they are to used for exhibition. Given all these difficulties and handicaps, photographers may deliberately choose gloss finishes as a mark of the outstanding quality of their work.

Further reading

Further information on the photographic process and materials thereof is to be found in *Basic photographic materials and processes* (Stroebel *et al*, 1989), and even more detail in the same authors' (1986) *Photographic materials and processes*. See also Vetter (1992). For practical darkroom technology, see Anchell (1994, 1997). Covington (1991) and Mobberley (1999) are of interest in relation to the photography of dim light.

19
Drawing

The oldest method of image capture is drawing, and the method is still relevant to modern data recording. The merits of drawing, as distinct from photography, are:

- A solid object too thick to be all in focus at once can be drawn, the focus of the microscope being changed during the procedure as necessary.
- An object too large to be accommodated in one field can be drawn, the microscope field being moved as necessary.
- Important but low-contrast taxonomic features (eg fish scales) can be emphasised.
- Incomplete, fractured or imperfect specimens can be more readily reconstructed in a drawing.
- The process of drawing, if not too finicky or mechanical, focuses one's mind wonderfully on the shape (form) of the structures in the subject.
- A drawing, executed with proper materials, is a permanent record suitable for archival purposes.

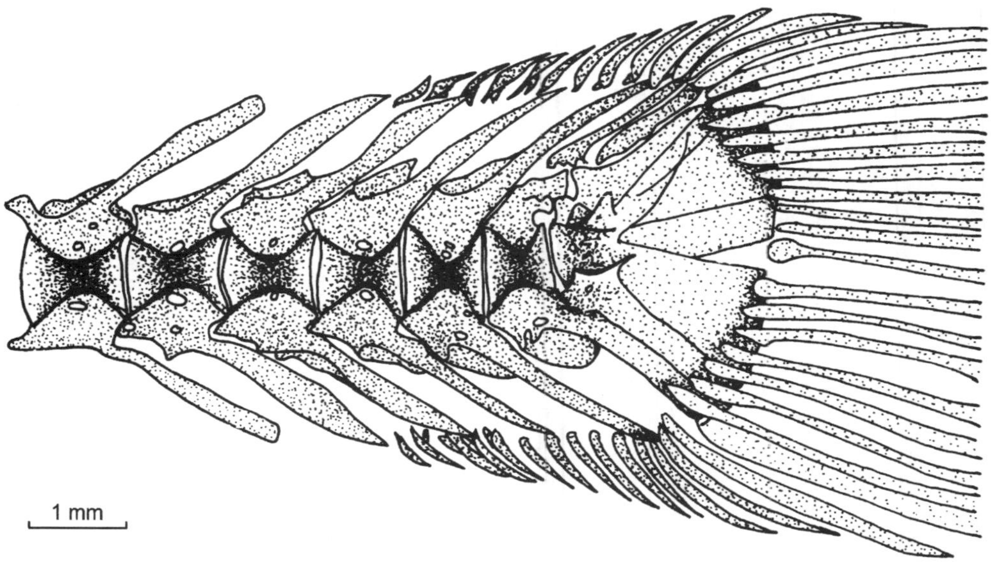

Fig 19.1. Drawing made with the apparatus shown in Fig 19.2, reproduced natural size. Caudal fin (skeleton and terminal vertebrae) of fish, *Atherina boyeri*. Specimen cleared and stained with Alizarin. By convention, the head faces to the left. The specimen is about 4 mm thick. The original drawing was made in black ink on tracing paper. Shading was achieved by stippling. For reproduction here, the drawing was scanned as a transparency. The scale bar has been re-drawn using *Photoshop* software (see Chapter 17). Preparation and drawing by Margaret Shepherd, Macquarie University, reproduced with permission.

The process of drawing by looking into a microscope and drawing what one sees, with the unaided eye requires some training, much practice, and possibly a special talent. The process is greatly facilitated by a drawing apparatus or a projection system. Drawings can also be produced by tracing from a photograph or computer monitor, or by computer conversion from a digital image (see Chapter 17). In all cases, the reproduction scale is established using a stage micrometer.

Figures 19.1 and 19.3 show examples of drawings from a fish specimen that is large, thick, and of low contrast, and therefore ideal for this kind of approach.

Drawing apparatus

A drawing apparatus (Fig 19.2), formerly known as a *camera lucida*, is an optical device that enables the microscopist to observe simultaneously the microscope image and (by way of a beamsplitter) an image of the pencil on the drawing paper. The image can thereby be traced onto the paper. A range of attachments was discussed by Oldfield (1994). The best are interposed between the objective and the eyepiece, so that binocular vision is maintained. The two superimposed images must be matched in intensity, but during the process of drawing each individual image can be subdued or emphasised by dimming of the microscope or desktop illuminators.

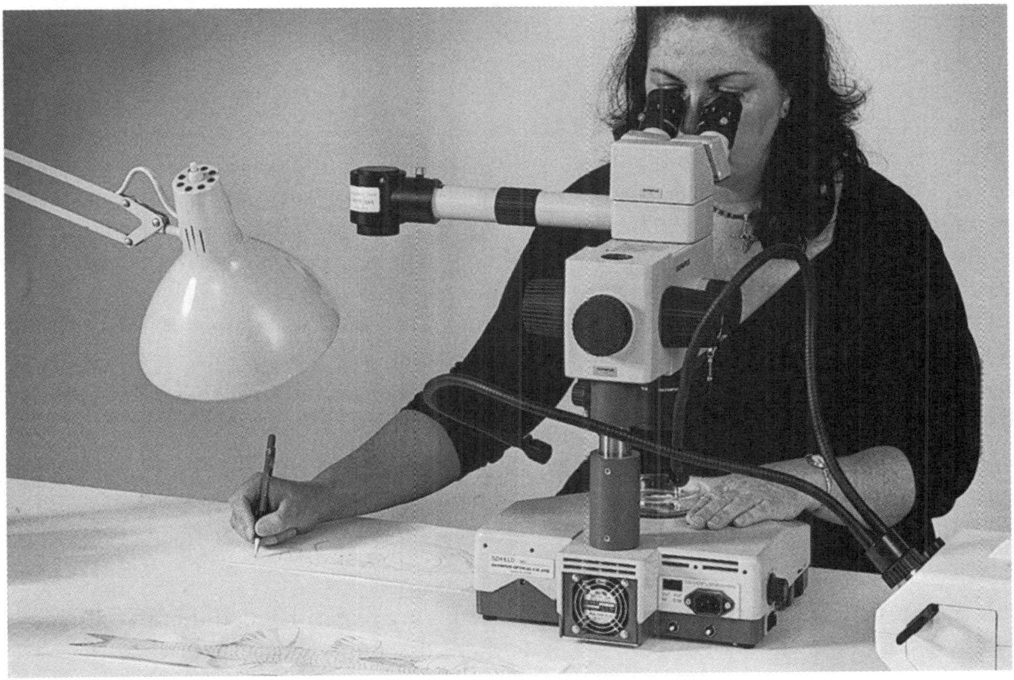

Fig 19.2. A modern Olympus drawing attachment (camera lucida) for a stereomicroscope, inserted below the binocular head. An image of the drawing, as seen in a mirror at the end of the lateral arm, is superimposed on the microscope image. To see superimposed images of paper and specimen, it is important to match the brightness of the respective illuminations.

Projection

An image can be projected onto a sheet of paper attached to a vertical screen or wall. This normally requires a projection prism or mirror attached over the eyepiece to reflect the image sideways. Unfortunately, the process of reflection alters the image, reversing it to form a 'mirror image'. Also, one's hand and pencil obscure the projected light beam.

Drawing from photographs

A photographic print can of course be traced. Alternatively, a soft light print can be made, and the outlines drawn onto the print with a waterproof ink. Finally, the silver image is removed with a solution of iodine in potassium iodide.

Equipment for drawing

An important consideration is the archival quality of the materials (paper, pencil, inks, etc) used. Paper need not be pure white; a wide range of tones (light to dark) and hues (colour) is available. A light cream or other tint is less strain to the eye, and may give a more artistic result. Artists' materials are commonly sold in different grades of quality, usually designated as being for artists, students, and children, respectively. For professional use (including that of students) we recommend only the artists' quality.

Paper

Paper is classified mainly according to the smoothness or roughness of its surface, its thickness (quantified as grams per square metre, gsm), its colour, and its archival qualities.

The smoother the paper, the finer the detail that can be drawn; the rougher, the greater the range of density obtainable with a pencil. Pen-and-ink requires a smooth surface, otherwise the pen does not travel smoothly over the paper. The process of smoothing paper during manufacture by passing between polished steel rollers is called calendering. *Hot pressed* (HP) paper is relatively smooth, *cold pressed* (usually called NOT, ie not hot pressed!) is rough; *supercalendered* paper is very smooth.

Ordinary paper has a thickness corresponding to about 80 gsm, medium thickness artists' papers weigh about 200 gsm, and thick paper 300–350 gsm. For drawing, the lighter papers are adequate, and about 150–200 gsm is generally ideal. Thicker paper is better for wet techniques such as watercolour and gouache.

Acid-free rag paper is essential for archival purposes. Paper which is not acid-free may cause the image to fade. Cheap paper such as newsprint (and paper commonly used for publications these days) is made from wood fibres rather than cotton or linen (flax) fibres, and yellows with age.

Bank paper, now more commonly called photocopying paper, is good quality thin paper, about 80 gsm, quite suitable for both pencil and ink. Its archival quality is doubtful.

Cartridge paper is a thicker, tough paper, originally used to hold gunpowder. It is relatively inexpensive, takes pencil well, but may be a little too rough for pen-and-ink.

Bristol board is cardboard with a very smooth, very white surface that accepts extremely fine detail and is ideal for pen-and-ink or detailed pencil studies.

Water-colour paper is high-quality, thick paper, suitable for use with a brush. There are numerous varieties, differing in the surface (rough or comparatively smooth), archival quality and colour. Its surface is typically too rough for use with a pen.

Tracing paper is thin, translucent and withal quite tough. As its name implies, its prime application is for tracing, eg from a photograph or from a monitor screen, but it can be used for any type of drawing. This paper has a grey, smooth matt surface that happily accepts both pencil and ink. It is widely used.

Alternatives to paper

Acetate sheet is a thin, tough, transparent plastic that will accept ink, and is commonly used for overhead projection. It cannot be used with ordinary pencils.

Digitising tablets consist of a flat board and a stylus, both connected to a computer. The tablet has embedded sensors which detect the coordinates of the stylus, and transmit this information to the computer. Digitising tablets can be used for tracing or for locating points, either on a photograph (placed on the tablet) or a microscope image (using a drawing device). They replace the mouse of a computer. Using a digitising tablet and a computer, drawings can be made, and the full power of graphics software is available for shading, colouring, adding labels, etc.

Pencils

Pencils consist of a stick of pigment in a holder of wood or metal. The pigment is mixed with a binding material to keep it together. The common pigment is graphite (called 'lead' for historical reasons, the predecessors of pencils being rods of lead or silver). Pencils come in different degrees of hardness (Table 19.1). The harder the pencil, the finer (sharper) the point that can be obtained. The softer the pencil, the darker the line that is obtained. Hard pencils come in a range graded from 9H (the hardest) to H; medium-hardness pencils are F and HB; soft pencils are B to 8B (the softest), followed by EB and EE which are particularly soft and dark.

Conventional pencils are made with a surround of wood, that is cut away as required. There exist also mechanical or clutch pencils made of metal, in which the 'lead' is separate and is extruded from the body of the pencil as required. For the better class of such pencils, the full range of hardnesses is available.

Table 19.1. Pencil types

Type	Characteristics
Black 'lead'	Contains graphite. The common pencil. Available in a range of hardnesses. Lightfast
Coloured	Medium hardness. Lightfastness depends on quality
Pastel	Very soft. Good colours. Artists' quality pastels usually lightfast. Requires spray fixation to prevent smudging
Charcoal	Very soft. Black or dark grey, lightfast. Requires spray fixation to prevent smudging

Sharpening, traditionally carried out with a penknife, is usually done with a manual or electric sharpener. Different sizes of cones in the sharpener accommodate pencils of different diameters. Special sharpeners are required for the leads of clutch pencils. Final sharpening to a fine point (for hard pencils) is best done with a piece of fine sandpaper, that is placed on the table and the pencil sharpened against it. Sandpaper blocks are sold for the purpose.

Eraser

Normal erasers are rubbery blocks that are used to abrade paper surfaces, to remove pencil marks. Harder and more abrasive erasers are used to remove ink marks. Kneadable erasers are gentler on the paper, and can be moulded to any desired shape, such as a point. Besides removing errors, the sharp edge or point of an eraser can be used to draw white or pale grey lines through areas that have been shaded. Kneadable erasers can be used to get a 'smudge' effect.

Pens and ink

Pen-and-ink, being very difficult to erase, is best done on top of a preliminary pencil sketch. The pen may be an old-fashioned conventional penholder and nib, still available with a wide variety of nibs from artists' supply houses. Special pens (eg *Rotring*) exist for graphic work, designed to give lines of uniform thickness, the range of nib widths being typically 0·1–1·0 mm. Fountain pens are generally not suitable because they tend to clog up if used with drawing inks. Ball-point and felt-point (fibre-nib) pens are not usually recommended for this purpose.

There are several types of ink available. Indian ink is black, permanent, and waterproof when dry, but cannot be used in a fountain pen. Fountain-pen inks may not be lightfast (blue-black is usually best), and are not suitable for archival purposes. Coloured inks are usually not lightfast, and are not suitable for archival purposes. Photocopies and laser printer printouts on archival-quality paper are of archival quality, because they use carbon particles to form the image. Ink-jet printers, at the time of writing (1999), use inks that are not permanent, and give an image life said to be about two years under good conditions.

Colour

Watercolour and gouache are very suitable for this kind of work. The difference between them is that watercolour is transparent, whereas gouache is opaque. Watercolour must be applied to a white paper, on which it gives (in the hands of an expert) an unrivalled luminous effect. Artists' grade watercolour is of archival quality. Gouache can be applied to paper of any tone or colour, and is particularly suitable for painting large flat areas of uniform colour. Many gouache colours, intended for graphic design, are not lightfast, and are not suitable for archival purposes. For purposes of microscopy, any required colour can be mixed from just three tubes of watercolour: phthalocyanine blue (= cyan), quinacridone magenta, and a pure yellow. For gouache, white is needed also. Watercolour and gouache are usually applied with brushes, which are available in a bewildering variety of hair, length, shape, and size. One or two good brushes are better than any number of poor ones. The test of a good round brush is that when wet the hairs meet in a point (the shop should provide water for this test). In European tradition, hairs should be quite springy; softer, less springy hairs are used in some brushes to save expense, and are the norm for Chinese-style painting. Watercolour can also be applied with a pen.

Coloured inks are convenient, can be applied with pen or brush, and can be mixed to obtain various colours. Drawing inks are waterproof when dry. Coloured inks may not be lightfast, and are not suitable for archival purpose. Coloured felt pens are not lightfast, and are suitable for ephemeral use only.

Coloured pencils are convenient, but even artists'-quality pencils tend to give rather poor results compared to other media.

Technique

The paper should be supported and held firmly; this is best achieved by taping to a board. If the paper is not completely flat, or if is to be used for wet techniques, it should be wet-mounted onto a drawing board, as follows. The paper is soaked in water, drained, smoothed out onto the board, taped down firmly with glued paper tape around the edges, and allowed to dry.

A *drawing* is made up primarily of lines, such as those made with a pencil or pen. A *painting* is made up primarily of areas, as are painted with a brush.

The thickness of lines is important. Often, thicker lines should be used for important boundaries; however, the outside edge of a rounded object should be underemphasised, to assist the illusion of roundness. Lines that vary in thickness along their length give character to the drawing, and may also suggest three-dimensional form. Curved lines are more easily drawn with the hand inside the curve than with it outside.

Areas can be filled, if desired, in various ways, to represent tone (light to dark), colour or texture. Shading is important in representing three-dimensional objects such as are seen in a stereomicroscope; it is important to imply a consistent direction of illumination (preferably from the top left or top right of the picture). Fill, using a drawing implement such as a pencil, is accomplished by stippling or hatching. Stippling is a pattern of dots, usually randomly arranged (see Fig 19.1). Hatching is a pattern of parallel lines more or less closely spaced according to the density required. Higher densities are achieved by cross-hatching, consisting of two or more layers of hatching with the strokes in different directions. In colour, hues can be combined by using dots or strokes of different colours. Given a painting implement such as a brush, areas can be filled with uniform or graduated greys or colours. The side of a pencil lead can be used as a tool for shading. Soft lead pencil, charcoal and pastel can be smudged out with the tip of a finger or a small piece of rolled-up paper. A thin, essentially uniform layer of paint is known as a wash. Indian ink can be diluted with water to obtain a range of greys.

The techniques of watercolour and gouache are too complex to describe here. There are numerous books on the subject, eg those of Appellof (1992), Parramón (1976) and Williams (1993).

It is usually convenient to make the drawing of a size of the order of 15 cm on a side. If the picture is to be reproduced at a smaller size, such as that of the illustrations in this book, detail will inevitably be lost in the process of reproduction. It is therefore helpful to bear in mind the intended demagnification. If, say, the final picture is to fit a column 65 mm wide (as in the half-column illustrations in this book), and the drawing is made 195 mm wide, ie 3 times bigger, one can reckon that nothing drawn smaller than $3 \times 0{\cdot}1$ mm $= 0{\cdot}3$ mm will reproduce clearly in the final image. Time and effort can be saved, therefore, by not drawing smaller detail!

Mechanical assistance

For drawing straight lines, of course one uses a ruler. Circles, or arcs of circles, can be drawn with compasses. For other curves, one can employ a kind of curved ruler, known as a French curve. These typically come in sets of three or four, each with a variety of complex curves that vary along their length. One draws the desired curve in sections, by finding portions of the French curve that match successive lengths of the desired curve. Alternatively, there are flexible rulers, that can be bent to the desired shape; sharp curves (small radii) are not obtainable with these. When using a computer, graphics programs usually offer a Bezier algorithm to draw smooth curves of any desired shape ('bezigon' in *Claris Office*; 'pen tool' in Adobe *Illustrator* and *Photoshop*).

Further reading

There are many books on the techniques of drawing, and of painting in watercolour, and more seem to be published every month. Some that may be helpful in the present context include those of Jastrzębski (1985) on scientific illustration; Borgman (1977), Camp (1981), Capon (1984) and Gill (1973) on drawing; Appellof (1992), Parramón (1976) and Williams (1993) on watercolour; and the well-known general work by Jaxtheimer (1962).

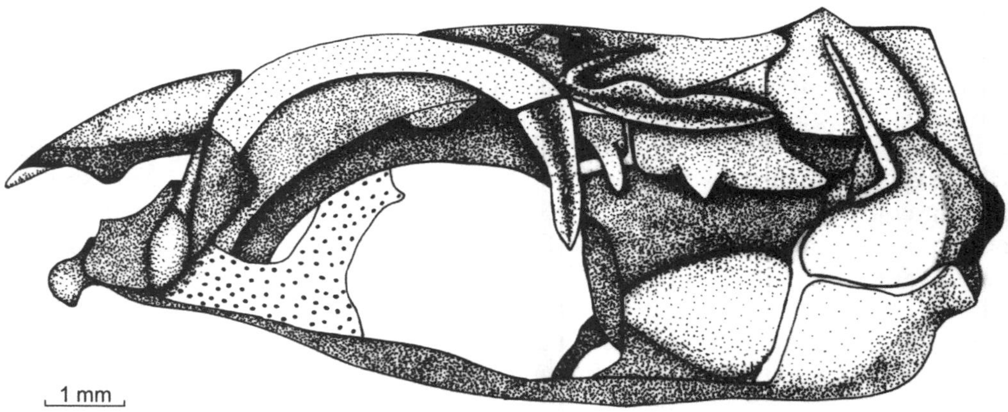

Fig 19.3. Drawing made with the apparatus shown in Fig 19.2. Brain case of fish, *Atherina boyeri*. By convention, the head faces to the left. The original drawing was made in black ink on tracing paper, and measured 70 mm × 160 mm. Shading was achieved by stippling. The scale bar has been re-drawn using *Photoshop* software (see Chapter 17). Preparation and drawing by Margaret Shepherd, Macquarie University, reproduced with permission.

Part VI

Appendices

There a glossary of digital terms on p 207; for other words, the Index should enable you to find the place in the text where the word is defined.

A1
Care and maintenance of equipment

Cleaning

Dust should be kept off the microscope as much as possible, and the optical surfaces cleaned from time to time. Dust accumulation can be minimised by keeping the microscope and the camera under a cover when not in use. *Caution: if the cover is plastic, it must not be allowed to touch a hot lamphouse, or the cover will melt.* It may be possible to keep the microscope in a box with doors, like a cupboard. Dust is a particular nuisance in fluorescence microscopes, because the dust (especially paper fibres) is often fluorescent.

The cause of blemishes in the optical image can best be diagnosed by checking the microscope systematically, commencing at the light source and ending at the eyepieces and camera. In the normal course of microscope use, when looking at the objective back focal plane, be observant of any indication of dust, fingerprints, oil, or asymmetries or irregularities of the image of the light source. Although the blemish may become apparent in this way, it is not always easy to locate precisely. One useful technique is to place a piece of tracing paper (say) on the stage: if the marks can still be seen, the offending plane is above the tracing paper; if the marks can not be seen, the problem is below the paper. Repeating this test with the paper held in different planes should help to confine the area in which the problem exists.

Surfaces that are particularly likely to create imaging problems when they are dusty or dirty, are the objective front lens (remove each objective from time to time, and look at it carefully with a stereomicroscope), and all glass/air surfaces, even the internal ones, of the photographic eyepiece. Remove the objective and look *through* it, from both ends; ensure that internal components are clean and free from blemishes; look for evidence of *balsam starts* – the separation of cemented optical components. Ask a competent technician to show you how to clean lens surfaces; any trained salesperson will be delighted to encourage such care by one of their customers. In many photomicrographic attachments and built-in systems, dirt, bits of film etc, find their way onto glass surfaces that are in the path of an image that cannot be scrutinised by the user, because at some stage in the optical path the rays go to the film, not the observer. The manifestation of this dirt is a set of marks positioned in precisely the same positions on successive negatives or transparencies. Occasionally, the dirt can be very difficult to find, and if it is located on beamsplitters involved with the viewfinding optics, it is quite risky to brush these surfaces with anything but the very lightest touch.

Cleaning of optical surfaces is required from time to time, particularly after the use of immersion oil. Coated surfaces must be treated with particular care. Dust must always be removed first (as otherwise it may grind into the surface), using a blower, jet of compressed gas, a mini-vacuum-cleaner and/or brush. Take care not to blow the particles onto other parts of the optical system. A soft brush may be needed to dislodge adherent particles.

Cleaning with solvent. Any bad contamination will require cleaning with a soft linen rag, chamois leather, or paper tissue. Dust-free material is essential. We prefer soft paper tissue to 'lens tissue', because it is softer, even though it tends to shed paper fibres that have to be blown off. Cottonwool is no longer recommended, unless it is guaranteed pure cotton and not a mixture with synthetic fibres. For dry (non-immersion) systems, distilled water is probably the solvent of first choice. An organic solvent is frequently required, and is essential for cleaning immersion systems. There is some uncertainty as to what is the most suitable solvent; it must be a solvent for organic non-polar compounds (such as are used in immersion oil), non-toxic and not dangerously flammable, and should be sufficiently volatile to evaporate quickly without leaving a greasy film behind. Mixtures of ether and ethanol (50:50 by volume), or of ether, ethanol and chloroform (48:48:4 by volume), are effective, but highly flammable and with toxic vapours. Xylene, which has been widely used, is toxic and carcinogenic; the proprietary solvent *Histolene* is a preferred alternative. A trade solvent (such as Shell *X-55*), or a commercial window-cleaning fluid, may be used. Co-author Fred has found isopropyl alcohol quite effective. Co-author Ron has a strong preference for *Windex* as the solvent, applied with a cottonwool bud (or a well-washed cotton handkerchief for larger surfaces).

The complete cleaning of small, concave lens surfaces such as the front lenses of some objectives is particularly difficult. Final cleaning is best accomplished with a freshly broken surface of polystyrene foam (*Styrofoam, Styropore, Poresta*), using a coaxial rotating motion (Pabst, 1974): any xylene used for preliminary cleaning *must* be allowed to evaporate completely first, so as not to dissolve the polystyrene. (Co-author Ron is far too conservative to subject his lenses to this treatment!) Professional optical technicians make use of small pieces of extremely clean chamois cemented onto an 'orange stick'. The wood is chosen because it is free from resins, and it is soft enough to avoid scratching the glass.

The back lens of an objective may accumulate dust or dirt and will need occasional blower treatment. The rest of the objective should be touched by trained staff only.

Eyepieces may get dust even *inside* the unit. It is reasonable, with great care, to unscrew the field and eye lenses, attempting to clean only those surfaces that are seen to be in need of cleaning. It is a cardinal rule *not* to clean a surface that is already clean. However, the act of screwing the metal parts back together may loosen pieces of varnish that had sealed the eyepiece; much patience is needed.

Fungal growth (mould), once it has become established on a glass surface, is almost impossible to remove successfully. The fungus etches into the coated surface, so that re-grinding and re-polishing are needed to maintain optical performance. More often than not, a replacement rather than a repair is cheaper. Air-conditioning cannot be guaranteed to prevent the growth of fungus, but it will slow it down. A de-humidifier is less expensive, and possibly just as effective. It is useful to copy the measures that Indonesian households adopt to prevent fungal growth on leather goods stored in a cupboard in the home. The cupboard has holes top and bottom, and a continuously burning 15 W bulb (at the bottom) that generates a flow of air through the cupboard. Extreme measures are also taken to keep the cupboard free from dust (that carries the fungal spores). The major manufacturers make specially tropic-proof equipment intended for use in the tropics. Storage of lenses under desiccated conditions (0%

relative humidity) is not necessarily correct practice, because the dryness may induce breakdown of the lens cements.

Routine maintenance

General servicing of the microscope should be carried out regularly by a trained technician; this usually means having the instrument serviced by the manufacturer or manufacturer's representative.

The lubrication of moving metal parts may best be left to a technician, but the technician should be alerted long before the parts have tightened or jammed. The specific lubricant to be used will depend on the metals and on the temperatures commonly sustained. If lubrication is attempted, always first clean the surfaces so that they are free from grease and dirt, and finally wipe off any excess lubricant.

Fluorescence microscopes require basically the same maintenance procedures and general care as any optical microscope. The arc lamp (mercury burner) needs careful attention. The lamp must be replaced when its bulb blackens significantly. *Caution: examine it only when cold, and never while switched on!* The lamp fitting will include (with its installation instructions) a guarantee for a nominal lifespan, generally about 200 hours. It is unwise to exceed this running time in spite of the cost of the lamp, because, although the demise of filament bulbs may be accompanied by a bright flash of light, mercury burners can go out with a bang, an implosive one! Modern rectifier units for an arc lamp include a timer to keep track of the burning time. Otherwise, a logbook should be established. The brightness and uniformity of the lamp is better guaranteed throughout its life if it is not subject to repeated switching on and off. It may be helpful to establish a practice that the minimum burning time is at least 1, possibly 2, hours. As with any newly installed light source, inevitable fingerprints on the glass or quartz envelopes should be carefully wiped off before the arc is ignited.

Excitation filters should be inspected regularly (annually, at least) to see whether they need replacement. The life of excitation filters is limited, particularly if they are subjected to overheating. The effect of excessive irradiation is usually to render the filter denser or more opaque, possibly in an irregular fashion, giving reduced transmission and an uneven field of illumination. Barrier filters are commonly made of several layers cemented together; sometimes the cement becomes partially unstuck, degrading the image.

A2
Troubleshooting

This appendix is intended as a guide to finding the source of faults in the microscope and camera systems. Faults in the microscope are discussed first, since they should be noticed before any photographs are taken. Faults only apparent in the photographs are discussed in the second section. Some suggestions for cures are given.

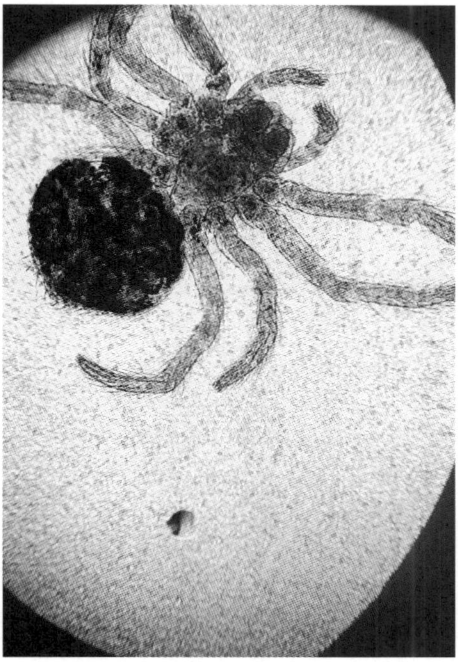

Fig A2.1. A compendium of faults! Spider, whole specimen. Field size 3·6 mm × 2·5 mm. This picture shows the following faults: (1) ground-glass of illuminator in focus (due to the condenser being too low), (2) field unevenly illuminated (same reason), (3) vignetting of field by field diaphragm (set too small), (4) vignetting of field by filter (not centred), (5) dirt on slide (the blob near the bottom), (6) poor composition.

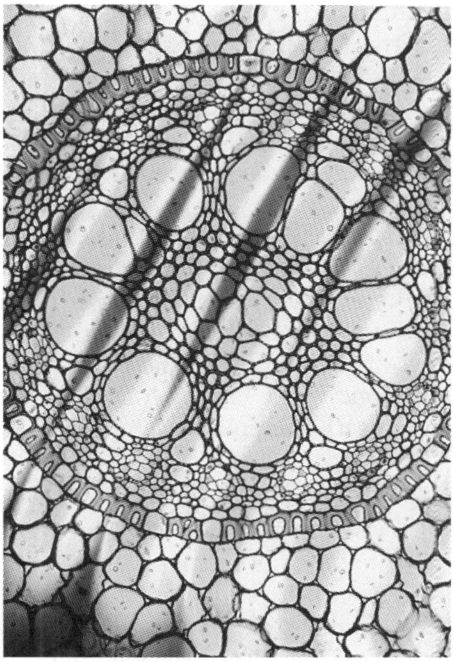

Fig A2.2. More faults! A botanical specimen, *Iris* root, transverse section, field size 1·0 mm × 0·7 mm. An image of the lamp filament appears in focus, because the condenser is too low. Also, the filament is not correctly centred. See also Figs 6.4 (curvature of field) and 6.7 ('reverberation' due to the illumination aperture being too small).

Faults in the microscope image

The lamp will not light

Faulty electrical connection: test each electrical connection, commencing at the power point. *Caution: the electricity is lethal!* In Britain, Singapore, etc.: check the fuse in the plug.

Blown fuse in the power unit: disconnect from the mains, check the fuse and replace if necessary. Why did the fuse blow?

Unserviceable lamp: replace the lamp.

Power unit not functioning: refer to manufacturer.

Nothing is visible in the microscope

The lamp has not lit (see above).

The mirror house arrangement does not allow the light from the lamp to reach the specimen (is it set for trans- or epi-illumination?).

(Trinocular body) The beamsplitter knob is set to reflect all the light away from the eyepieces.

The light is so much reduced that the image is invisible (see below, The image is too dim).

The nosepiece is positioned between objectives (no objective properly in place).

(Epi-illumination) The shutter in the epi-illuminator is closed.

(Transillumination) The condenser is not focused.

(Transillumination) The specimen is opaque.

(Darkground condenser) The condenser is set too low (or too high, less likely).

(Fluorescence) The barrier filter slide is improperly positioned.

(Polarisation) The polars are crossed (correctly!) and the specimen is not visible.

The specimen is not visible

The specimen is not under the objective.

The specimen is not in focus.

(Fluorescence) Wrong filter combination for the subject.

The objective has been damaged.

(High power) The slide is upside-down.

The specimen cannot be focused

The (dry) objective has oil on it.

(High power) The slide is upside-down.

(Low power) The objective has too long a working distance.

The wrong kind of objective is in use (eg infinity-corrected instead of finite tubelength, or vice versa).

The operator is using the fine-focus only, instead of the coarse-focus control.

The fine-focus control has come to the end of its mechanical movement.

The image is too dim

A neutral-density filter or polariser is present.

The condenser (or epi-illuminator) aperture diaphragm is partially closed.

The objective aperture diaphragm is closed.
(Trinocular body tube) The beamsplitter set to send only part of the light to the eyepieces (diverts portion of light up phototube).
The lamp is old, blackened inside, needs replacing.
The lamp is not properly centred.
The lamp is not at full current.
The lamphouse collector lens requires focusing.
The eyepiece magnification is too high.
The wrong collector lens in the lamphouse (not suitable for the lamp installed).
Inappropriate use or omission of auxiliary lens in illumination system.
(Darkground condenser) Condenser not focused correctly (too low or too high).
(Epi-illumination) The objective numerical aperture (NA) is too low.
The substage condenser is not focused.
No oil, or insufficient oil on the condenser.
The specimen is too thick.
Auxiliary lens for high/low magnification wrongly set.
(Substage condenser) Top component of condenser swung out, fully or partially.
(Substage condenser) Wrong kind of top (low NA).
(Substage condenser) Phase-contrast rings present.

Fluorescence only:
Wrong filter combination.
Wrong barrier filter (cutoff wavelength too long).
Wrong excitation filter (wavelength not suitable for fluorophore).
Two incompatible excitation filters present simultaneously.

The illumination of the field is uneven

Lamp incorrectly centred.
Collector lens not focused correctly.
Diffusing glass required in lamphouse.
Darkground condenser not focused correctly.
Field diaphragm opening too small.
Nosepiece improperly positioned, not at indexed position (objective not properly in place).
(Fluorescence) The excitation filter slide (if present) not positioned correctly (push it in).
(Polarisation) The analyser and/or compensator are not positioned correctly.
Condenser not centred.
Bubble in the oil on the condenser.

Only one side of the image is visible, or stronger than the other side, with a clear line of demarcation

The beamsplitter or sliding mirror of the trinocular body tube is at an intermediate position (pull it fully out or push it fully in as appropriate).
(Fluorescence) The barrier filter slide is incorrectly positioned as above (push it in).
(Polarisation) The canalyser and/or compensator are incorrectly positioned as above (push it in).

(Fluorescence only) Excitation light coming through to eye
No barrier filter.
No excitation filter.
Mismatched filter set (wrong barrier filter or wrong excitation filter or both).
(Red background) Red-stop filter omitted.
Filters positioned for dia-illumination, lamp for epi-illumination or vice versa.
Excitation filter broken (light comes through break).
(Darkground condenser) NA of objective too great for condenser .
(Oil-immersion objective with iris) Iris too widely open.

Substage condenser cannot be focused high enough
Specimen slide is too thick (exceeds 1·2 mm).
Condenser has slipped down in its mount.
Long-working-distance condenser required.

Image is of poor contrast
Field diaphragm too wide.
Masking by neighbouring artefacts (try reducing the field diaphragm).
Wrong type of immersion fluid (oil? water? glycerol? silicone? air?).
Bubbles in immersion fluid.
Dirt on objective.
(High NA dry objective) Wrong thickness of coverslip.
(High NA dry objective) Correction collar wrongly set.
(Epi-illumination) Dirt on mirror surface in illuminator.
(Darkground condenser only) NA of objective greater than that of darkground condenser.

Fluorescence only:
The substage light-trap is not in place.
The specimen's fluorescence has faded.
Normal substage illuminator lamp left on.
Unsuitable excitation filter (excitation wavelength unsuitable for fluorophore, or not specific enough).
Improper filter combination (barrier and excitation filters do not match).
Try a longer-wavelength barrier filter.
Barrier filter with poor transmission characteristics.
Fluorescent barrier filter (bad design).
Red-stop (BG38) filter omitted from primary filter set.
Fluorescent immersion fluid.
Fluorescent foreign matter in optical system.
Objective fluoresces (unsuitable objective).
Specimen in fluorescent mountant (eg balsam).
Excitation filter broken (light comes through break).

Image is of excessive contrast
Aperture diaphragm closed down too much (see Fig 6.7, Reverberation).
Substage condenser too low.
Over-stained specimen: try same-colour filter (see Chapter 15).

Image blurred, or not sharp enough
Not in focus.
Dirt on optical system, probably front surface of objective.
Dry objective has immersion fluid or mountant on front surface.
Immersion objective used dry, or with wrong fluid (Chapter 6).
Bubble in immersion fluid.
Barrier filter faulty (cement may have come loose).
Condensation on ocular (from observer's breath).
Ocular and objective do not match (eg of different make).
Coverslip of incorrect thickness (see Chapter 6).
Correction collar on objective incorrectly set for coverslip thickness (see Chapter 6).
Fault in objective.
Poor-quality objective.
Poor-quality condenser.
Inappropriate use of intermediate magnifier.

The image is not sharp all over
Poor quality objective (field not flat; see Chapter 6).
Slide tilted on stage.

Spots, flecks or blurs which remain in the field when specimen is moved
Dirty lens surface. Try rotating the ocular or objective: corresponding rotation of the spots identifies the dirty component (see Appendix A1).

Faults in photographs

Prints
Before looking for a fault in the microscope, check the negative.

Pictures unsharp all over
Focusing procedure incorrect (operator error).
Focusing apparatus inadequate (try a focusing telescope).
Stage slipping down during exposure.
Objectives of inadequate quality.
Vibration in camera or microscope during exposure.
Grainy film (this has a characteristic grainy appearance).
Finder eyepiece dislodged from correct position.
Finder graticule not used for final focusing.
Finder not adjusted to operator's eye (is the graticule sharp?).
Over-enlargement (useful magnification exceeded)

Pictures unsharp at corners
Objective inadequately corrected (use a flat-field objective).
Wrong projective.

Colour pictures seem wrong colour

Colour shift due to long exposure (reciprocity failure).

(Excessive blue)'Artificial light' colour film used with daylight-type illumination or for fluorescence.

Wrong barrier filter (fluorescence only).

Improper processing of film.

(Prints) inappropriate filters used for printing.

Background grey, blue, amber, etc, not white: underexposure.

Blue cast: lamp current too high, unsuitable colour filter, use of daylight film with a system balanced for artificial light, use of Type A film with system balanced for Type B, reciprocity failure, incorrect printing.

Amber (brownish-yellow) cast: lamp current too low, unsuitable colour filter, use of artificial-light film with a system balanced for daylight film, use of Type B film with system balanced for Type A, reciprocity failure, incorrect printing.

Casts of other colours: reciprocity failure or incorrect printing, possibly combined with one of the above.

Pale, washed-out colours: overexposure of transparency film, underexposure of negative (print) film.

Dye bleeding from stained specimen into mountant.

Pictures consistently underexposed

Film speed set wrongly on control box.

Wrong correction for proportion of field bright/dark (Chapter 16).

No correction, or insufficient correction, for reciprocity failure (Chapter 16).

Meter needs recalibrating.

Subjective appearance (decrease speed setting to suit).

Exposure-compensation dial set for underexposure.

Pictures consistently overexposed

Film speed set wrongly on control box.

Wrong correction for proportion of field bright/dark.

Excessive compensation for reciprocity failure.

Meter needs recalibrating.

Subjective appearance (change speed setting to suit).

Exposure compensation setting set for overexposure.

Dark corners (vignetting)

Field diaphragm set too small.

Uneven illumination of field.

Illumination system not centred properly.

(Low powers) Unsuitable condenser (remove top lens, or change the condenser).

Poor focusing of condenser.

> ***'If all else fails, try reading the instructions!'.***

A3
Exercises

These exercises are meant partly as such, and partly as topics for discussion. They are numbered according to the chapter to which they are most closely linked: eg 2.3 is the third question relating to Chapter 2.

1.1 What film should be used if colour prints are the primary aim?

1.2 Should your spectacles be worn when using the microscope?

2.1 Using a 40× objective, no intermediate magnification, and a 3·3× projective, what is the total magnification?

2.2 An object measuring 100 μm in diameter is to be recorded on a 35 mm film frame, which measures 24 mm × 36 mm. What overall magnification is required?

2.3 What overall magnification is required for the same object using the 4×5 inch format?

2.4 See how many objectives you can find, and interpret the markings on each.

2.5 The majority of modern objectives have an RMS screw thread mount. Does this imply that they are all fully interchangeable?

2.6 Can a photograph be taken using only an objective, ie without an eyepiece?

3.1 A stage micrometer has a ruling of 1 mm divided into 100 equal parts. If, on a photograph, 73 stage micrometer divisions are enlarged to a size of 14.6 cm, what is the magnification of the print?

3.2 The graticule (reticule) in an eyepiece is not sharply focused. How is this corrected?

3.3 If a daylight colour transparency film is to be used, what steps must be taken with the light source, and filtration (if any) for a correct colour balance to be ensured?

3.4 How is colour correction best judged?

4.1 What are the meanings of SLR, TTL, OTF as applied to 35 mm cameras?

4.2 In patch-stop darkground, is condenser immersion necessary? Or desirable?

5.1 How should a transparency be marked for correct orientation in a projector?

6.1 A perfectly flat specimen such as a polished metallurgical specimen shows out-of-focus edges in the microscope image. Why? Will the effect show in a photograph? How can the fault be corrected?

6.2 The image of a black particle shows coloured fringes, green in one focus, magenta as the focus is changed slightly. Should this be present in a planachromatic objective?

6.3 How is an oil-immersion objective identified?

6.4 An objective bears the notation 160/0.17. Does this mean that the thickness of the coverslip should be exactly 0·17 mm?

6.5 What and where is the back focal plane of an objective? How can it be seen?

6.6 An objective is labelled 'HI', and has an NA of 1·32. What image defects might be expected if the objective is used without immersion? What image defects might be expected if the condenser is not immersed when using that lens?

7.1 As the condenser iris is closed, what effects can be expected in the image?

7.2 A condenser is labelled 'aplanatic-achromatic', with an NA of 1·4. Can it be used without immersion oil on it?
7.3 Is a setting other than the '7/8ths position' of the aperture diaphragm ever justified?
7.4 If a condenser of inferior optical quality is used for photomicrography, what image defects are likely to occur?
7.5 Most condensers have an iris diaphragm as part of their construction; what is the function of the iris?
7.6 If such an iris diaphragm (above) is closed, will it affect the image intensity?
7.7 How should variation of light intensity be controlled?
7.8 If the field iris diaphragm is not adjusted for each objective, in what way is the image affected?
7.9 If the aperture diaphragm is not adjusted for each objective, in what way is the image affected?
8.1 Distinguish between shortpass, longpass, and bandpass filters, giving examples.
8.2 Distinguish between the characteristics of an 80A blue colour correction filter and a blue excitation interference filter for fluorescence.
8.3 What is the colour temperature of a 12V 100W halogen lamp as used in the microscope?
8.4 If artificial light colour film and a halogen lamp at full current are being used, what colour correction is needed?
8.5 Where should a colour filter be placed in the light path?
9.1 Where in the optical path should a patch stop or Rheinberg filter be placed?
9.2 With conventional metering, will photographs in darkground tend to be overexposed or underexposed?
10.1 How is a phase-contrast objective identified? Is it reasonable to use such a lens for normal brightfield work?
10.2 In spite of best efforts at preparation of a specimen, its image is considerably lacking in contrast. What optical procedures will enhance the contrast? What photographic procedures will enhance the contrast?
10.3 In a polarisation system with crossed polars, even where there is no specimen, the field is grey rather than black. Why might this be so?
10.4 Strain-free objectives are a more costly recommendation for polarisation microscopy. Does this mean that normal objectives can not be used?
10.5 In a DIC system, movement of the beam combiner is incapable of bringing the background to a very dark grey. What are the likely causes of this?
10.6 What alternatives are there to Nomarski DIC if the specimen is held in a plastic container?
10.7 Can the normal range of objectives be used for DIC?
10.8 Has DIC replaced darkground and phase-contrast techniques?
11.1 Green fluorescent objects appear bright yellow in a transparency. Why?
11.2 For fluorescence photographs, should daylight or artificial light colour film be used? If daylight film is used for fluorescence, where should the 80A daylight colour correction filter be placed?
11.3 The fluorescence image with a 10× objective is unacceptably very dark. Will it be a waste of time looking at the fluorescence with a 40× objective?
11.4 What is the function of a dichromatic mirror?
11.5 How is a dichromatic mirror specified?

12.1 A very reliable photomicrographic system produces negatives that are considerably overexposed with photography in the infrared. Why?
12.2 Can normal lenses be used for infrared work?
12.3 Is a special light source required for infrared microscopy?
13.1 Why are CMO stereomicroscopes preferred to the Greenough variety for photomicrography?
14.1 What are the advantages of telescopic aerial image focusing?
14.2 What is implied by 'automatic reciprocity correction'?
15.1 For the photography of spherical specimens such as pollen grains, what steps might be taken to extend the depth of field for photography?
15.2 An old specimen has acquired objectionable brown stains in the mountant; how can the stain be minimised in a B&W photograph? or emphasised?
15.3 What microscopical procedures might be adopted for the rapid identification and pictorial display of (green) chloroplasts?
16.1 An excellent specimen with a very considerable area of bright background has produced a colour transparency that is much too dark. Does this mean that it was overexposed or underexposed?
16.2 If exposed at its correct ISO rating, will a B&W Polaroid photomicrograph of a completely empty microscope field appear completely white, light grey, or dark grey? And what happens if the exposure is taken with a green filter?
16.3 A well-stained specimen has about 25% of the field clear (ie no specimen); what exposure compensation should be given?
16.4 A poorly-stained specimen has about 25% of the field clear (ie no specimen); what exposure compensation should be given?
17.1 What alternatives (or combinations) might be considered for a publication record of features in a poor-contrast specimen in which there is continuous movement?
18.1 A professional transparency colour film is several months older than its 'use-by' date. Will this be a problem?
18.2 What are the advantages of chromogenic B&W films?
18.3 What storage conditions are recommended for film, for a matter of weeks?
19.1 Make a drawing of an object seen in a microscope.
A1.1 What are the hazards in using solvents for lens cleaning?
A2.1 Experiment with intentionally putting some of the microscope's adjustments out of kilter, and see what happens.

(Some answers are given below, commencing on the next page)

Answers (partial)

1.1 Slide film for the best, but expensive prints; negative film for much cheaper prints of lesser quality. Consider also digital imaging.

1.2 Generally, yes. Many spectacle wearers find them a nuisance at the microscope but a necessity for the careful manipulation of equipment, and for note-taking.

2.1 $40 \times 3{\cdot}3 = 132$.

2.2 About 23 mm $\div$ 0·100 mm = 230×, eg 40×objective and 5× projective.

2.3 About 100 mm $\div$ 0·100 mm = 1000×, eg 100×objective and 10× projective.

2.5 No. There is very considerable variation in parfocal distance (32 or 45 mm) and tubelength correction (160 mm and infinity).

2.6 Yes, but with some objectives only.

3.1 200× linear magnification.

3.2 The eyelens of the eyepiece should be focused for each individual user, possibly for each eye.

3.3 Usually, the lamp must be run at full voltage, and an 80A colour correction filter should be interposed.

3.4 A grey should be rendered grey, not yellow or blue.

4.1 Single lens reflex, through-the-lens, off-the-film.

4.2 Not necessarily; it is an additional option, but only to be considered if the condenser is an immersion condenser.

5.1 A distinct mark at the bottom left of the transparency mount, as the slide is to appear on the screen.

6.1 Field curvature of the optical combination will show in the photograph, especially if a large print is contemplated; reduce the effective NA or use a planefield objective with a photo eyepiece.

6.2 Yes; it is normal longitudinal chromatic aberration in an achromatic objective.

6.3 HI, oil, Imm, and/or a black ring.

6.4 Not necessarily. The distance between the upper surface of the coverslip and the point of focus within the specimen should be 0·17 mm; therefore the correct coverslip may need to be much thinner.

6.5 Back focal plane of an objective: where parallel rays from the condenser are brought to a focus, usually within the upper barrel of the objective. It shows the effective NA of the objective. Seen by removing an eyepiece and looking down the tube of the microscope.

6.6 Objective without oil will give an unacceptable, soft image; if the condenser is not of equivalent NA to the objective, contrast will be increased at the expense of potential resolving power.

7.1 Reduced NA, therefore poorer resolution, increased contrast, lower intensity, increased depth of field.

7.2 Yes. But only with immersion will its superior correction be achieved, and its NA will only be about 0·9.

7.3 Very definitely yes! Perfect microscopy applies only to perfect specimens.

7.4 Overall colour cast due to condenser chromatic aberration, the colour changing with condenser focus.

7.5 Control of effective NA.

7.6 Yes, the image darkens when the aperture iris is closed below the objective NA.

7.7 For colour work, with neutral density filters, for B&W work the transformer may prove more convenient if yellowing of the light source can be tolerated.
7.8 Either the field is not fully illuminated, or image contrast is decreased through flare.
7.9 Either the resolution is compromised, or image contrast is decreased through flare.
8.1 UV-transmitting filter, yellow glass filter, and green interference filter.
8.3 3200 K, but only if at full current.
8.4 None, except for prolonged exposures or low lamp current.
8.5 Between the light source and the specimen, but not close to a field iris diaphragm.
9.1 As close as possible to an aperture plane.
9.2 Overexposed, but this may be countered by reciprocity failure, ie underexposure, with long exposures.
10.1 A dark phase ring in the back focal plane of the objective. Yes, although the image will be somewhat soft.
10.2 Reduce the effective NA, but at the expense of resolution; consider optical contrast techniques eg darkground/phase/polarisation/DIC; photographically, use a film or developer of higher contrast. High-performance objectives may help; filtration, especially green, can help with B&W. Consider computer image enhancement.
10.3 Polars not crossed correctly; poor-quality polars; glass lenses or prisms with strain; plastic specimen support.
10.4 They will work very well for most studies.
10.5 Polariser not oriented correctly; or an isotropic (plastic) specimen support.
10.6 Oblique illumination, darkground, phase contrast, Hoffman modulation contrast.
10.7 Generally, no, only strictly specified designs; this is likely to change with modern instrumentation of more 'universal' design.
10.8 No; each technique complements the other, and has its place in a general microscopy laboratory.
11.1 Overexposure; also possibly colour changes with extended exposure.
11.2 We recommend daylight film. A blue colour-correction filter is not required.
11.3 In epi-fluorescence, the intensity increases with objective NA, so the intensity with a 40× objective can be expected to be very much brighter than with a 10× objective.
11.4 To selectively reflect specified lower wavelengths onto a specimen, and to transmit all other wavelengths.
11.5 Generally by the cutoff wavelength at which reflection (lower wavelengths) and transmittance (higher wavelengths) occurs.
12.1 Exposure meters are not designed to work in this range of the spectrum, but recalibration might be possible.
12.2 Apochromatic objectives are to be preferred to minimise focusing problems.
12.3 Halogen lamps have a very considerable output in the infrared. The recommendation is that the infrared be filtered out for normal microscopy.
14.1 Bright images, not impaired by the structure of a ground-glass screen.
14.2 An automated lengthening of exposure to compensate for loss of film sensitivity during long exposure intervals.

15.1 Decreasing the effective NA, or focusing through the specimen during an extended exposure. Perhaps scanning electron microscopy is more appropriate.
15.2 Minimised with a yellow filter, or emphasised with a blue, or possibly blue-green, filter.
15.3 Blue excitation fluorescence; red/blue filtration in B&W; computer discrimination and image enhancement.
16.1 Underexposed.
16.2 A medium (18% reflectance) grey, even with filtration if the exposure meter responds as the film does to different wavelengths.
16.3 Negative film: +1, +2 stops; transparency film: $+^2/_3$, $+1^1/_3$ stops.
16.4 Negative film: 0, +1 stop; transparency film: $-^2/_3$, 0, $+^2/_3$ stop.
17.1 Microscopy with darkground, phase or DIC; vital staining; film with medium to high ISO; electronic flash; video microscopy.
18.1 Yes, if the film has been stored incorrectly. Possibly not, if it has been kept refrigerated.
18.2 Very fast and economical turnaround in a '1 hour' processing mini-lab.
18.3 4 °C, implying refrigeration.
A1.1 Many are carcinogenic, flammable or explosive, and may dissolve lens cements.

References

Acharia, K. (1975) Stereophotography. *Industrial and Commercial Photography* **15** (12), 31.

Anchell, S.G. (1994) *The darkroom cookbook*. 207 pp. Focal Press, Boston and London.

Anchell, S.G. (1997) *The variable contrast printing manual*. 193 pp. Focal Press, Boston.

Anon (1973) *Medical infrared photography*. Kodak Publication N-1. 76 pp. Eastman Kodak Company, Rochester, NY.

Anon (1984a) *How to improve photography through the microscope*. 83 pp. Olympus Optical Corporation, Tokyo.

Anon (1984b) *Mastering composition and light*. 104 pp. Kodak Limited, Mitchell Beazley Publishers, Salvatore Editores.

Anon (1988) *Conservation of photographs*. Kodak Publication F-40. 156 pp. Eastman Kodak Company, Rochester, NY.

Anon (1990) *Kodak photographic filters handbook*. Kodak Publication B-3. 161 pp. Eastman Kodak Company, Rochester, NY.

Appellof, M. E. (1992) *Everything you ever wanted to know about watercolour*. 399 pp, Watson–Guptill Publications, New York.

Arnold, C.R., Rolls, P.J. & Stewart, J.C.J. (1971) *Applied photography*. Focal Press, London.

Beyer, H. (Ed.) (1977) *Handbuch der Mikroskopie*, 2nd edn, 495 pp. VEB Verlag Technik, Berlin.

Blaker, A.A. (1989) *Handbook for scientific photography*, 2nd edn. 287 pp. Focal Press, Boston and London.

Bollinger, A. & Fagrell, B. (1990) *Clinical capillaroscopy*. 166 pp. Hogrefe & Huber, Toronto, Lewiston, Bern, Göttingen and Stuttgart.

Borgman, H. (1977) *Drawing in ink. Drawing for reproduction.* 159 pp. Watson–Guptill Publications, New York.

Bracegirdle, B. & Bradbury, S. (1995) *Modern photoMICROgraphy.* 94 pp. Bios Scientific Publishers, Oxford.

Briscoe, M. H. (1990) *A researcher's guide to scientific and medical illustrations*. Chapter 11. Springer-Verlag, New York.

Camp, J. (1981) *Draw: how to master the art*. 256 pp. Andre Deutch Ltd, London; reprinted (1985) by Book Club Associates, London.

Capon, R. (1984) *Basic drawing*. 120 pp. B.T. Batsford Ltd, London; reprinted by Book Club Associates, London.

Casida, L.E. (1968) Infrared color photography: selective demonstration of bacteria. *Science* **159**, 199–200.

Clark, W. (1946) *Photography by infrared*, 2nd edn. 472 pp. John Wiley, New York; Chapman & Hall, London.

Clements, B. & Rosenfeld, D. (1979) *Photographic composition*. 260 pp. Van Nostrand Reinhold, New York. (Paperback edn; originally published 1974 by Prentice-Hall.)

Corle, T.R. & Kino, G.S. (1996) *Confocal scanning optical microscopy and related imaging systems*. 335pp. Academic Press, London.

Covington, M. (1991) *Astrophotography for the amateur*. 168 pp. Cambridge University Press, Cambridge.

Cowen, B.C. (1969) A factual survey of fully automatic cameras currently available for use with the microscope. *Proceedings of the Royal Microscopical Society* **4**, 71–73.

Cox, G. (1995) Mass storage and hard copy. In: Pawley, J.B. (Ed) *Handbook of biological confocal microscopy*, 2nd edn, Chapter 35, pp 535–548. Plenum Press, New York and London.

Croy, O.R. (1968) *Creative photomicrography*. 151 pp. Focal Press, London.

Davies, A. & Fennessy, P. (1998) *Digital imaging for photographers*, 3rd edn. 167 pp and CD-ROM disc. Focal Press, Oxford.

Delly, J. & Brown, J. (1980) Light and SEM stereomicrography. *Optical Spectra* **14** (12), 32.

Delly, J.G. (1988) *Photography through the microscope,* 9th edn. 104 pp. Kodak Publication P2. Eastman Kodak Company, Rochester, NY.

Dragesco, J. (1988) Reciprocity failure of photographic emulsions before and after hypersensitization by forming gas: a densitometric study. *Journal of the British Astronomical Association* **98**, 249–254.

Editors of Time-Life Books (1972) *Caring for photographs*. 192 pp. Time-Life International.

Elkin, L. & Park, R.B. (1975) Chloroplast fluorescence of C4 plants. I. Detection with infrared colour film. *Planta* **127**, 243–250.

Farrell, G.M. (1969) *Annals of Applied Biology* **63**, 265–275.

Ferwerda, J. G. (1987) *The world of 3-D: a practical guide to stereo photography*, 2nd edn. 300 pp. 3-D Book Productions, Borger, The Netherlands.

Gibson, H. (1980) *Photography by infra-red: its principles and applications, 3rd edn.* 545 pp. John Wiley, New York.

Gill, R.W. (1973) (*The Thames and Hudson manual of) Rendering with pen and ink*. 368 pp. Thames & Hudson, London.

Gu, M. (1996) *Principles of three-dimensional imaging in confocal microscopes*. 337 pp. World Scientific, Singapore.

Hanke, R. (1979) *Filter-Fascination*. 159 pp. Hama, Monheim.

Herman, B. (1998) *Fluorescence microscopy*, 2nd edn. RMS Handbook No 40. 170 pp. Royal Microscopical Society / Bios Scientific Publishers, Oxford.

Hind, H.L. & Randles, W. B. (1913) *Handbook of photomicrography*. 292 pp. George Routledge & Sons, London.

Inoué, S & Spring, KR (1997) *Video microscopy: the fundamentals*, 2nd edn. 741 pp. Plenum Press, New York and London.

Jastrzębski, Z.T. (1985) *Scientific illustration. A guide for the beginning artist*. 319 pp. Prentice-Hall Inc, Englewood Cliffs, NJ.

Jaxtheimer, B. W. (1962) *How to paint and draw*. 408 pp. Thames & Hudson, London.

Judge, A.W. (1950) *Stereoscopic photography: its application to science, industry and education, 3rd edn*. 480 pp. Chapman & Hall, London.

Kapitza, H.G. (1994) *Microscopy from the very beginning*. 41 pp. Carl Zeiss, Oberkochen.

Lawson, D. (1972) *Photomicrography*. 494 pp. Academic Press, London and New York.

Lester, H.M. & Richards, O.W. (1954) Stereos through the microscope. In: Morgan, W.D. & Lester, H.M. (Eds.) (1954) *Stereo Realist manual*, Chapter 13, pp. 335–359. Morgan & Lester, New York; Fountain Press, London.

Lillie, R.D. (1977) *H.J. Conn's Biological stains*, 9th edn. 692 pp. Williams & Wilkins, Baltimore, MD.

Longmore, T.A. (1955) *Medical photography*, 5th edn. 990 pp. Focal Press, London and New York.

Loveland, R.P. (1970) *Photomicrography: a comprehensive treatise*, vols I and II. 1039 pp. Wiley, New York, London, Sydney and Toronto.

Luey, Beth (1987) *Handbook for academic authors.* 226 pp. Cambridge University Press, Cambridge.

Mobberley, M. (1999) *Astronomical equipment for amateurs*. 266 pp. Springer, London.

Moneta, G., Brülisauer, M., Jäger, K. & Bollinger, A. (1987) Infrared fluorescence microscopy of skin capillaries with indocyanine green. *International Journal of Microcirculation: Clinical and Experimental* **6**, 25-34.

Morgan, W.D. & Lester, H.M. (Eds.) (1954) *Stereo Realist manual*. 400 pp. Morgan & Lester, New York; Fountain Press, London.

Morton, R. (1984) *Photography for the scientist*. 542 pp. Academic Press, London.

Oldfield, R.J. (1994) *Light microscopy, an illustrated guide*. 160 pp. Wolfe Publishing, London.

Pabst, H. (1974) A new method of cleaning front lenses of objectives. *Leitz Scientific and Technical Information* **2**, 235.

Parramón, J. M. (1976) *Painting*, revised edn. 119 pp. Fountain Press, Kings Langley, Herts.

Parramón, J. M. (1984) *Composition in painting and drawing*. 112 pp. Parramón Ediciones SA, Barcelona, Spain (distributed by Fountain Press, Windsor, UK).

Patzelt, W.J. (1985) *Polarized light microscopy,* 3rd edn. 102 pp. Ernst Leitz, Wetzlar.

Pawley, J.B. (Ed) (1995) *Handbook of biological confocal microscopy*, 2nd edn. 232 pp. Plenum Press, New York and London.

Ploeg, M. van der, Bosman, F.T. & Duijn, P. van (1976) Pre-exposure of films in fluorescence photography. *Histochemical Journal* **8**, 201–204.

Pluta, M. (1988) *Advanced light microscopy*, vol 1, *Principles and basic properties*. 464 pp. Elsevier, Amsterdam, Oxford, New York and Tokyo; PWN–Polish Scientific Publishers, Warsaw.

Pluta, M. (1989) *Advanced light microscopy*, vol 2, *Specialised methods*. 484 pp. Elsevier, Amsterdam.

Poore, H. R. (1967) *Composition in art.* 96 pp. Dover Publications, New York. (Unabridged republication of work originally titled *Pictorial composition and the critical judgement of pictures*.)

Puchtler, H., Meloan, S.N. & Paschal, L.D. (1980) Infrared fluorescence microscopy of stained tissues: principles and technic. *Histochemistry* **68**, 211–230.

Ray, S.F. (1994a) *Applied photographic optics: lenses and optical systems for photography, film, video and electronic imaging*, 2nd edn. 586 pp. Focal Press, Oxford.

Ray, S.F. (1994b) *Photographic imaging & electronic photography*. 307 pp. Focal Press, Oxford.

Richardson, T. (1997) Do you, your slides and your CCD camera need sunglasses? *Proceedings of the Royal Microscopical Society* **32**, 101–105.

Robinson, P.C. & Bradbury, S. (1992) *Qualitative polarized-light microscopy*. 112 pp. Royal Microscopical Society/Oxford University Press, Oxford.

Ross, M. H. & Romrell, L. J. (1989) *Histology text and atlas*, 2nd edn. 783 pp. Williams & Wilkins, Baltimore, MD.

Rost, F.W.D. (1991) *Quantitative fluorescence microscopy*. 236 pp. Cambridge University Press, Cambridge.

Rost, F.W.D. (1992, reprinted with update 1996) *Fluorescence microscopy*, vol I. 253 pp. Cambridge University Press, Cambridge.

Rost, F.W.D. (1995) *Fluorescence microscopy*, vol II. 457 pp. Cambridge University Press, Cambridge.

Schade, K.-H. (1995) *Light microscopy*, 2nd edn. 70 pp. Verlag moderne Industrie, Landsberg/Lech. (Original in German, *Lichtmikroskopie*.)

Schott (nd) *Schott color filter glass.* Jenaer Glaswerk Schott & Genossen, Mainz.

Shillaber, C.P. (1944) *Photomicrography in theory and practice*. 773 pp. John Wiley, New York.

Shimizu, S. & Takenawa, H. (1994) Microscope objective design. In: Mulvey, T. & Shepherd, C.J.R. (eds) *Advances in optical and electron microscopy*, vol 14, pp 249–334. Academic Press, London.

Sluder, G. & Wolf, D.E. (Eds) (1998) *Video microscopy*. Methods in Cell Biology vol 56. 334 pp. Academic Press, London.

Smith, Bill (1985) *Designing a photograph*. 144 pp. Amphoto, New York, NY.

Stroebel, L., Compton, J., Current, I. & Zakia, R. (1986) *Photographic materials and processes*. 585 pp. Focal Press, Boston and London.

Stroebel, L., Compton, J., Current, I. & Zakia, R. (1989) *Basic photographic materials and processes.* 384 pp. Focal Press, Boston and London.

Tufte, E. R. (1983) *The visual display of quantitative information*. 196 pp. Graphic Press, Cheshire, CT.

Tufte, E. R. (1990) *Envisioning information*. 176 pp. Graphic Press, Cheshire, CT.

Tufte, E. R. (1997) *Visual explanations*. 156 pp. Graphic Press, Cheshire, CT.

Valyus, N.A. (1966) *Stereoscopy*. 426 pp. Focal Press, London and New York. (Translated by H. Asher, from *Stereoskopya*, Izdatel'stvo Akademii Nauk USSR, Moscow, 1962.)

Vetter, J.P. (Ed) (1992) *Biomedical photography*. 531 pp. Butterworth-Heinemann, Stoneham, MA.

Walker, M.I. (1971) *Amateur photomicrography*. 194 pp. Focal Press, London and New York.

Watts, J.T. (1982) The design of stereomicroscopes and macroscopes. *Proceedings of the Royal Microscopical Society* **17**, 192–195.

Wilhelm, H. & Brower, C. (1993) *The permanence and care of color photographs: traditional and digital color prints, color negatives, slides, and motion pictures*. Preservation Publishing Co., Grinnell, IO.

Williams, R. (1993) *The beginner's guide to painting watercolours*. 80 pp. Bison Books, London.

Willingham, M.C. & Pastan, I. (1978) The visualization of fluorescent proteins in living cells by video intensification microscopy (VIM). *Cell* **13**, 501–507.

Young, W.A., Benson, T.A. & Eaton, G.T. (1985) *Copying and duplicating in black-and-white and color*. Kodak Publication M-1. Eastman Kodak Company, Rochester, NY.

Zelanski, P. & Fisher, M.P. (1988) *The art of seeing*. 464 pp. Bay Books, Sydney and London.

Index

Italicised page numbers indicate the most important discussion of the subject.

Italicised bold page numbers indicate the most important discussion of the subject.

Italicised bold page numbers indicate the most important discussion of the subject.

Italicised bold page numbers indicate the most important discussion of the subject.

Italicised bold page numbers indicate the most important discussion of the subject.

Italicised bold page numbers indicate the most important discussion of the subject.

Italicised bold page numbers indicate the most important discussion of the subject.

Italicised bold page numbers indicate the most important discussion of the subject.